THE ENCYCLOPEDIA OF

VITAMINS, MINERALS AND SUPPLEMENTS

Second Edition

THE ENCYCLOPEDIA OF

VITAMINS, MINERALS AND SUPPLEMENTS

Second Edition

Tova Navarra, B.A., R.N.

Foreword by
Wendy Shankin-Cohen

☑®
Facts On File, Inc.

Facts On File, Inc.
132 West 31st Street
New York NY 10001

Library of Congress Cataloging-in-Publication Data

The encyclopedia of vitamins, minerals, and supplements / Tova Navarra; foreword by Wendy Shankin-Cohen.—2nd ed.
p. cm.
Includes bibliographical references and index.
ISBN 0-8160-4998-X (hc : alk. paper)
1. Vitamins in human nutrition—Encyclopedias. 2. Minerals in human nutrition—Encyclopedias.
3. Dietary supplements—Encyclopedias. I.
Navarra, Tova.
QP771.E53 2004
612.3'99'03—dc22   2003061662

Facts On File books are available at special discounts when purchased in bulk quantities for businesses, associations, institutions, or sales promotions. Please call our Special Sales Department in New York at (212) 967-8800 or (800) 322-8755.

You can find Facts On File on the World Wide Web at http://www.factsonfile.com

Text and cover design by Cathy Rincon

Printed in the United States of America

VB Hermitage 10 9 8 7 6 5 4 3 2 1

This book is printed on acid-free paper.

To "Vitamin JY"—Julia Yolanda Fleming—my granddaughter,
from your loving Nonni

Sickness is felt, but health not at all.
—French proverb

Prevention is better than cure.
—Latin proverb

Better is a dinner of herbs where love is,
than a stalled ox and hatred therewith.
—Proverbs 15:17

An apple a day keeps the doctor away.
—17th-century proverb

Der Mensch ist was er isst.
(Man is what he eats.)
—German philosopher Ludwig Feuerbach

"A loaf of bread," the Walrus said,
"Is what we chiefly need:
Pepper and vinegar besides
Are very good indeed."
—Lewis Carroll, from *Through the Looking-Glass, And What Alice Found There*

"Cravings? Of course you have cravings.
Your body is crying out for the nutrients it lacks!"
—Shoshanna Katzman and Wendy Shankin-Cohen, from *Feeling Light*

CONTENTS

FOREWORD

In a world filled with information, it becomes our task not to find more, but to sort through all that is available and make informed decisions about how to lead our lives.

The wealth of information that is now available to us is sometimes overwhelming. That is why this book needed to be written. Consumers of health supplements needed a reliable source to which they could turn with confidence and explore the options available to them. What was needed was one source that pulled it all together in a no-nonsense, easy-to-read, simple format. This encyclopedia serves that purpose not only for the layperson but also for the professional who is looking for sound and clear information. This valuable resource is written so that anyone from novice to expert will be able to access the material.

In my many years of speaking to people about their health, I have noticed that one of the most pressing issues concerns their confusion about all that they read and hear. Most people are left in a world of indecision about how best to achieve optimal health. It seems the more they read, the more uncertainty they experience, due to the number of conflicting opinions that are ever present in the media, on the Internet and in reference materials. This book will be a valuable addition to the library of anyone who wants to get the information they need without the confusion.

We would all love to believe that our health could be optimal without the addition of supplements. Unfortunately, our food sources do not provide adequate vitamins and minerals for optimal health. Our earth has been depleted of minerals, making the plants, fruits and vegetables that are grown in the soil also depleted of minerals. Our foods are picked too early and shipped for days before finally reaching our supermarket shelves, where they may sit for many more days before they are purchased. Those same foods may then sit in our refrigerators for an additional number of days before they are consumed. The result of all of this is the consumption of fruits and vegetables that are deficient in vitamins and minerals essential to good health.

Our foods are also often processed, refined, canned, frozen or otherwise modified before we consume them. Many of us rely on fast foods and fast meals in our busy and hectic world. The day of the home-cooked meal made with entirely fresh ingredients is a thing of the past for most of us. The further we get from nature's way of supplying us with food, the further we get from eating whole foods that provide us with a basis for healthy living. And although good nutrition and exercise remain the most important factors for maintaining good health and preventing disease, most of us don't get enough of either.

Technological advancements in many health fields are miraculous. We live in an age where organ transplantation, joint replacement and corrective eye surgery are almost commonplace. And yet chronic diseases such as diabetes, heart disease and cancer are on the rise. We know that many of these diseases may be partially or totally preventable. And yet very few strides have been made in the prevention of chronic illness.

In our search for ways to prevent disease and to maintain optimal health, we look at our less-than-perfect nutrition and ask, "What should we do?" The answer is to boost our nutrition by the consistent, knowledgeable and prudent use of supplements. Using supplements not only ensures that minimal nutritional requirements can be met on a daily basis, but it also provides the opportunity for restoring and maintaining optimal health.

In addition to supplements that help meet daily vitamin and mineral requirements, herbs are now part of our daily routine. Herbs, which have been used as standard treatments in many cultures all over the world for thousands of years, are now coming to the forefront as a viable way of assisting the body in healing itself; but again, confusion reigns. Certain herbs, such as echinacea, have become so popular that they are used almost as frequently as the common aspirin. This encyclopedia is a valuable aid in determining exactly what herbs are used for, as well as explaining possible interactions with pharmaceuticals and potential side effects.

Educating ourselves is a must if our desire is to feel well, avoid disease and promote a healthy immune system. In world that challenges us to live with daily stress and imperfect forms of food and exercise, it is only through our constant quest for knowledge that we can hope to keep ourselves healthy in mind, body and spirit. This quest may lead us down many different paths; some may be more beneficial than others. But if we stay the course of good nutrition, frequent exercise and sound sources of information, we afford ourselves the best chance of achieving the goal of wellness.

With this encyclopedia, Ms. Navarra has provided us with a reliable, sound source of information—a book that one will use again and again. We are all grateful to her for having given us such a valuable resource.

—Wendy Shankin-Cohen,
holistic health consultant and coauthor of
*Feeling Light—The Holistic Solution to
Permanent Weight Loss and Wellness*

PREFACE

This plain-language reference book on vitamins, minerals and food supplements provides non-judgmental information on nutritional options, as opposed to books dedicated to one nutritional philosophy. As a health professional, I present positive, negative and neutral views, if appropriate, of the many substances known to have some effect upon human well-being.

I acknowledge freely that a good number of these substances have their detractors. Therefore, I do not advocate taking any particular substance or combination of substances unless you are well informed and have confidence in the substance's known effects. Many people report that eating raw garlic cloves cures them of a sore throat. But please keep in mind that not every sore throat is just a sore throat, and not everyone's metabolism and mind-set are the same. If a sore throat is caused by cancerous lesions, or if a person is severely allergic to garlic, this choice of treatment may lead to tragic results.

The alternatives to the better-known vitamins and minerals, including substances used in traditional Chinese medicine, Ayurvedic (traditional Hindu) medicine, Native American and other herbal medicine and homeopathic medicine, were interesting to research and write about. The more familiar substances, such as vitamin C and iron, took on a headier scientific glow as this book neared completion. I noted that the books, periodicals and other materials I used in my research had valuable information, though none was truly complete in itself. Scientific opinions, such as those expressed in the controversy over vitamin C's effectiveness, sur-

prising media reports of liver damage caused by the herb chaparral and a death caused by an herbal tea, and political actions, such as the passing of the new law on supplements (see Appendix VI), often change the "supplement scene" unexpectedly in the public eye.

In addition to presenting entries on essential (that is, necessary to human life) and nonessential nutrients, I offer entries on herbal and other supplements that have long been considered nutritive and medicinal agents.

> No supplement can duplicate the complexity of the real substance, only be a mediocre second choice. Eating a variety of these healthful foods is the best way to assure getting the maximum impact of the plants' abundant gifts. Don't build your house with cardboard.
>
> So, eat well, eat colors, eat variety, eat seasonal foods, eat your family's ancestral foods, eat with a peaceful heart, eat when you're hungry, eat in moderation, eat whole unprocessed foods, eat wild and free-range foods, eat in gratitude for what it has taken to get the food to your table.
>
> —from "Food as Medicine: An Enlightened Approach to Eating," by Dale Bellisfield, R.N., clinical herbalist, Siegler Center for Integrative Medicine, Livingston, New Jersey

In the foreword to *Botanical Medicines: The Desk Reference for Major Herbal Supplements, Second Edition,* by Dennis J. McKenna, Ph.D., Kenneth Jones, Kerry Hughes, M.Sc., and Sheila Humphrey, B.Sc., Gregory A. Plotnikoff, M.D., M.T.S., write: "The most recent national survey documented that more than 44.6 million Americans use herbal remedies on a regular basis and that more than 90 million Americans had used an herbal remedy in the past 12 months. Thirty-six percent of those who use herbal medicines do so instead of prescription medicines and 31 percent do so with prescriptions. The leading reason for substitution is preference for a natural or organic product. Leading sources for information are, in order of preference, friends, magazines, product labels, and advertising. Ironically, health professionals are the least frequently consulted for information. At this time, there is a profound knowledge gap with significant public health implications." I discovered, at times to my horror, that there are thousands upon thousands of herbs in use, so I decided to feature the ones I thought were the most widely used, the most broad-spectrum and the most fascinating. Many herbal preparations prescribed by homeopaths, naturopaths and others are believed to be effective against the most common ailments of many cultures. Therefore, some entries may seem repetitive as remedies for the same problems. But varying dosages and combinations with other herbs that are not addressed in this book create the possibility of treating several different illnesses, from a simple cold to catastrophic diseases such as cancer.

My research uncovered a wealth of information. For example, without the mineral zinc, we would have a much-diminished sense of taste or smell; without salt, no neurotransmitters; without sugar, no energy; and so on. The study of how to use vitamins, minerals and supplements seems to be in its infancy, even though Hippocrates, the Ancient Greek "father of medicine," used diet and herbs as the staples of his treatments. Many of the substances described are cross-referenced, and I included several appendices offering related information to the text.

In 2004 the World Health Organization published guidelines on good agricultural and collection practices aimed at improving the quality and safety of herbal products and preserving the plants from which they come.

I sincerely hope everyone who opens this volume will find something of personal interest, valuable information and perhaps a new attitude on nutrition—say, that your body is a sacred temple and deserves not to be inundated with garbage, but lovingly fed nature's "gold."

ACKNOWLEDGMENTS

For this second edition of the *Encyclopedia of Vitamins, Minerals and Supplements,* I heartily thank James Chambers and the staff of Facts On File, Inc., for making my job as author a pleasure. I also acknowledge with sincere gratitude my coauthor for the first edition, the late Myron A. Lipkowitz, R.Ph., M.D., and my wonderful family, whose constant encouragement bolsters my spirit: Yolanda, Guy, Vincent, Julia, Amanda and Wesley Fleming; Johnny and Mitzi Navarra; Jacquie, Tony and Matthew Munoz; Dorothy Fox and Joe and Rose Treihart. Many thanks as well go to those dear colleagues and friends who go out of their way to "help the cause": Frederic C. Pachman, Paul Boyd, Dr. David Kaplan and Victor Zak, and to my friends Sallie and Stan Tillman, Trista Clayton, Betty Sorrentino, Hope and Brian Richardson, Mona Wichman, Leon Strollo, Chris and Vicki Reidemeister, Bunny Schuler, Gary Sorkin, and Dr. Andrea Campbell, who supplement my life with much joy.

INTRODUCTION

*Man's mind stretched to a new idea never goes
back to its original dimension.*

—Oliver Wendell Holmes

Americans are generally aware of the importance
of healthy eating, but about one third of the population remains unconcerned about their own
dietary habits, according to new survey results.
Overall, the findings from the new American
Dietetic Association survey of Americans' beliefs
about nutrition show that some nutritional information is reaching the public, but not all of it, and
not everybody is listening, a panel of experts said
here on October 20, 2002.

Since 1996, when *The Encyclopedia of Vitamins,
Minerals and Supplements* was first published,
nutrition has stepped into a limelight it has never
before enjoyed. First of all, the dietary supplement market is a nearly $6 billion annual indus-
try that skyrocketed to success after it was
significantly deregulated in 1994. Shelves in
supermarkets, pharmacies, department stores and
even convenience stores are lined with jars of vitamins and products containing various supplements. The mineral calcium has been cavalierly
added to many food, drug and supplement products, such as Tums and chocolate. Zinc sprang into
throat lozenges as a healing rather than just pal-
liative feature. Advertisers tout black and green
teas as a source of antioxidants, when only a few
years ago, the word *antioxidant* was barely a mainstream reference. Until fairly recently, many
Americans thought of herbs mainly in the context
of witches' brews or ancient folk remedies; now

herbal supplements of some sort are in constant
view and often wind up in our home cupboards
and refrigerators for daily use.

Prominent authors and health professionals,
such as Andrew Weil, are also doing their best to
educate and encourage Americans to eat and use
supplements wisely; in the process they are
mending the seeming rift that occurred between
the efforts of the late Adelle Davis and her ilk in
the 1960s and 1970s and a public that is now discovering the benefits of good nutrition. In a society that at one time hoped Popeye could motivate
kids to eat spinach, lots of people are more than
willing to drink thick, green, good-for-you glop;
eat seaweed, nettles and strange mushrooms; and
swallow big capsules of omega-3 fatty acids, acidophilus or beef-cartilage tablets.

Moreover, nutrition has become so integral a
factor in health these days that medical schools
have begun to include nutrition courses for student physicians, a subject heretofore left to the
realm of nursing, dietitians and other allied health
professions. The old adage "you are what you eat"
is being revisited as inherently medical, to the
point that large segments of American culture are
not only conscious of food values, but vigilant of
them as well. With the help of the Internet, nutrition has now become an important and popular
subject of study among professionals and laypeo-
ple alike.

Both old and new organizations provide
detailed information on nutrients, herbs, food and
related topics. For example, the National Institutes of Health established the Office of Dietary

Supplements (ODS), and the Council for Responsible Nutrition has been founded. The U.S. Food and Drug Administration (FDA) has published a guide to dietary supplements, and the Mayo Foundation for Medical Education and Research and other organizations post to their websites content on food and nutrition issues, including information on certain herbs that have been shown to yield biologically active compounds that could lead us toward a new generation of drugs. In addition, the recent development of "golden rice"—rice with built-in beta-carotene—promises to keep millions of children and adults in developing nations from various diseases and blindness caused by a lack of vitamin A.

Many discoveries and developments have taken place concerning the traditional roster of nutrients such as vitamin C, niacin, calcium, folic acid, selenium, vitamin B_6, vitamin D, vitamin E, iron, magnesium and zinc. Updated Dietary Reference Intakes (DRI) and Recommended Dietary Allowances (RDA) have been established, and the American way of eating is now being challenged by the latest Food Pyramid, which at last urges the intake of significant daily portions of grains and vegetables and the use of sugars and fats as sparingly as possible. This "Everest" is not an easy climb for a culture that loves fast, fattening and fun food.

New research has been conducted too, such as the Johns Hopkins University study of 310 HIV-positive men with adequate blood levels of vitamin B_{12} who stayed free of AIDS for eight years on average, compared to just four years for those deficient in the vitamin. Another study from several medical centers revealed that selenium does not prevent skin cancer, but it was discovered that it lowered the rates of several other cancers, including cancers of the colon, lung, prostate and rectum. Selenium apparently reduced the death rate of these cancers by 50 percent. Medical researchers had thought that megadoses of vitamin C could cause kidney stones, but this has been disproved. In a study of 45,000 men who took 1,500 milligrams of vitamin C a day, an increased risk of kidney stones was not observed.

Herbal supplements have also either blossomed into fads—evening primrose, boswellia, stinging nettle, chondroitin and glucosamine sulfate—or fallen into controversy—goldenseal, St. John's wort, ephedra (*ma huang*) and echinacea. Ephedra has been banned and phenylpropanolamine (Phen-fen), used as an over-the-counter weight-loss product, is now under federal investigation for harmful effects. Also newly spotlighted in a separate appendix are herb and prescription-drug interactions that may be harmful. An investigative arm of Congress, the General Accounting Office (GAO), has reported some potentially harmful effects, and this may create tighter federal regulations on firms that make unsubstantiated claims about the benefits of their products. Antiaging and weight-loss products, in particular, are under fire.

Long before President George H. W. Bush declared he hated broccoli and dubbed carrots "orange broccoli," people seemed to be in constant skirmishes over what foods are necessary for overall good nutrition. The American culture's affection for junk food and gourmet fare often manifests as meats, vegetables, fruits and starches that are hollandaised, glazed, grilled, creamed, sautéed, flambéed, candied, topped and glopped. Plain, wholesome food may represent "eating to live" rather than "living to eat."

In short, we have become nutritionally challenged, a society living on pizza, burgers and fries and wondering why *Time* magazine would run a cover story billed as "Girth of a Nation."[1] As S. J. Nielsen and B. M. Popkin wrote in the January 23, 2003, issue of *JAMA*,

> Americans are not only super-sizing their meals at the drive-thru but eating bigger portions at home, too. Researchers from the University of North Carolina at Chapel Hill analyzed three government surveys taken over two decades and reviewed answers to the average portion size consumed for specific foods, such as snacks, desserts and soft drinks. They also looked at whether the eating was done at home or out. Between 1977 and 1996, food portion sizes increased both inside and outside the home for all categories except pizza.

The problem is not only obesity; it's also mindset. People sport either a laissez-faire attitude, as in, "Let them eat chips," or a general ignorance of nutrients. There is little in between, except possibly for registered dietitians (and not even all of them), health-food "nuts" and some conscientious types who prefer to eat sensibly.

Knowing what to eat involves recognizing, at least to a certain extent, that some foods are more nutritious than others. Furthermore, nutrition is an individual matter, especially for people with diabetes, heart disease, irritable bowel syndrome or an uncooperative gallbladder, for example. Nutritionists working with cancer patients may champion the intake of huge portions of ice cream with hot fudge and real whipped cream, or extra dollops of mayonnaise on a bologna sandwich— all hideous in terms of "good" nutrition. The rationale? Many of these patients have lost the desire to eat at all, so whatever appeals to them and offers the greatest number of calories may help keep up their energy and weight. The same principle applies to stubborn or fussy children whose parents allow them to live on cocktail wieners, if that's what they want, just to ensure they will eat *something.*

As if the daily routine of eating well weren't enough of a battle, the concept of food supplements compounds the confusion. Never mind the cost, but to take, or not to take?

The major studies conducted indicate mostly controversial results. A recent study in Finland, done under the auspices of the National Cancer Institute (NCI), tested beta-carotene supplements' effect on approximately 29,000 male smokers. Earlier studies suggested that people who regularly ate foods containing large amounts of beta-carotene were at low risk of developing lung cancer. But the Finnish study gave a startling result. The incidence of lung cancer in the Finnish men who took the supplement was 18 percent higher than in those who did not.

Also in the Finnish study, vitamin E was implicated as a possible troublemaker. It lowered the risk of prostate cancer as expected, but increased the death rate from hemorrhagic strokes.[2] On the other hand, studies have shown that calcium supplements (even in the form of Tums and other antacid tablets) do help prevent osteoporosis, vitamin C does lessen the wrath of many infections,

vitamin A helps improve night vision and many other nutrients are tried and true in a variety of situations. The consensus today is that vitamin E helps address anemia, sterility, and any other ailment involving the need for oxidative protection of red blood cells. (*Stedman's Medical Dictionary,* 27th ed. Baltimore: Lippincott Williams & Wilkins, 2000.)

In general, people favor taking some form of supplement to their diets; vitamins, minerals, herbs and other substances and combinations are ingested to give us what our diets may not, even though vitamin and mineral supplements do not necessarily substitute for eating a healthful variety of foods (see Appendix 1, USDA Food Pyramid). Popping a stress-formula B-vitamin capsule, a garlic pill or a vitamin C tablet hooks directly into our cultural taste for things instant, easy, painless and, it is hoped, efficient.

In the 1950s, jars of "One-A-Day" multiple vitamins were snapped up by young moms eager to provide their families with a "magic bullet" that would compensate for any unwitting nutritional lack. It was a postwar era characterized by children who, despite Popeye's prowess-in-a-can, refused to eat spinach and turned up their noses at liver, rutabaga and brussels sprouts as well.

Moreover, food-processing and the supermarket emerged as enormously successful industries during that time. The corner grocer with his fresh produce became less popular as housing developments in suburban areas blossomed. The American family grew more interested in the modern conveniences of large freezers and processed foods. The Wonder Bread advertising campaign of 40 years ago comes to mind as an example: "Wonder Bread helps build strong bodies 12 ways." Nutritionists and home economics teachers tried to tell us then that "enrichment" with 12 nutrients was necessary because the grain's original nutrients had been processed out of the product that ended up in our lunch boxes.

Youngsters following the example of older siblings and media role models promptly spurned whole-wheat bread—or any grainy kind that was good for you—because white bread somehow tasted better than brown bread. (White bread was also soft, and the taste blended with the flavor of whatever was on it or between two slices of it.) I remember Miss Sharp, my fifth-grade home economics teacher, who said, "Put a white slice on top of the sandwich and a brown one on the bottom, and when you eat, hold the white side toward you." One must admire her gift for compromise.

Miss Sharp also made each girl in her home-economics class (the boys took wood shop) eat a teaspoonful of wheat germ during a decade when the unappetizing key word was "germ." Grimaces shot around the room. I was the only girl who liked it, and I still eat it to this day. That experience in the 1950s influenced me to thrive on a merry assortment of both health and junk foods. I must also admit that, although I am not a disciplined supplement-taker, I believe in the nutritive and healing potential of vitamins, minerals and herbs and have experienced a fair amount of personal success in their use. Cranberry pills and marshmallow-root capsules from the health-food store, for instance, ended years of taking ineffective prescription medications for chronic bladder and urethral infections that had become the bane of my existence.

No doubt Miss Sharp would approve were she still around. Today, her baby-boomer pupils are middle-aged and may be junk-food junkies and the parents of finicky eaters. And conflicting ideas about the requirements of "good" nutrition struggle on. So many people became enamored of fast foods that nutritionists conducted scientific analyses of the nutrients (and dietary disadvantages) offered by the Whopper, the Big Mac, and other fast-food offerings.

Among the thornier questions are: How will the issue and study of nutrition become more significant in the future? Will the government's new Food Pyramid (see Appendix I) truly guide a nation that embraces as great a gastronomic diversity as ours? Is there a spirituality of nutrition evolving, a philosophy of mind-body connection that may encourage people to become more vegetarian and take supplements with educated discretion?

Perhaps the only answerable question is the last, because the concept of mind-body connection has finally engaged itself as part of our health-care infrastructure. According to recent surveys in women's and other consumer magazines, people generally believe that one's way of thinking affects his or her physical state. That the media repeatedly call the increasing interest in vitamins, minerals and supplements "the vitamin craze" (see Bibliography for the *Time* magazine April 1994 article of that name) indicates the overall American disposition toward better nutrition, despite an appetite for empty calories, fats, sweets and poor sources of nutrients.

There are and always will be skeptics, however, including some who may have worthy points of view. In the *New York Times Magazine,* Nicholas Wade wrote:

> Nature doesn't yield its secrets easily. As with the oracle at Delphi, its answers may conceal a dangerous ambiguity. . . . It's tempting to infer that vitamins are the cause of better health. . . . But beneath that beguiling message, all that these observational studies really tell us is that there is an association between vitamins and health benefits. For a biologist, that's the statement of the puzzle, not its solution.
>
> Scientific trials will in time provide the verdict on vitamin supplements. For all who assumed the answer was already known, the Finnish trial offers two lessons. One is that science can't be rushed. The other is not to put all your bets on those convenient little bottles: back to broccoli and bicycles.[3]

While Wade suggests the benefit of the doubt, Dr. Victor Herbert, a professor of medicine at New York City's Mount Sinai Medical School, set forth an uncompromisingly negative stance. He said taking supplementary nutrients creates nothing more than "expensive urine."[4] Many physicians, not trained in nutrition (or mind-body connection, for that matter), would agree. They tell their clients the food they eat supplies them with all the nutrients they need, which could possibly be true if people dutifully ate their carrots, broccoli, wheat germ and such.

But it isn't true, because people insist on eating what they like. They are not complying with basic nutritional information. This is largely attributed to the variations of food quality, ability to prepare nutritious meals, loss of nutrients in cooking, and general factors, including individual body types and needs, medications used, amount of stress experienced according to one's lifestyle, and lack of knowledge of supplements. According to *Alternative Medicine: A Definitive Guide,* edited by Burton Goldberg, Larry Trivieri Jr., and John W. Anderson (Berkeley, Calif.: Celestial Arts, 2002) "an estimated 80 percent of adult Americans take nutrition supplements . . . no longer just a fad, but part of a growing trend as people start to take a proactive approach to their own health." But there are risks, and people are frequently baffled by conflicting reports on supplements. *Consumer Reports* (September 1994) says, "The ups and downs of nutrition advice have come to seem as capricious as the fluctuations of the stock market."[5] The article continues with evidence in favor of antioxidants—vitamin C, vitamin E and beta-carotene—that help protect us from the potentially destructive activities of the body's naturally produced molecules called free radicals. The article, which still holds true, also discusses evidence that for certain people the taking of certain supplements may be harmful.

Because most scientists and health professionals have established that we must obtain vitamins from outside sources to maintain good health, there is a clear need for extensive research and controlled clinical studies that take a multitude of factors into account, such as:

(a) understanding what a balanced daily diet is, given an individual's ethnicity, age, circumstances and history;

(b) understanding emotional and spiritual aspects, known to some as "psychic vitamins," in our lives that may affect the individual metabolism of nutrients; and

(c) studying nutrients, including herbal sources, as substances that prevent and treat disease.

The broccoli study is one example. Broccoli and other cruciferous vegetables, including cabbage, cauliflower and brussels sprouts, contain the chemical compound sulforaphane. According to the findings of Dr. Paul Talalay, Dr. Gary H. Posner and other research scientists at Johns Hopkins University in Baltimore, Maryland, sulforaphane blocks the growth of cancerous tumors in rats and stimulates the production of anticancer enzymes in mouse cells. These intriguing results were originally published in the March 1992 issue of *The Proceedings of the National Academy of Sciences,*[6] and subsequent research has confirmed the findings.

From this, scientists speculate that broccoli may provide a key to preventing colorectal cancer in humans. Sulforaphane in the *Brassica* genus of vegetables, whose most potent star is broccoli, is being tested at Fox Chase Cancer Center in Philadelphia, Pennsylvania, under the auspices of Dr. Paul F. Engstrom, senior vice president for population science, and Dr. Margie Clapper, who holds a Ph.D. in molecular and cell biology. The clinical trial with human participants seeks to determine the role of broccoli in preventing colorectal cancer.

"We're looking at individuals who are at high risk for colorectal cancer," Dr. Clapper said. "The criteria are those undergoing routine colonoscopy, those with a history of colorectal cancer who completed treatment at least two years ago, those with a history of colon polyps, and people with a family history of colorectal cancer."

Individuals with active colorectal cancer, colitis or radiation enteritis are among those not eligible for the broccoli trial. A sulforaphane treatment for active cancer may take years to emerge, if ever. The big questions for the clinical study are how much broccoli must a participant eat, and will it help if he or she actually likes broccoli.

Owing much to the techniques of pharmacy, participants do not eat any broccoli whether they like it or not. They take as a dietary supplement six broccoli tablets per day, two with each meal. Yes, broccoli tablets, made from real broccoli by a well-known supplement manufacturer. Available over the counter, they are green, malodorous and equivalent to approximately 30 grams of the vegetable, a typical restaurant serving of cooked broccoli. The cumulative dosage for participants is three grams a day.

In addition to taking the broccoli tablets, participants agree to undergo two flexible sigmoidoscopies, during which physicians can obtain colon tissue for biopsy, and give two blood samples before and after the study.[7]

Slowly but surely, the Fox Chase research exemplifies, skeptics are beginning to agree with those who believe in eating the most beneficial foods and food supplements. As nutrition takes center stage, the proverbial "food fight" over supplements will revert to a foolishness of the past. The latest consensus is that cruciferous vegetables, including broccoli, cabbage, cauliflower, turnips, and others, do, indeed, contain anti-cancer and antioxidant vitamins and a type of flavonoid that activates liver detoxification enzymes. (*Alternative Medicine: A Definitive Guide,* Berkeley, Calif.: Celestial Arts, 2002)

Ironically, we may need first to step back in time and follow the culinary example of our biblical ancestors. The Bible is replete with references to the cultivation, preparation, consumption and significance of food, such as: ". . . A land of wheat, and barley, and vines, and fig trees, and pomegranates; a land of oil olive, and honey; A land wherein thou shalt eat bread without scarceness, thou shalt not lack any thing in it . . ." (Deuteronomy 8:8).

Basic food came from the earth, the sea and the animals. If one favored St. Benedict's philosophy of moderation in all things, basic foods taken in moderation (including meat, to the dismay of vegans) would constitute the next step toward a revitalized view of modern nutrition.

Furthermore, the Bible advocates using plants not only as food but as agents of healing:

"Along both banks of the river, fruit trees of every kind shall grow; their leaves shall not fade, nor their fruit fail. Every month they shall bear fresh fruit, for they shall be watered by the flow from the sanctuary. Their fruit shall serve for food, and their leaves for medicine" (Ezekiel 47:12).

If familiar vitamins and minerals have wreaked havoc in the supplement wars, lesser-known herbal supplements, also used as remedies for illness, increase the confusion about what to take or not to take. As swiftly as "One-A-Day" multiple vitamins were accepted, many people now run to the health-food store to purchase any number of novel products. "Biochavan," for example, is an Ayurvedic (traditional Hindu) herbal supplement designed to nourish, promote longevity and cater specifically to the needs and/or deficits of the various body types upon which the practice of Ayurvedic medicine is based.

It is sobering to know that people from the time of the ancient Egyptians (and possibly before recorded history) used aloe, poppy, caraway seeds, garlic and hundreds of other plants as both food and medicine. In the last few years, Americans have been leaning, if cautiously, toward tapping into the rewards of good nutrition as they were experienced by our ancestors. We are looking more carefully at natural instead of processed foods. Holistic concepts and practices now in the American mainstream—yoga, among others—teach us about the body's innate power and desire to resist damaging invaders and heal itself. While it is advisable to investigate products before ingesting them, such as powders made of deer antler and shark cartilage sold as treatments for certain maladies, it is also advisable to keep an open mind to foods and other substances that have actually been part of our culinary and pharmaceutical heritage for thousands of years.

Fears pertaining to nutrition still loom large: world hunger and malnutrition; the future effects of managed care on preventive and alternative health-care options; certain herbal teas making headlines as killers; dietary or health-food backlash; supplement quackery; the cruelty of animal testing; and other dilemmas. But we might as well seek as intelligently as we can the opportunity to fortify our bodies without sacrificing the pleasures of food and drink—whether a sumptuous prime rib or a plain broiled flounder, an artichoke parmigiana or a portobello mushroom, a calming cup of warm milk with nutmeg or a goblet of wine. In the presence of these, One-A-Days risk being forgotten in the fridge, and memories of Miss Sharp's home-economics class endure only as a rudimentary connection between nutrition and tastebuds.

—Tova Navarra

Notes

1. Elmer-Dewitt, Philip. "Fat Times." *Time,* January 16, 1995, pp. 58–65.
2. "Taking Vitamins: Can They Prevent Disease?" *Consumer Reports,* September 1994, pp. 561–567.

3. Wade Nicholas. "Method and Madness: Believing in Vitamins." *New York Times Magazine,* May 22, 1994, p. 20.

4. Toufexis, Anastasia. "The New Scoop on Vitamins." *Time,* April 6, 1992, p. 54

5. "Taking Vitamins: Can They Prevent Disease?" *Consumer Reports,* p. 561

6. Prochaska, Hans J., Annette B. Santamaria, and Paul Talalay. "Rapid Detection of Inducers of Enzymes That Protect Against Carcinogens." *The Proceedings of the National Academy of Sciences,* vol. 89, March 1992, pp. 2394–2398.

7. The two-year study, funded by the National Cancer Institute, was completed in April 1995.

ENTRIES A–Z

A, vitamin A fat-soluble vitamin essential for growth and bone development in children, for vision (especially in low light), for healthy skin and mucous membrane surfaces, for reproduction and the integrity of the immune system. Vitamin A consists of several active compounds, including alpha-carotene, beta-carotene, retinal (retinaldehyde), retinol (vitamin A_1), retinoic acid and the carotenoids. Natural sources of vitamin A are egg yolks, fish-liver oils, liver, cream, butter, green leafy and yellow vegetables, pineapples, prunes, cantaloupes, oranges and limes. The richest sources include cod-liver oil, butter, butterfat in milk and egg yolk. Vitamin A can also be synthetically produced.

Documented reports of "night blindness" more than 3,500 years ago indicate a positive response to foods rich in vitamin A. In ancient Egypt, there was evidence that juice prepared from cooked animal livers was placed in the eyes of those with poor night vision. This practice has persisted to modern times in some societies. Later, in the third and fourth centuries B.C., Hippocrates prescribed eating beef liver for the treatment of night blindness.

Early in the 20th century, Englishman Frederick Gowland Hopkins discovered a growth-stimulating substance in milk. Later, a German researcher named Stepp identified a substance he had labeled "minimal qualitative factors" as a lipid. In 1913, E. V. McCollum and Marguerite David demonstrated an essential growth factor for rats in butter and egg yolk, which they called "fat soluble A."

Simultaneously, Osborn and Mendel, working in New Haven, Connecticut, found a similar fat-soluble substance in cod-liver oil and butter.

Moore, an English scientist, demonstrated that beta-carotene obtained as a colored substance from plants was transformed in the human body to a colorless form of vitamin A, which was then stored in the liver. It was not until 1930 that Karrer and his group in Switzerland determined the chemical structures of vitamin A and beta-carotene. In 1935, Wald defined a biochemical in the retina that he termed retinene, later renamed retinal.

Beta-carotene

A provitamin, precursor chemical or building block that the human body converts to vitamin A, beta-carotene is one of many pigments called carotenoids that give the deep coloring found in orange or green vegetables and fruits. Although there are more than 500 naturally occurring carotenoids, only about 50 have provitamin A activity, or the ability to be converted to retinol.

Beta-carotene is the only carotenoid that can be converted to significant amounts of vitamin A, and only about one-sixth is converted in humans. Dietary fat is required for the adequate absorption of carotene. The deeper the orange coloring of a carrot, the higher the concentration of beta-carotene.

In an Arizona study, 26 to 49 patients with oral leukoplakia, a premalignant lesion, were given 60 milligrams daily of beta-carotene for six months, resulting in a significant reduction in the size of their lesions. However, excessive ingestion of beta-carotene and other carotenoids from dietary sources or supplements may cause a yellowing of the skin. Fortunately, the skin pigmentation is reversible with reduction in the quantity of beta-carotene consumed. There is no evidence that natural sources of beta-carotene are more effective than synthetic sources (see CANTHAXANTHIN, GOLDEN RICE).

Retinol

The major vitamin A compound is found naturally in eggs, dairy products, liver and fish-liver oil. The compounds require proteins for their absorption from the intestines. Etretinate, a synthetic retinoid, appears to be effective in the treatment of psoriasis. Half of 32 patients being treated for advanced cervical cancer had a 50 percent regression in the size of their tumors when treated with oral 13-cis-retinoic acid and alpha interferon.

Vitamin A Deficiencies

The most common vitamin A deficiencies are caused by disorders of impaired fat absorption. These conditions include: (1) preschool-age children with cystic fibrosis, malabsorption syndromes or obstruction in the biliary system; (2) impaired storage or transport of the vitamin in cirrhosis and abetalipoproteinemia (an inherited metabolic disorder involving the synthesis of low-density cholesterol); and (3) increased metabolic demands during infancy, pregnancy and breastfeeding or with hyperthyroidism. Dietary deficiency of only vitamin A is rare and is usually combined with other vitamin deficiencies.

Nyctalopia, or night blindness, is the initial indication of inadequate vitamin A. With continued vitamin insufficiency, xerophthalmia (dryness of the conjunctiva and cornea) and keratomalacia (softness of the cornea) occur with perforation and ultimately cause blindness. This is especially common in the children of underdeveloped countries, where vitamin-A deficiency may be responsible for an estimated 250,000 cases of blindness annually. Although most symptoms of vitamin A deficiency improve with vitamin-A supplementation, there may be a permanent stunting of growth if the epiphyseal, or growth, plates close prematurely in bones.

Data collected from the 50,828 women enrolled in the Nurses' Health Study by researchers at the Brigham and Women's Hospital in Boston suggest that consuming foods high in vitamins A and C may reduce the incidence of cataracts. Antioxidant-rich vegetables such as spinach, sweet potatoes and squash appear to protect the eyes by preventing oxidation of proteins in the lens that lead to the formation of cataracts.

Measles seems to have a poorer prognosis in children who are vitamin A deficient. Children with severe measles infections should be given vitamin supplementation (see MEASLES AND VITAMIN A DEFICIENCY).

One study of AIDS patients demonstrated that individuals with vitamin A deficiency died sooner than those with normal levels of the vitamin (see AIDS AND VITAMIN DEFICIENCY).

Toxicity

Vitamin A excess can be toxic to a developing fetus. More than 15 mg of beta-carotene per day may impair fertility. Liver damage may result in a child from as little as the adult Recommended Daily Allowance (RDA) for a certain number of years and in adults from as little as five times the RDA for seven to 10 years. Chronic toxicity in infants and children causes pseudotumor cerebri (increased pressure in the brain that acts like a brain tumor), tinnitus (ringing in the ears), bulging fontanelles (swelling of the soft spot in the infant skull), increased cerebrospinal fluid, bone pain, lethargy, pruritus (itching), scaly rashes, cracks in the corners of the mouth, hyperostosis and metaphyseal cupping (abnormal bone growth) and paronychia (infections in the nail edges). Eye changes include diplopia (double vision), papilledema (swelling of the optic nerve), optic atrophy (wasting of the optic nerve) and eventually blindness.

In adults, chronic toxicity of vitamin A may cause vomiting, skin changes, irritability, headache, diminished menstrual bleeding, weakness and psychiatric disorders. Depression and symptoms suggestive of schizophrenia can be so severe that individuals have been placed in mental hospitals. Liver and spleen enlargement have been seen along with elevated levels of calcium in the blood. Chronic vitamin-A toxicity causes drying of the skin and mucous membranes, hair loss, brittle nails, loss of appetite and muscle, bone and joint and abdominal pains. Enlarged spleens and anemia may also result. Fatal anaphylactic shock (the most severe form of allergic reaction) and death have been reported following intravenous administration of vitamin A.

It has been estimated that almost 5 percent of vitamin A–supplement users in the United States exceed the 800 to 1,000 mcg recommended dietary allowance (RDA) of retinol approved by the Food and Nutrition Board of the National Research Council in 1980.

Teratogenicity (Birth Defects)

Doses greater than the RDA of 6,000 international units (I.U.) or 1,800 retinol equivalents of vitamin A should never be taken by pregnant or lactating women. Serious birth defects have been reported in infants born to mothers who took as little as 25,000 I.U. of vitamin A daily during conception and the first trimester of pregnancy. The Food and Drug Administration considers this vitamin to be in Pregnancy Category X, or having the potential for serious birth defects if taken in excess during pregnancy (see PREGNANCY VITAMIN AND MINERAL REQUIREMENTS).

Dosage

The liver stores several months' supply of vitamin A in well-nourished individuals. Protein and possibly zinc may be involved in the utilization of the liver stores. Healthy breast-feeding infants, children and adults generally do not require vitamin A supplementation. Rarely should adult doses exceeding 25,000 I.U. daily be taken unless a deficiency is especially severe. See Table 2 for U.S. RDA for vitamin A.

Although breast milk normally supplies adequate vitamin A, infants of poorly nourished mothers should receive 1,400 I.U. of vitamin A daily for the first six months. Although milk is labeled as fortified with vitamins A and D, studies by the Boston University School of Medicine found wide variance in vitamin content of milk tested in both regular containers of whole milk and infant formulas. Investigators identified vitamin D toxicity in eight children and fear that incorrect amounts of these vitamins in the milk may result in vitamin deficiencies or cases of toxicity. Only a third of milk samples tested had a vitamin content within 20 percent of the amount stated on the label. Seven of 10 samples had more than twice the amount stated.

The International Center for the Prevention and Treatment of Major Childhood Diseases reported that a single large dose of vitamin A (50,000 to 200,000 I.U. each) reduced death by 26 percent in a group of 3,700 malnourished children in India and Nepal.

Water-soluble vitamin A is six times more readily absorbed than an oily preparation and also more toxic to the same degree.

Drug Interactions

Cholestyramine, the cholesterol-lowering drug, and mineral oil may reduce absorption of vitamin A. Oral contraceptives (birth control pills) significantly increase blood levels of vitamin A.

TABLE 1 DOSAGE REQUIREMENTS FOR VITAMIN A DEFICIENCY STATUS

Severe deficiency with xerophthalmia (see above) without xerophthalmia	Age > 8 500,000 I.U./day for 3 days, then 50,000 I.U./day for 2 weeks
	Age > 8 100,000 I.U./day for 3 days, then 50,000 I.U./day for 2 weeks, then 10,000 to 20,000 I.U./day for 2 months
	1 to 8 years 5,000 to 10,000 I.U./day orally for 2 months or 17,500 to 35,000 I.U./day intramuscularly for 10 days
	Infants 7,500 to 15,000 I.U./day intramuscularly for 10 days

TABLE 2 U.S. RDA FOR DIETARY VITAMIN A SUPPLEMENTATION

Age	Daily Requirement	
	Retinol Units (RE)	International Units (IU)*
Birth to 1 year	375	1,875
1 to 3 years	400	2,000
4 to 6 years	500	2,500
7 to 10 years	700	3,300
Adolescent and adult males	1,000	5,000
Adolescent and adult females	800	4,000
Special circumstances		
Elderly	no changes required	
Pregnant females	no additional requirement	
Lactation, initial 6 months	1,300	6,500
after 6 months	1,200	6,000

[RE = Retinol equivalents: 1 RE = 3.33 IU of vitamin A or 10 IU of beta-carotene]
*The Recommended Dietary Allowances (RDAs) assumes more than half of the vitamin A intake will come from beta carotene, thus the values given are based on 1 RE = 5 IU. (Sources: National Research Council Recommended Dietary Allowances 10th edition and *The Essential Guide to Vitamins and Minerals* by Elizabeth Somer, M.A., R.D.)

abrus (rosary pea, love pea, Indian licorice, wild licorice vine, prayer-beads, weather plant or vine, coral-bead plant, red-bead vine, crab's eye, precatory bean) A plant of the family Leguminosae, *Abrus precatorius,* whose whole seeds are used to treat fever, malaria, headache, dropsy and intestinal worms. *Abrus* is the Greek word meaning delicate, which describes the leaves of the plant; the other names refer to the seeds. As long as the seeds are completely intact, they are harmless or considered by herbologists to be therapeutic. However, the ingestion of a cracked seed, or even the absorption through the skin of the contents of cracked seeds used for necklaces and the like, may be fatal. Abrus is used in traditional Chinese medicine.

absorption The process by which nutrients enter the circulatory system from the gastrointestinal tract. In order for vitamins and minerals to reach the bloodstream, they must dissolve in the stomach or intestines and diffuse across the membranes lining the digestive tract. Nutrients that fail to be absorbed may pass through the digestive tract and be excreted in the feces and therefore provide no nutritional value. The U.S. Pharmacopoeia (USP) establishes standards for the composition of drugs. Products that meet its rigid requirements assure the consumer that water-soluble products will dissolve within 30 minutes if uncoated or 45 minutes if coated. However, some products are designed for a prolonged release in order to reduce adverse effects. Evidence is lacking that chelated or bioflavonoid forms of vitamins work faster or are better absorbed than less expensive forms.

A dissolution test measures how soon a supplement dissolves in liquid and is more stringent than a disintegration test, which measures how long it takes for a product to break into tiny pieces.

acanthopanax (spiny panax) The plant of the family Araliaceae used in traditional Chinese medicine. From the Greek words *akantha,* or thorn, *pan,* or all, and *akes,* or remedy, acanthopanax is also known as thorny panax (panacea). *Acanthopanax gracilistylus* root bark is considered a tonic for weakness and for the treatment of rheumatism, impotence, lumbago and syphilis. The entire *Acanthopanax davidii* plant is used to treat mechanical injury, and the leaves of the *Acanthopanax trifoliatus* are used in preparations to treat tuberculosis, partial paralysis and bleeding in the lungs.

acidophilus (*Lactobacillus acidophilus*) A bacterium occurring naturally in the intestines that assists in the digestion of proteins, reduces blood cholesterol levels, fights fungal infections and augments nutrient absorption and distribution. Acidophilus also helps the body combat the effects of harmful substances by reinforcing the intestines' balance of what are called "friendly" bacteria or "good flora." For example, a *Candida* (yeast) infection is the result of an excess of coliform, instead of lactobacillus, bacteria that provided an accommodating climate in which *Candida* flourished. An acidophilus supplement has an antibacterial effect, thus defeating the coliform bacterial environment and restoring intestinal health.

Acidophilus is also found in yogurt, kefir, cheese, buttermilk and other "soured milk" or fermented-milk products. Nondairy acidophilus includes DDS Acidophilus, Neo-Flora, Kyo-Dophilus and Primadophilus and is available in powdered, tablet or capsule form in health-food stores and pharmacies. When a food containing the "good bacteria" of yogurt cultures is heated, the bacteria are destroyed. Frozen yogurt products do not contain the beneficial *lactobacillus acidophilus* culture.

See also YOGURT.

acne Inflammation of the sebaceous glands and hair follicles that causes pustules and other skin eruptions, especially during adolescence. Pitting and scarring of the skin may result. Vitamin A has been used to treat acne for many years. However, oral forms can be toxic in the high doses required for significant improvement. Isotretinoin (13-cisretinoic acid), or Accutane (trade name), is a very potent synthetic derivative of vitamin A. Unfortunately the drug has a great many adverse effects and is teratogenic (causes birth defects) if taken early in pregnancy. Tretinoin (all-trans-retinoic acid) or Retin-A, is another vitamin A derivative that is useful in treating acne when applied topically. Beta-carotene, which is converted to vitamin A in the body, is nontoxic and may also improve acne.

Selenium and vitamin E in one study showed significant improvement in acne and also seborrheic dermatitis (a form of severe dandruff). Pyridoxine (vitamin B_6) may also have value for severe acne, but large doses may cause toxicity to the central nervous system and must be used cautiously.

See also A, VITAMIN.

aconite (aconitum, monkshood, fu tzu) A north-temperate herb, of the family Ranunculaceae, with thick roots and flowers that resemble the garb of Benedictine monks. Monkshood was known to the Greeks in mythology and ancient times as containing a poisonous juice of various uses, including for poisoning the wells and other water supply of encroaching enemies, for criminals to drink as a death penalty and on one Greek island as a euthanasia method for the ill elderly.

In folklore, a concoction of monkshood and deadly nightshade was believed to enable witches to fly. Some herbologists believe the concoction may induce a sensation of flight, which fostered the fables.

Used in China for more than 2,000 years, aconite, including *Aconitum carmichaelii, chinensis* and *transectum,* has many benefits when the plant parts have been dried. Among them are treatment for pain, colds, chills, vomiting, rheumatoid arthritis, loss of appetite and kidney inflammation. Aconite is also considered a stimulant, heart tonic, narcotic, mild laxative and local anesthetic.

acorn The oak tree nut encapsulated in a woody covering with indurated bracts, like tiny "jewelry settings," from which the acorn grows. Of the *Quercus* species, shelled and ground acorns are made into a meal that can be used as a food or drink. Herbalists claim that acorns are nutritive, containing flavonoids, sugar, starch, albumin (a protein) and fats, to individuals with wasting diseases including tuberculosis and AIDS, as well as medicinal for those with diarrhea.

acrodermatitis enteropathica An inherited disease resulting in an inability to absorb zinc. Infants with this disorder have poor appetite, severe diarrhea, impaired night vision, hair loss, skin rashes,

depressed immunity and bizarre neurological and psychological disturbances. These children fail to thrive and if untreated may die. Family members share a tendency to have diminished zinc levels as well.

Zinc is poorly absorbed from cow's milk, and manifestations of acrodermatitis enteropathica were initially recognized when symptoms of zinc deficiency appeared in infants fed cow's milk. These infants improved when switched to more easily digested breast milk.

See also ZINC.

Active-H. See HYDROGEN.

adder's tongue (lamb's tongue, snake leaf, rattlesnake violet, erythonium, dog-tooth violet, serpent's tongue, yellow snowdrop) A perennial, flowering herb, *Erythonium americanum,* that grows in rich soil all over the United States, whose bulbs and leaves are used as an emetic (to induce vomiting) and as a poultice for scrofula and other skin conditions.

additives Chemicals or substances added to foods, medications or supplements as coloring or flavoring agents, preservatives, sweeteners or to improve consistency. Adverse reactions are rare from the approximately 2,800 substances approved by the Food and Drug Administration (FDA). An estimated 12,000 other chemicals enter the food supply unintentionally.

One important and potentially life-threatening reaction can occur in persons susceptible to the preservatives known as sulfiting agents. These additives can cause asthma or life-threatening anaphylaxis (allergic shock), with symptoms including a flushed feeling, drop in blood pressure and tingling sensations.

Dyes approved in the Food, Drug and Cosmetic Act (FD&C) of 1938 are derivatives of coal tar. Tartrazine or FD&C yellow dye number 5 is frequently implicated as a cause of hyperactivity in children and asthma. However, less than 10 percent of individuals suspected of having adverse reactions to these additives reacted when challenged in a controlled study. Asthmatics who are allergic to aspirin may also react when exposed to the dye tartrazine.

Butylated hydroxanisol (BHA) and butylated hydroxytoluene (BHT) are used in low doses as antioxidants (see ANTIOXIDANTS) in grain products, including breakfast cereals, and have not been shown to cause any allergic problems. However, since antioxidants are thought by some to prevent cancer and herpes infections and to retard aging, they are often used in megadoses in various health-food preparations that may be toxic.

The azo dye amaranth (FD&C red number 5) was banned by the United States in 1975 because of suspected carcinogenicity. Aspartame (Nutrasweet) is often blamed for adverse effects, but except for a few cases of urticaria (hives), there is no scientific proof of ill effects. Tartrazine is also frequently implicated in causing hives. However, well-controlled studies such as those at the Scripps Clinic and Research Foundation have rarely confirmed these suspicions. The dyes do play a role as sensitizers, or allergens, in allergic dermatitis. They are often suspected of inducing adverse effects both in the skin and when ingested. Skin reactions are relatively common; when dyes are used in foods and supplements, they are rarely proven to be the source of the adverse effect.

adonis (false hellebore, pheasant's eye, ox-eye, red Morocco, rose-a-rubie, sweet vernal) An anemone-like, early spring plant native to Russia, Hungary and Bulgaria, *Adonis vernalis,* prepared as a powder and used in Russian folk medicine for treating menstrual problems, edema and fever, and in homeopathic medicine for cardiac disorders, including arrhythmia and general weakness. Individuals with potassium deficiency or on digitalis-based medication, such as Lanoxin, should avoid adonis. Adonis may potentiate both the effectiveness and side effects of calcium supplements, diuretics, quinine, laxatives and steroids, including prednisone and hydrocortisone.

agastache (huo xiang, wrinkled giant hyssop) The herb *Agastache rugosa* of the family Labiatae, native to China, Japan, northern Vietnam and Laos, used in traditional Chinese medicine for treating fever, headache, nausea and vomiting, diarrhea, gas, colds and cholera. *Agastache* is Greek for "many-spiked," which describes the plant's flowering spikes.

agave (American agave, spiked aloe, American century, century plant, flowering aloe) A perennial plant, *Agave americana,* of the tropical regions of America and in some parts of Europe, considered to be an antiseptic, diuretic and laxative. It has been used in the treatment of liver disease and pulmonary tuberculosis.

aging See NUTRITION AND AGING.

agrimony (xian he cao, sticklewort, burr marigold) A fruit-bearing, yellow-flowered herb with toothed leaves, of the genus *Agrimonia* of the rose family. Available in powdered or capsule form, agrimony is thought to relieve gastrointestinal disorders and to strengthen the liver, gallbladder and kidneys. Agrimony, which contains vitamins B and K and other nutrients, is also said to inhibit any type of bleeding. In Chinese traditional medicine, agrimony, especially *Agrimonia eupatoria* and *pilosa,* is used to treat dysentery, stomach pain, and vomiting of blood, bleeding in the uterus, blood in the urine and stool and exhaustion.

AIDS (acquired immunodeficiency syndrome) and vitamin deficiency Some individuals with AIDS, in addition to many other health deficits, seem to lack the ability to absorb nutrients including vitamins and minerals that leads to malnutrition. Studies conducted by researchers at Johns Hopkins University, Baltimore, Maryland have found lower levels of vitamin A in individuals who test positive for HIV. Those with AIDS and vitamin A deficiency died up to six times more rapidly than those who had normal vitamin A levels.

See also A, VITAMIN.

ailanthus (tree-of-heaven, varnish tree, copal tree) The tree *Ailanthus altissima,* of the family Simaroubaceae, indigenous to China, whose root bark and fruit are used in Chinese traditional medicine to treat dysentery, piles, bloody stools, vaginal discharge, premature ejaculation and tapeworm, and to increase menstrual flow.

akebia (mu tong, five-leaf akebia, chocolate vine) The vine *Akebia quinata* or *trifoliata,* of the family Lardizabalaceae, whose stem, fruit stalk and root are used in Chinese traditional medicine. Native to China, Japan and Korea, akebia is thought to relieve fever and inflammation of the skin, induce the secretion of breast milk in a new mother, induce perspiration and increase menstrual flow. The fruit stalk is used as a purgative.

alanine A natural amino acid, $C_3H_7NO_2$, that is considered nonessential.
See also AMINO ACIDS.

albizia (mimosa tree, silk tree) An ornamental tree, *Albizia julibrissin,* of the family Leguminosae, grown from Iran to Japan and cultivated in other countries, whose bark and flowers are considered medicinal by traditional Chinese practitioners. The bark is said to tranquilize, relieve pain, improve circulation and treat insomnia, bleeding, fractures and lung cancer. The flowers are used as a general tonic.

alcoholism The excessive, debilitating intake of alcoholic beverages, accompanied by a decreased desire for food. The substitution of alcohol for food causes multiple nutritional deficiencies and interferes with the absorption of nutrients when they are ingested. Beriberi, Korsakoff's syndrome and Wernicke's disease, all disorders of thiamine deficiency, are prevalent in alcoholism. Riboflavin, vitamin B_{12}, magnesium, potassium and selenium are other vitamins and minerals that are frequently deficient in alcoholics.

Women who drink more than two alcoholic drinks daily have a 25 to 50 percent increased risk of hip fractures. A group of white men between the ages of 49 and 61 years with a history of alcohol abuse for at least 10 years was found to have spinal bone densities averaging 58 percent of the normal density. The cause for these findings has not been determined.

alder (holly, winterberry, feverbush, black alder, brook alder, striped alder) A deciduous shrub, *Ilex verticillata,* common to swamplands of northeastern America and England, whose bark and fruit are used in the preparation of infusions or decoctions to treat worms and dyspepsia. An excessive quantity of the berries may be poisonous.

alehoof (ground ivy, cat's foot, gill-go-by-ground, turn hoof, hay maids, alehoof, gill-creep-by-ground, creeping Charlie, gillrun, hedge maids, turnhoof) A flowering perennial herb, *Nepeta hederacea,* found in the eastern states, on the Pacific coast and in Europe, whose leaves and flowering herb are used as an appetizer, astringent, digestive, diuretic, stimulant and tonic. Ground ivy is commonly thought to relieve diarrhea, colds, sore throat, bronchitis, headache, hypoacidity, neurasthenia and liver problems. Large quantities of ground ivy can be poisonous.

aleurites (tung: oil tree, China wood-oil tree) A tree indigenous to central Asia and cultivated elsewhere, *Aleurites fordii,* of the family Euphorbiaceae, known to have insecticidal properties. The oil, used in the manufacture of India ink, is also claimed to treat boils, burns and other topical anomaly, according to traditional Chinese medicine. The immature fruits are used to treat anemic conditions and the absence of menses.

alfalfa An edible herb grass, succulent perennial and legume, *Medicago sativa,* containing calcium, magnesium, phosphorus, potassium, iron, essential enzymes, choline, sodium and vitamins A, B_6, D, K and P, cited for its beneficial effects against arthritis, intestinal ulcers, liver disorders, eczema, asthma, anemia, bleeding gums, gastritis, hemorrhoids, burns, fungal infections, cancer and hypertension, among other problems. In Arabic, alfalfa means "father" and as herbalist, acupuncturist and author Michael Tierra, of California, says, perhaps this refers to alfalfa's "patriarchal" function as a highly esteemed restorative tonic. The chlorophyll content of alfalfa is thought to contribute to its potency. While alfalfa sprouts may be purchased at most supermarkets and eaten raw in salad, alfalfa is also available as a liquid, especially recommended to be taken during a fasting period.

Known as Mu-Su in Chinese medicine, alfalfa is effective as a raw green food, powder or tea. Its vitamin P (rutin) is reported to build the strength of capillaries and reduce inflammation of the stomach lining, thus it is used an antiulcer treatment. Alfalfa is said to increase the flow of mother's milk and relieve low back pain. Alfalfa tea contributes to the digestive process for sugars, fats, starches and protein. Native Americans, who introduced the plant as a fresh green after it was brought from Europe to the United States in the mid-1800s, also ground alfalfa seeds into flour and added it to breads, gruel and other foods. People of the Great Plains region of America often referred to alfalfa as buffalo grass.

According to Ayurvedic medicine (*ayu* means life and *veda* means knowing in Sanskrit, the classical language of India and Hinduism), alfalfa is used as an anti-inflammatory, a natural pain reliever (for sciatica, for example) and as an agent that cleanses the large intestine of toxins.

algae   The Latin word for seaweed. Algae belongs to a group of aquatic plants—subphylum Algae of the phylum Thallophyta, the lowest division of the animal kingdom—including pond scums, stoneworts and seaweeds that contain chlorophyll. Ranging in size from microscopic to massive and found in salt or fresh water or moist places such as swamps, algae have no roots, stems or leaves. Kelp and Irish moss are forms of algae.

Blue-green algae, which grows in brackish water, has not been approved for sale in the United States. However, harvested wild, it is marketed as an organic food containing vitamins and all the amino acids and as beneficial in the daily diet. Some marketers and distributors of blue-green algae claim that algae increases energy; alleviates stress, anxiety and depression; relieves hypoglycemia, fatigue, constipation and allergies; and improves digestion, memory and immune functions.

According to the late nutritionist and author Adelle Davis, whose best-selling books of the 1950s to the 1970s influenced the public view and study of nutrition, algae in the form of kelp constitutes a treatment for an inadequate supply of iodine to the thyroid gland, which regulates metabolism, especially in areas affected by fallout from bomb testing. Kelp and other seaweeds contain iodine that is necessary for healthy thyroid functioning and pro-

tection against radioactive material easily absorbed by, and thus damaging to, the thyroid.

See also IRISH MOSS; KELP.

alisma (ze xie, water plantain, mad-dog weed)   The North American and East Asian herb *Alisma plantago-aquatica,* of the family Alismataceae, considered to have anticancer properties and the ability to lower blood sugar in animals. In traditional Chinese medicine, the underground stem is used to treat hypertension, diabetes, kidney inflammation, venereal diseases, vertigo, lumbago and painful urination.

allergy to foods   See FOOD ALLERGY.

allium (garlic)   The plant *Allium sativum,* of the family Amaryllidaceae, of European origin and cultivated all over the world. The garlic bulb, divided into cloves, is popular as both a food flavoring and medicinal/nutritive agent. Eastern and Western medical disciplines recognize the value of garlic as a natural antibiotic for colds, sore throat, phlegm in the respiratory tract, asthma, bronchitis, abscesses and tuberculosis. Garlic is also known to reduce high blood pressure and cholesterol.

The ancient Egyptians used garlic to cure headaches, tumors, heart disorders and intestinal worms. Ancient Olympic athletes ate garlic to increase their energy. In the first century A.D., garlic was prescribed by Dioscorides, chief physician to the Roman army, as an anthelmintic (intestinal worm-killing) agent. Garlic may also have anticarcinogenic properties and is used as an antidote against various toxins. First known to be used in Chinese medicine during the reign of Emperor Huang Ti, garlic has been gaining popularity and credibility by researchers as an agent that promotes immune-system support and fights viruses.

allspice   An aromatic spice, *Pimenta officinalis,* prepared from the berries of the West Indian tree *Pimenta dioica* (the allspice tree), of the myrtle family. According to herbalists, allspice has medicinal properties similar to those of cloves: it warms the body, increases circulation, promotes digestive health, and treats nausea, vomiting and intestinal gas.

See also CLOVE.

aloe A member of the Lily family, *Aloe vera*, also known as "the burn plant," and whose name in Sanskrit, *kumari*, means goddess. Indigenous to East and South Africa, the succulent aloe is grown in the West Indies, tropical areas, some Mediterranean countries and in the southwestern and southeastern United States. While the aloe plant's gel has long been used as a topical remedy for minor burns, sunburn and abrasions, insect bites, diaper and heat rashes and rashes from poison ivy, oak or sumac, aloe may also be taken internally. Herbalists and nutritionists often use crystallized aloe in extract form as a laxative and "cleanser" for the liver, kidneys and spleen.

In Ayurvedic (Indian) medicine, aloe is considered a general liver tonic, a pain reliever of muscle spasms associated with menstruation, a mild laxative, a blood purifier and therefore beneficial to the liver, gallbladder and stomach, and a balancer of *vata, pitta* and *kapha*—the Ayurvedic aspects of human constitution, or body types.

However, the internal use of aloe, which contains a substance called anthraquinone, has come under question because it has been known to cause gastrointestinal cramping.

The National Aloe Science Council, a trade association created in 1972 by 30 manufacturers of aloe products, plans to establish scientific studies, ethics and standards for the production of aloe, including as juices and drinks, to satisfy the requirements of the Food and Drug Administration (FDA).

Alstonia bark (Australian quinine, Australian fever bush, devil tree, fever bark, pali-mara) Native to the Australian evergreen tree *Alstonia constricta,* this herb is used to treat diarrhea, malaria, rheumatism and fever, because of its small amount of reserpine, an ingredient also found in medications for hypertension.

alum root (American sanicle, crane's bill) The root of an herb of the genus *Sanicula* (of the carrot family) used in folk medicine as an astringent for sore throats or canker sores or as an anodyne (pain reliever) and anti-inflammatory for diarrhea, hemorrhoids, ulcers and excessive menstruation.

aluminum A mineral with no known nutritional benefit and which may be harmful to bone or the brain tissues. High levels of aluminum in the diet may interfere with the absorption or utilization of other essential minerals, including calcium, phosphorus, magnesium, selenium and fluoride. Muscle pain and weakness and bone deterioration are signs of aluminum toxicity. Studies in rats suggest that aluminum accumulation in the brain may be a cause of Alzheimer's disease. Sources of dietary aluminum include food additives, acidic foods cooked in aluminum pans that absorb or leach the mineral and some antacids.

See also ALZHEIMER'S DISEASE.

Alzheimer's disease Progressive and irreversible disorder, characterized mainly by loss of memory, named for the German neurologist Alois Alzheimer (1864–1915). As the dementia worsens, it results in loss of the control of body functions and eventual death.

Although the cause of Alzheimer's disease is unknown, scientists have implicated both aluminum and zinc deposits in the brain as possible causes. Failing appetite in Alzheimer's patients may result in severe vitamin deficiencies, and they should be given supplements.

amalaki An Ayurvedic herb thought to rejuvenate tissue, relieve gastrointestinal irritation and stabilize blood sugar–related problems.

amaranth (love lies bleeding, red cockscomb, pile wort, prince's feather, velvet flower) A common weed, *Amaranthus hybridus,* of the family Amaranthaceae (also listed as *Amaranthus hypochondriacus* of the family Americanceae), whose seeds and greens (called pigweed in the West because it is fed to pigs) are used as food and other parts as medicinal preparations for the treatment of throat, stomach and intestinal ulcers, dysentery, diarrhea and bleeding. Amaranth greens are said to taste like spinach and contain iron, other minerals and vitamins A and C. The greens are also considered valuable as an acid neutralizer to a diet high in acid-producing grains, beans, meat and milk products.

American Cancer Society guidelines on diet and nutrition To help people make educated choices about nutrition, the Society publishes nutritional guidelines to advise the public on dietary practices that may reduce the risk of cancer. The guidelines are meant to be practiced as a whole, creating a total dietary pattern to follow for lowered cancer risk. (1) maintain a desirable body weight; (2) eat a varied diet; (3) include a variety of vegetables and fruits in the daily diet; eat more high-fiber foods such as whole grain cereals, legumes, vegetables and fruits; (4) cut down on total fat intake; (5) limit consumption of alcoholic beverages, if you drink at all; limit consumption of salt-cured, smoked and nitrite-preserved foods. (Used with permission, American Cancer Society, Inc.)

American Dietetic Association position statements   The philosophy and requirements set forth by the American Dietetic Association pertaining to public policy on nutrition, including:

(1) It is the position of the American Dietetic Association that the U.S. government establish a national policy on enrichment and fortification of the food supply that protects against nutrient insufficiencies and toxicities.

(2) To assure the American public safe, nontoxic dietary supplements, it is the position of The American Dietetic Association that dietary supplements be regulated like foods and that all associated health claims be based on significant scientific agreement.

See Appendix V for the latest complete text.

American Nutraceutical Association   See NUTRACEUTICALS.

amino acids   A group of organic compounds considered the "building blocks" of proteins. Of the nearly 80 amino acids found in nature, about 20 are required for human growth and metabolism. Essential amino acids are those provided by foods; nonessential amino acids are produced naturally by the body and therefore not required through food intake. The essential amino acids are histidine, isoleucine, leucine, lysine, methionine, cysteine, phenylalanine, tyrosine, threomine, tryptophan and valine. The nonessentials are alanine, aspartic acid, arginine (nonessential in adults but essential in infants because infants' bodies can-

not produce enough of the compound in time to meet the metabolic demand), citrulline, glutamic acid, glycine, hydroxyglutamic acid, hydroxyproline, norleucine, proline and serine.

Examples of complete proteins, that is, those containing all the essential amino acids, are milk, milk products, eggs and meat. Vegetables, grains and gelatin are incomplete proteins. In a normal adult maintaining a constant weight, the recommended daily protein intake is about 0.8 grams per kilogram of body weight, or about 46 grams of protein per day for women and 56 grams per day for men.

During digestion, amino acids transfer from the walls of the intestine and the portal vein into the blood. From the blood they move through the liver into the bloodstream, and are then distributed to the tissues as required so the tissues can produce their own protein. Amino acids not needed by the body for the building and repair of tissue are broken down into ammonia, carbon dioxide and water, producing heat and energy. They may also become the end products of digestion, such as urea, which is eliminated by the body.

One component of all proteins is the gas nitrogen, found in compounds including ammonia, nitrites and nitrates and essential to plant and animal life as a tissue builder. The physical state of nitrogen balance refers to an equal amount of nitrogen ingested and excreted daily by the body. The Western diet, tends to foster a negative nitrogen balance. However, the body can withstand a

TABLE 3 20 AMINO ACIDS SPECIFIED BY THE GENETIC CODE	
Alanine	*Leucine
Arginine	*Lysine
Asparagine	*Methionine
Aspartic acid	*Phenylalanine
Cysteine	Proline
Glutamic acid	Serine
Glutamine	*Threonine
Glycine	*Tryptophan
*Histadine	Tyrosine
*Isoleucine	*Valine

*Essential amino acids

negative nitrogen balance for a certain period because body proteins and other compounds containing nitrogen are continuously being synthesized and degraded as amino acids and reutilized to satisfy any needs.

Inadequate intake of proteins, responsible for the growth and repair of cells, may lead to nutritional disorders including kwashiorkor and marasmus, commonly seen in African and Asian countries. Anorexia nervosa, an eating disorder characterized by extreme slenderness and malnourishment because of a lack of protein and calories, is often the result of compulsive dieting. Lack of protein may also result in anemia, a reduced number of red blood cells (and therefore reduced oxygen circulation) stemming from defective nucleoprotein synthesis, iron deficiency and other causes.

Ovolactovegetarians, who eat eggs, milk and cheese, can obtain sufficient amounts of essential amino acids, but vegans, who eat only vegetables and grains, may be at risk of protein deficiency.

Requirements

Allowances are expressed as protein but reflect requirements for amino acids. Proteins and other compounds containing nitrogen are continuously being synthesized and degraded as amino acids are reutilized. However, some amino acids are lost in a process called oxidative catabolism. Metabolic breakdown products of amino acids such as urea, creatinine and uric acid are excreted in the urine. Nitrogen is also lost in hair and nails and as skin sloughs. Therefore, a continuous supply of amino acids is required. During the metabolic processes the keto acid portion of the compounds are utilized for energy or converted to carbohydrate or fat.

Deficiencies

Inadequate nutrition is the major cause of protein and therefore amino acid deficiency, a cause seldom seen in the United States.

Supplementation

Many unproven claims have been attributed to amino acid supplements, either in balanced formulations or as individual products. Allegations range from strengthening the immune system to reducing dependency on drugs. Additionally, there may be as yet unrecognized risks associated with these supplements, and they should not be used except under the supervision of a physician or university-trained nutritionist.

High protein intake or unbalanced diets seem to suppress the appetite. A combination of phenylalanine, valine, methionine and tryptophan taken by a group of obese persons one half-hour before lunch reduced their food intake by almost 25 percent. In a group of normal weight individuals, tryptophan alone suppressed the appetite.

Phenylalanine and tyrosine may be low in persons suffering from depression. These amino acids are involved in the manufacture of the neurotransmitters dopamine, norepinephrine and epinephrine (adrenaline). Tryptophan is converted to another important neurotransmitter serotonin. Interestingly, antidepressant drugs such as fluoxetine (Prozac) exert their effect by blocking the utilization of serotonin. Amitriptyline (Elavil) and other tricyclic antidepressants act similarly by blocking the action of both norepinephrine and serotonin at the level of the neurons. As the compounds appear to terminate the activity of these nerves, depression is counteracted.

Caution must be used in taking individual amino acid supplements because the risks have not been adequately defined at this time.

Toxicity

There is no strong evidence that ingestion of excessive amino acids is harmful in persons with normal kidney function.

amino acid chelates A method of combining amino acids with a metal such as iron. Advocates for the use of chelated minerals claim that they improve absorption of poorly absorbed minerals three to five times over the absorption of unchelated minerals. Detractors of these compounds feel they are not worth the extra expense. In addition, when minerals are taken with meals, they are naturally chelated by the digestive system.

amomum (sharen, round cardamon) An herb native to Java, *Amomum compactum*, and *illosum*, of the family Zingiberaceae, whose seeds are used as an aromatic spice. In Asian medicinal practices, the cardamom fruit is used to expel gas, prevent vomiting and stimulate stomach secretions.

amorphophallus (devil's tongue, snake palm)
The tropical herb *Amorphophallus riveri,* of the family Araceae, whose stem is used in Chinese medicine to treat poisonous-snake bites and whose flowering stalk is used to reduce fever.

ampelopsis A deciduous plant native to China and Japan, *Ampelopsis japonica,* of the family Vitaceae, whose roots are considered by Chinese traditional practitioners to be an anticonvulsant, purgative, cooling and anti-inflammatory. The roots are also used to expel phlegm.

amygdalin (also known as laetrile or "vitamin B$_{17}$") A potentially toxic substance extracted from the pits of apricots and falsely reputed to cure cancer. This substance is not a vitamin and has no nutritional value. Initially promoted by Ernst Krebs, a biochemist, in 1952, the drug was found worthless in clinical trials by the National Cancer Institute and other scientific organizations. Since there is no known need for this substance, it does not meet the criteria to be classified a vitamin (see VITAMIN). In addition, the product contains 6 percent cyanide and has caused chronic cyanide poisoning and death. Despite this, many cancer sufferers desperate to find a cure turned to illegal or foreign sources of the drug. Perhaps the greatest tragedy was that many individuals with potentially treatable cancers delayed conventional therapy until it was too late.

amylase Also known as amylolytic enzyme, amylase is one of the colloid enzymes that split or hydrolyze starch, as in pancreatic, salivary and vegetable amylase. Amylolysis is the enzymatic breakdown of starch into sugar during digestion. Plant amylases are called beta-amylases; amylases found in animals are called alpha-amylases.

andrographis (creat) The Asian herb, also considered a weed, *Andrographis paniculata,* of the family Acanthaceae, used in Chinese medicine to treat flu, pneumonia, bronchitis, whooping cough,

hypertension, bites, burns and infection of the gallbladder.

anemarrhena (zhi mu) A native northern Chinese plant, *Anemarrhena asphodeloides,* of the family Lilliaceae, best known in Chinese medicine for its extract, which yields steroidal saponins, anti-inflammatory agents effective against lumbago. The underground stem is used for preparations to treat congestion and thirst as a result of fever, excessive perspiration, pneumonia, chronic cough, measles, vertigo, nausea and vomiting related to pregnancy, and premature ejaculation. Large doses of the medicinal underground stem of the plant are toxic and may inhibit cardiac function.

anemia Diminished number of erythrocytes, or red blood cells, or in the quantity of hemoglobin caused by decreased production or blood loss.
See also ANEMIA, MACROCYTIC; ANEMIA, MICROCYTIC.

anemia, macrocytic A type of anemia characterized by below-normal numbers of red blood cells that are larger than normal size. The red blood cells, or erythrocytes, are recognized by their increased mean corpuscular volume (MCV) and mean corpuscular hemoglobin (MCHC). Pernicious anemia, a vitamin B$_{12}$ deficiency, and folate deficiencies are types of macrocytic anemia.
See also B$_{12}$, VITAMIN; FOLIC ACID.

anemia, microcytic A type of anemia characterized by below-normal numbers of red blood cells that are smaller than normal size. The red blood cells, or erythrocytes, are recognized by a diminished mean corpuscular volume (MCV) and mean corpuscular hemoglobin (MCHC). Iron deficiency is the most common cause of this type of anemia.
See also IRON; PYRIDOXINE.

anemone Temperate herb of the family Ranunculaceae containing glycoside ranunculin, a poison. The sap of the anemone causes skin irritation and blisters and, when taken internally, may cause various problems ranging from severe gastrointestinal and kidney inflammation to respiratory failure. The *Anemone hupehensis* (Japanese anemone) is used in Chinese medicine, however, to treat ringworm and lymphatic tuberculosis, and the roots of the *Anemone cernua* are used to treat sore throat, toothache, stomachache and bone fractures and pain. *Anemone chinensis* roots are used to treat diarrhea.

angelica (dang gui, holy ghost plant, root of the holy ghost, archangel, masterwort, purple angelica, alexanders) The genus *Angelica atropurpurea* of herbs of the Ammiaceae family used as a flavoring oil. In powdered form or capsules, angelica is touted by nutritionists (though not proven by scientists) to be an effective heart-strengthener and for use against heart and lung disease. *Angelica archangelica* is also claimed to remedy gastrointestinal problems, including indigestion and gas, and to have the ability to create a distaste for alcoholic beverages. In addition, angelica is said to be effective against menstrual irregularity, colds and coldness.

anise The herb *Pimpinella anisum,* a member of the Umbellifer family, whose leaves, stalks and seeds are used as a licoricelike flavoring and as a salad ingredient. Cultivated by the ancient Egyptians, Greeks and Romans and touted by Chinese, Japanese and other herbalists, anise is said to have a therapeutic effect on intestinal gas, indigestion, bad breath, coughing and congestion, and a property that increases breast milk. Anise is also known as a mild diuretic.

antacids as calcium supplements Agents that neutralize excessive acid in the stomach and intestines. Tums and Rolaids, among the over-the-counter antacids, contain calcium carbonate and are widely promoted as calcium supplements.

antibiotics and vitamin interactions See Appendix III.

anticarcinogens See CANCER PREVENTION; CANCER TREATMENT WITH VITAMINS.

anticonvulsants and vitamin interactions Drugs used in the treatment of seizure disorders, including phenytoin (Dilantin), carbamazepine (Tegretol), phenobarbital and primidone, that interfere with the absorption or action of certain vitamins. Phenytoin, phenobarbital and primidone compete with the absorption of folic acid, thus long-term use may cause a folate deficiency. However, the consumption of large doses of folic acid may block the effectiveness of phenytoin, increasing the likelihood of seizures.

Calcium-containing antacids may interfere with the absorption of anticonvulsants, and the doses should be staggered to prevent this. Osteomalacia (the increased softness of bones as a cause of deformities, such as the adult form of rickets) has been associated with phenytoin and is thought to be due to the drug's interference with vitamin D metabolism.

antioxidants Substances, including vitamins A, C and E and the trace elements selenium, manganese and zinc, thought to protect the cells from destructive oxidation by free radicals. Free radicals are compounds naturally produced in the body. They contain one or more unpaired electrons, or electrical charges, and are therefore unstable. To achieve stability, free radicals "borrow" or "steal" electrons from stable compounds. This process allows formerly stable compounds to become reactive and cause the oxidation that may interfere with normal cell function and possibly mutate cells.

Peroxides are among the free radicals that are byproducts formed when fat molecules react with oxygen. Free radicals are also formed by radiation and are present in air pollution, ozone and cigarette smoke. Other examples of oxidation are the rusting of iron and the browning of apples and lettuce left exposed to the air. Oxidation also occurs when cooking fats become rancid.

Fatty cell membranes are choice targets for attack by free radicals. These substances alter cell functions by interfering with the transport of nutrients, oxygen and water into the cell and the removal of waste materials. Free radicals may also assault nucleic acids and the genetic code in each cell. The resulting cell damage may disrupt growth or repair of damaged or aging tissues. Some researchers implicate free radicals as a cause of premature aging.

In a six-month study at the Washington University School of Medicine, 11 young men were given supplemental antioxidants consisting of 600 International Units (IU) of vitamin E, 1,000 milligrams of vitamin C and 30 milligrams (50,000 IU) of beta-carotene daily. A nine-man control group was given a placebo (an inactive lookalike) supplement. After running for 35 minutes on a treadmill at the beginning and end of the study, free-radical production was measured in each group. The vitamin-users produced 17 to 36 percent fewer free radicals than the control group.

Antioxidants have been promoted as cancer-preventing agents. Unfortunately, this has yet to be proven. In one study involving more than 850 people, mostly men, known to have had at least one benign polyp in the colon, subjects were given antioxidant supplements for four years. There was no difference in the recurrence of polyps among the group that took beta-carotene, vitamins C and E, all three vitamins or a placebo. Colon polyps begin as benign growths, but some have the potential to become malignant if they are not removed.

Evidence from a Harvard University study looks promising for vitamin E's ability to modify the incidence of heart disease. However, vitamins A, C and E may be more appropriately considered redox agents. Although antioxident in the physiologic quantities present in food, they are pro-oxidant in the larger quantities found in some supplements. Therefore, more research is needed to determine if there is any benefit from taking large doses of these vitamins.

See also ASCORBIC ACID; BETA-CAROTENE; CARDIO-VASCULAR DISEASE PREVENTION AND ANTIOXIDANT VITAMINS; E, VITAMIN; EYE DISEASES.

antithiamine factors (ATF) Substances in the diet that diminish the bioavailability (the ability of body tissues to utilize a substance present in the diet) of thiamine in the diet. Inadequate thiamine causes beriberi, a potentially fatal vitamin-deficiency disease. There are two types of ATF: thermolabile (destroyed by heat) and thermostable (ability to withstand heat). Thiaminase I is found in the viscera of freshwater fish, some saltwater fish, shellfish, in ferns and some plants and some bacteria. Thiaminase II is found in some bacteria

and fungi. These substances break down the thiamine during food preparation, storage or as the vitamin passes through the gastrointestinal tract. Frequent ingestion of raw freshwater fish and shellfish may cause thiamine deficiency. However, cooking prevents this process.

Thermostable ATF are found in ferns, tea, betel nut, some other plants, vegetables and animal tissues. Ascorbic acid, or vitamin C, prevalent in citrus fruits, improves thiamine status in those who habitually chew tea leaves or betel nut.

See also BERIBERI; THIAMINE.

anxiety and stress Illness as well as physical and emotional stress that may deplete the body of some vitamin storage. Many advocate the use of megadoses of supplements, especially niacin and the other B-complex vitamins, for conditions ranging from minor anxiety and depression to schizophrenia and major depression. The large doses recommended by some are not only of unproven benefit, but may actually be toxic.

See also MEGAVITAMINS.

apple A tree of the *Malus* species, cultivated throughout the world and whose fruit, flowers, buds, leaves, twigs and bark are used as a food, beverage, and medicine. Apple seeds are toxic and are not recommended for consumption. Herbalists and naturopaths (practitioners of natural treatments) claim that apples, which contain malic and tartaric acids and potassium, sodium, magnesium and iron salts, help dissolve kidney or gallbladder stones. Chinese practitioners also claim that apple cider and other preparations are effective against diabetes, hypoglycemia, nausea and vomiting, fever and influenza. French herbalist Maurice Méssegué, author of *Of Men and Plants: Autobiography of the World's Most Famous Plant Healer* (Macmillan, 1973), used an apple blossom infusion as a treatment for sore throats and colds.

apricot seed (ku xing ren) The seed of the fruit of the tree *Prunus armeniaca*, of the Rosaceae family, whose kernel is said to provide a lung tonic, according to Chinese traditional medicine, but is also thought of as a source of laetrile, or "vitamin

B17," or amygdalin, not considered a true vitamin. Once praised as an anticancer agent, laetrile is not considered therapeutic or nutritive, and it contains cyanide, which in large doses may be lethal.

See also AMYGDALIN.

aquilaria (chen xiang, eagle-wood tree) A tropical tree, *Aquilaria agallocha,* of the family Thymelaeaceae, whose wood is grated and used in the preparation of Chinese medicines for rheumatism, smallpox and illness related to childbirth.

arbutus, trailing (gravel plant, winter pink, mountain pink, wild May flower, gravel laurel) A small evergreen plant, *Epigaea repens,* of the Ericaceae family, considered by Native American herbalists to be effective in the treatment of debilitated bladder, diarrhea and bloody or infected urine.

arctium (cuckold, great burdock, edible burdock) Derived from the Greek word *arctos,* meaning bear, a flowering, fruit-bearing weed, *Arctium lappa,* of the family Compositaea, found in Asia and Europe. American Indians and Europeans used the plant as an antibacterial agent. In the Middle Ages, it was considered a remedy for gallstones and kidney stones. In Chinese medicine, arctium leaves are used for dizziness and rheumatism, and the fruit and seeds are used for colds, sore throat, pneumonia, scarlet fever, smallpox, mumps, measles in the early stage and skin eruptions such as pimples and St. Anthony's fire. The roots are a mild laxative and can induce sweating and urinary flow.

areca (da fu pi, pinang, catechu, betel nut, betel palm) A flowering, fruit-bearing palm tree, *Areca catechu,* of the family Palmae, whose ripe seeds are used in Chinese medicine to treat diarrhea, indigestion, lumbago and urinary tract problems. The seeds also increase menstrual flow and expel tapeworms and roundworms. The areca kernel is flavored and chewed by people throughout the Old World tropics as a narcotic. It turns their saliva bright red.

arginine A nonessential amino acid produced by the breakdown of proteins and used to treat ele-vated ammonia levels in liver failure. Arginine supplementation seems to play a role in treating chronic inflammatory conditions. Following major surgery, it has been shown to reduce the patient's need to stay in the hospital. Arginine is necessary for the synthesis of polyamine and nucleic acid and can stimulate the secretion of the hormones prolactin, insulin, growth and glucagon.

Arginine is promoted by some as a way to increase sperm count, muscle tone and physical stamina and alertness. It should be avoided in growing children because it could cause joint and bone deformities. Excessive doses of supplements may cause thickening of the skin.

arnica (leopard's bane, mountain tobacco) A flowering plant, *Arnica montana,* of the family Compositae, prescribed in minute doses as an internal tonic by herbalists and homeopaths. Arnica oil and liniment are used freely, however, for bruises and other injuries such as aches, strains and painful skin problems in which the skin has not been broken.

arsenic Nonmetallic element with a garlicky odor. Although it has been used in some medicinal preparations in the past, it is rarely used today. Although no human deficiency has been identi-fied, some scientists feel arsenic and other trace minerals (see TRACE ELEMENTS) may play a role in human enzyme systems. Arsenic has been proven to be essential for normal growth and reproduction in rats, minipigs, chicken and goats. An estimated 0.4 mg to 0.9 mg daily intake of arsenic is far below amounts known to be toxic.

arsesmart (walter pepper, peach-wort, dead arssmare) An American plant, *Polygonum hydropiper,* of the family Polygonaceae, used in Native American medicine as a stimulant, diuretic and diaphoretic (to induce sweating). Homeopaths prescribe arsesmart for amenorrhea, colic, cough, diarrhea, dysentery, eczema, epilepsy, gonorrhea, gravel, hemorrhoids, cardiac problems, hysteria, laryngitis, ulcers and splenic ailments.

In Russian medical and herbal literature, poly-gonum is recognized as an effective herbal treat-ment for various problems.

Polygonum contains oil, several minerals and rutin and vitamins C and K. Folk-medicine practitioners believe it also stops bleeding.

arthritis Inflammatory disorder of the joints. The deformities common to severe rheumatoid arthritis can be crippling, and medical treatment is often inadequate for the relief of pain and does little if anything to prevent worsening of the disease. In addition, medical treatment may have many serious adverse effects. The antioxidant vitamins, omega-6 fatty acids (fish oil) and other supplements are promoted as "cures" for arthritis, but remain unproven. Double-blind clinical trials with these products are difficult because the pain of arthritis waxes and wanes even if no treatment is given.

See also ANTIOXIDANTS; BOSWELLIC ACID; CHONDROITIN; GERMANIUM; GLUCOSAMINE; OMEGA-3 FATTY ACIDS; OMEGA-6 FATTY ACIDS.

artichoke (blessed thistle, garden artichoke, globe artichoke) A perennial plant, *Cynara scolymus*, of the thistle family, whose flower heads are eaten as a vegetable and whose leaves and root are considered medicinal by herbalists. Extracts from these parts are said to have healing properties in cases of arteriosclerosis, liver dysfunction, postoperative anemia, chronic protein in the urine and indigestion.

arum (cocky baby, dragon root, starchwort, gaglee, Portland arrowroot, ladysmock) A perennial plant, *Arum maculatum*, whose arrowhead-shaped leaves are poisonous when eaten, but whose rootstock is considered a diaphoretic and expectorant.

asafoetida (devil's dung, gum asafetida) The plant *Ferula assafoetida*, of the Umbelliferae family, whose gum resin is often used in place of garlic in parts of Asia because it does not leave an offensive odor on the breath as garlic does. An ingredient in Worcestershire sauce, asafoetida is said to be effective in the treatment of coldness, respiratory distress including coughs, mood swings, hysteria, weak digestion, intestinal gas, yeast (*Candida albicans*) overgrowth, hypoglycemia and food allergies.

In Ayurvedic medicine, a pinch of asafoetida cooked with lentils is said to aid digestion. It also is thought to relieve gas in the intestines, relieve pain and remove toxins.

asarum (hazelwort, asarabacca, public house plant, asarabacca, wild nard) A European perennial plant, *Asarum europaeum*, whose rootstock and leaves are considered medicinal, mainly as an emetic (to induce vomiting).

ascorbic acid (vitamin C) A water-soluble compound that acts as a coenzyme, a reducing agent and antioxidant. The word *ascorbic* is derived from the Latin, meaning "without scurvy." Humans, other primates, guinea pigs and some birds lack the enzyme (L-glu-conolactone) that forms ascorbic acid in the body. The inability to manufacture ascorbic acid is due to an inborn mutation in carbohydrate metabolism. In most other animals, the vitamin is synthesized from glucose. Inadequate dietary supply of the vitamin causes scurvy.

History of Vitamin C

Scurvy is the oldest recognized nutritional-deficiency disease. Symptoms include loss of energy; pain in legs and joints; anemia; spongy, bleeding gums; bad breath; loosening of teeth; subcutaneous hemorrhages and bleeding from mucous membranes; and muscle pain. It is also characterized by abnormal formation of bones and teeth. Scurvy can be cured by vitamin C.

From the 16th through 18th centuries, scurvy was responsible for the death of one-half to two-thirds of the crew on prolonged ocean voyages during which the diet consisted only of cereals and meat. In 1747 British naval surgeon and physician James Lind recommended that limes and lemons be included on board ships of the British navy. Although the navy initially ignored Lind's recommendation, it finally complied, and British sailors became known as "limeys."

Actions

Vitamin C supplies electrons to enzymes that require metal ions. It also acts with the substances prolyl and lysyl hydroxylases in the manufacture of collagen. Collagen is the proteinaceous, fibrous material—or "body cement"—found in the connective tissues of the body, including skin, bone, ligaments, cartilage and dentin of teeth and comprising approximately 30 percent of body protein.

Some scientists feel that vitamin C (and vitamin E) may protect against carcinogens such as nitrosamine. This chemical is formed in the body from nitrates and nitrites found in processed meat products such as lunch meats and hot dogs.

Data from the Prospective Basel [Switzerland] Study and other studies seem to support the premise that the antioxidant properties of vitamin C and other nutrients may prevent some cancers. However, there is no conclusive evidence that they are curative.

Deficiency

Signs and symptoms of scurvy occur after about three to 12 months of a severe lack of dietary vitamin C. As the deficiency worsens, splinter hemorrhages develop near the tips of nails, gums become swollen, purple and bleed. Wounds fail to heal, bleeding may occur spontaneously from any part of the body, ankle and leg edema occurs, and there is diminished urinary output. A classic sign of scurvy is the formation of thick hair follicles with surrounding redness or bleeding.

Some authors on nutrition claim that vitamin C increases sperm count, motility and viability. Lack of vitamin C may have some deleterious effect on sperm, particularly in the case of severe deficiency.

Vitamin D deficiency results in imperfect formation of or inability to form the calcified lattice, or framework, of bone tissue. This poor bone structure is also characteristic of scurvy. In the presence of coexisting vitamin C and D deficiencies, important symptoms and X-ray findings of scurvy may be masked or modified, causing confusion in the diagnosis.

Possible but Unproven Benefits

English researchers have found that 1,000 milligrams per day of vitamin C given to healthy persons inhibit a destructive process in proteins known as glycosylation. Since this process is thought to cause diabetic complications, investigators speculate that complications may be delayed or prevented by vitamin C.

Vitamin C, along with folic acid, carotenoids and fiber, has been linked to a reduced incidence of breast cancer in a study of 626 patients in New York State. However, high-fiber intake rather than vitamin C and beta-carotene seemed to reduce colorectal cancer risk in a Canadian study.

Boston researchers found that vitamin C and A supplements taken for many years appeared to reduce the incidence of cataracts (see A, VITAMIN). Many nutritionists recognize that a balanced intake of multiple fruits and vegetables is probably a much better approach to reducing cancer risks than the use of any supplement, because different cancers seem to be protected by different vitamins or other factors.

Dosage and RDA

The U.S. recommended dietary allowances (RDA) for vitamin C are 35 mg daily from birth through one year of age, 40 mg from one to four years, and 60 mg over age four, including pregnant and lactating women. Scurvy usually responds to doses of 250 mg daily until signs of the disorder have begun to disappear. Then 100 mg daily prevents recurrence. Requirements increase up to 500 percent during periods of environmental stresses, such as exposure to extremes in temperature, burns, trauma and surgery. Cigarette smokers have a 50 percent increased need for vitamin C to maintain normal blood levels. Women taking oral contraceptives also have an increased need for the vitamin.

There is probably no significant benefit from taking natural rather than synthetic vitamin C (see NATURAL VITAMINS). Timed-release vitamin C may be less effective in raising vitamin C levels than regular, less expensive tablets.

There is evidence that doses of vitamin C need to be taken every 12 hours rather than once daily, because the body eliminates large doses in that time and timed-release formulas in about 16 hours.

Citrus fruits, tomatoes, potatoes and leafy vegetables are good sources of vitamin C. Much of the natural vitamin C in foods, however, is lost during storage and certain cooking processes, or is present in forms not bioavailable.

The Vitamin C Controversy and Dr. Linus Pauling

Nobel Prize–winning scientist Dr. Linus Pauling (1901–1994) believed there are wide variations in the vitamin requirements of animals and man.

Pauling and others have claimed large amounts of vitamin C are not only beneficial, but strengthen the immune system. Vitamin C supplementation has been shown to prevent or cure colds. The idea that it cures cancer is still controversial. However, the popularity of the vitamin indicates a discernible success rate in prevention or treatment of colds and other infections. There may be some cancer-protective properties of vitamin C.

A virtual war over vitamin C has existed for years between "establishment" scientists (including many physicians) and nutritionists. The scientists demand proof that megadoses, which can approach 10 grams of vitamin C per day, have any benefits. In addition, scientists believe megadoses may be harmful (see Toxicity below). To counter unsubstantiated claims by Dr. Pauling, the Mayo Clinic ran scientifically controlled studies that failed to prove any lasting benefits of vitamin C in a group of cancer patients.

New, more optimistic studies include an analysis of carotenoid and vitamin A, C and E intake for the prevention of age-related macular degeneration (AMD), conducted by Dr. Johanna M. Seddon of the Department of Ophthalmology of the Massachusetts Eye and Ear Infirmary, Harvard Medical School, Boston, Massachusetts, and colleagues. Another study, conducted from 1993 to 1994 by the University of Medicine and Dentistry of New Jersey, in Newark, New Jersey, indicated that elderly people who eat well and take daily multivitamins generally have stronger T-lymphocytes, the white blood cells that fight infection.

Furthermore, luminaries such as Kenneth Cooper, M.D., of the Cooper Aerobics Center in Dallas, Texas; Bruce Ames, Ph.D., professor of biochemistry at the University of California; William Castelli, M.D., director of the Framingham Heart Study; Dean Ornish, M.D., director of the Preventive Medicine Research Institute in Sausalito, California; Walter C. Millett, M.D., and Margo N. Woods, D.Sc., director of the nutrition unit at Tufts University School of Medicine, among others, have reported that they take vitamin C in doses ranging from 50 to 3,000 mg per day.

Toxicity and Other Adverse Effects

Vitamin C increases the absorption of iron. Elevated iron levels can be dangerous in some individuals and may even increase the risk of cardiovascular disease (see IRON). Even if large doses of vitamin C are not toxic to most persons, the process by which the body eliminates the excess vitamin may be. Theoretically, with doses of 1,000 to 10,000 mg per day, great quantities of urine are produced to eliminate the 99 percent of vitamin C not utilized. If insufficient fluids are not replaced, the vitamin C may crystallize and damage the kidneys. In order for vitamin C to be eliminated by the kidneys, this acidic substance must be neutralized. Calcium salts may be required in the process, possibly causing the formation of kidney stones. Large doses of the vitamin may cause water to be pulled into the colon from the circulatory system, thus causing diarrhea.

Vitamin C reacts to tests for diabetes and may give a false impression that blood sugar is too high, causing patients to increase insulin doses. This increased dose may result in insulin shock. The acidity of chewable vitamin C tablets, if used regularly and in large quantities, can dissolve tooth enamel.

Persons taking large doses of vitamin C should not suddenly stop taking it, but gradually taper the dose. Advocates of megadoses of vitamin C claim that the deep yellow color of urine indicates saturation of the body tissues, assuring adequate vitamin supply. However, the skeptics rebut this theory by saying the excess is at best a waste of money and at worst, actually harmful.

ash tree (weeping ash, European ash, American white ash)   A tree, *Fraxinus excelsior,* of the Oleaceae family, of the north temperate zone and extending into southern regions including Mexico and Java, whose bark and leaves are used by herbalists in the treatment of gout, arthritis, rheumatic pain, obesity, dropsy and fevers. Homeopathic application of ash includes the treatment of uterine problems. In Russia, Manchuria and China, ash leaves and bark are made into a tea thought to stimulate circulation in the extremities.

ashwagandha ("Indian ginseng")   An Ayurvedic preparation of the roots and leaves of the *Withania somnifera* plant, with its active constituents known as *withanolides*. The standardized measure of withanolides is 4.5 mg per tablet. Ashwagandha has been widely used as an "adaptogen," a term coined by advocates and manufacturers of natural dietary supplements that refers to an agent that helps the body adapt to physical, emotional and environmental stresses for optimal well-being.

asparagus (sparrowgrass) A popular spring vegetable, *Asparagus officinalis,* of the Liliaceae family, whose shoots are eaten and whose root is said to provide a respected "Yin tonic," which, in Chinese traditional medicine, refers to its healing properties for tuberculosis, AIDS, female hormonal and reproductive problems, dryness of the lungs and throat, and to promote love and compassion (possibly attributable to its steroidal glycosides). Asparagus shoots are considered useful for bladder infections. As a general body tonic, asparagus root is said to fight fatigue, various forms of "burnout" or exhaustion and knee, joint and back aches.

asthma and supplements Ascorbic acid (vitamin C) and other vitamins promoted for the treatment of asthma and allergic rhinitis (hay fever). Some studies have demonstrated improvement in spirometry (lung function tests), the standard for measuring response to asthma treatment. However, results are inconsistent, and benefits have not been seen in all studies.

Botanical, or herbal medicines that may be prescribed for asthma, allergies and other respiratory disorders include cat's claw, cordyceps, echinacea, ephedra, evening primrose oil, ginkgo biloba, green tea, kava, reishi, schisandra and St. John's wort. A source of remedies, dosages, studies and contraindications is *Botanical Medicines: The Desk Reference for Major Herbal Supplements,* second edition, by Dennis J. McKenna, Ph.D., Kenneth Jones, and Kerry Hughes, M.Sc.

astragalus (huang qi) An herb, *Astragalus membranaceus,* or *cochinchinensis,* of the family Lilliaceae, whose roots contain betaine, B-sitosterol, choline, dimethoxy-isoflavane, glucoronic acid, kumatak-

enin and sucrose, thought to be of use in the treatment of chronic lung weakness. In Chinese medicine astragalus in tonic form is used to protect the immune system, as a diuretic to reduce edema (excessive tissue fluids), and as an anhidrotic, an agent that inhibits perspiration. The herb is also used to promote healing and adrenal gland function, increase metabolism and fight fatigue.

atherosclerosis See CARDIOVASCULAR DISEASE PREVENTION AND ANTIOXIDANT VITAMINS.

athletes' needs See EXERCISE AND SUPPLEMENTS.

atractylis (bai zhu, atractylodes) An herb of Manchuria, Korea, northern and eastern China and Japan, *Atractylis ovata* (also *macrocephala*), of the Compositae family, whose roots are used in Chinese medicine to treat indigestion, skin problems, fever, nervousness, loss of appetite, chronic bronchitis, cough, night blindness, diarrhea and anemia associated with pregnancy.

aurantium (zhi ke) The fruit of the plant *Citrus aurantium,* used in Chinese medicine to tonify and disperse the body's energy, called *qi* (pronounced "chee"), especially in counteracting spasms and symptoms including poor digestion, muscle weakness, a feeling of heaviness and water retention.

averrhoa Originally a Malayan plant, *Averrhoa carambola,* of the Oxalidaceae family, whose fruit, commonly known as starfruit, is used in Chinese medicine to increase the flow of urine, treat wounds and stop bleeding. The starfruit was named for the Arabian physician Averrhoes (1149–1217).

avidin A protein in egg white that binds to biotin (of the Vitamin B complex) and prevents its absorption. A biotin deficiency may result if large amounts of raw egg white are ingested.

B₁, vitamin   See THIAMINE.

B₂, vitamin   See RIBOFLAVIN.

B₃, vitamin   See NIACIN.

B₅, vitamin   See PANTOTHENIC ACID.

B₆, vitamin group   See PYRIDOXINE.

B₁₂, vitamin (colbalamin, cyanocobalamin, hydroxocobalamin)   A component of the vitamin B complex essential to the growth and repair of all body cells. Vitamin B_{12} is a generic term for several cobalt-containing compounds, of which cyanocobalamin is the most stable form. Synthetic vitamin B_{12} contains a cyanide group not found naturally.

This water-soluble vitamin is derived from certain microorganisms. In the stomach, hydrochloric acid and pepsin release cyanocobalamin from dietary protein to which it is tightly bound. Parietal cells in the gastric mucosa (stomach lining) secrete a substance called intrinsic factor. The vitamin then binds to salivary R proteins and, after passing into the small intestine, is altered by pancreatic enzymes at the level of the jejunum. For simplification, the small intestine, or bowel, is a long tube, approximately 22 feet in length. The upper two-fifths is called the jejunum and the remaining three-fifths the ileum. In the jejunum, cyanocobalamin binds to a substance called intrinsic factor. The resulting intrinsic factor-cyanocobalamin complex formed is resistant to proteolysis (further breakdown by digestive enzymes) and passes unchanged until it adheres to special receptors on mucosal cells lining the distal ileum (the lower end of the bowel). It is at this level that vitamin B_{12} is absorbed.

Discovery

In the early 1800s, the word *pernicious* (meaning deadly or fatal) anemia was first used to describe a serious disease affecting older adults. Death usually occurred within two to five years. The 1926 discovery by George Richards Minot that nutrients in liver cured pernicious anemia led to the isolation of the vitamin (later termed B_{12}), for which Minot, William Parry Murphy and George Whipple received a Nobel Prize in 1934. Others, including Edwin Cohn and William Castle, were also involved in this important medical advancement.

The initial treatment for pernicious anemia was one pound of raw liver daily. The researchers reasoned that there must be extrinsic, or external, and intrinsic, or internal, factors involved in this anemia. These factors turned out to be vitamin B_{12} and intrinsic factor, respectively (see above).

Uses of Vitamin B_{12}

In addition to its growth and repair abilities, the vitamin is essential for the formation of mature red blood cells and central nervous system function. It interacts with folic acid coenzymes and is involved in the synthesis of DNA and methionine, an essential amino acid.

Experiments with laboratory mice suggest that vitamin B_{12}, when combined with vitamin C, may inhibit the formation of cancerous tumors in mice. Mice given either of the vitamins alone were not protected from developing tumors. Early studies suggested that vitamin C supplements might destroy vitamin B_{12} in the body. However, later, better designed studies showed that the presence of vitamin C actually promotes the absorption of cynocobalamin. The hydroxo-cobalamin form of B$_{12}$ may be preferred for the treatment of vitamin B$_{12}$ deficiency, since optic neuropathies (disorders of the optic nerve) may worsen with the use of the cyanocobalamin compound.

Dietary Sources

Vitamin B$_{12}$ is produced only by bacteria and must be obtained from animal products or fermented foods such as miso from fermented soybeans. The average American diet supplies an estimated 5 to 15 mcg daily. However, this amount of the vitamin B$_{12}$ is sufficient only if intrinsic factor (see above) is available and adequate calcium is present.

Deficiencies

Dietary deficiencies are rare except in strict vegetarians. Whether from inadequate dietary intake or from inadequate secretion of intrinsic factor (required for the absorption of B$_{12}$ from the small intestine) by the stomach, anemia occurs from insufficient vitamin B$_{12}$. The classical type of anemia that results from a lack of intrinsic factor is termed "pernicious." This anemia is caused by improper replication of the genetic code. Anemia is recognized by decreased numbers of larger-than-normal red blood cells called macrocytic cells. Less frequently, white blood cells and platelets are diminished, which increases susceptibility to colds, other infections, poor blood clotting and bruising.

Manifestations of anemia include fatigue, a feeling of weakness, dizziness (lightheadedness or vertigo) and tinnitus (ringing in the ears). In severe cases there may be palpitations, angina (chest pain) and congestive heart failure (shortness of breath). Due to its slow and gradual onset, anemia may be quite advanced before the individual becomes pale, has a rapid pulse, slight fever and appears to have mild jaundice (yellowing of the skin and the whites of the eyes). In late stages, the heart, liver and spleen may become enlarged.

Faulty formation of epithelial cells lining the gastrointestinal tract causes nausea, vomiting, diarrhea, anorexia (poor appetite) and poor absorption of food, possibly resulting in malnutrition. There may be skin rashes and a sore tongue that appears smooth, beefy and red.

Most troublesome, however, may be the irreversible neurologic disorders caused by vitamin B$_{12}$ deficiency before characteristic anemia occurs. Nerve damage is characterized by disorientation, numbness, tingling, confusion, agitation, irritability, dimmed vision, dizziness, delusions or hallucinations. B$_{12}$ is essential to the production of myelin, the substance that covers and protects our nerves. Destruction of this sheath, called demyelination, is the first step in a process that, if uninterrupted, may result eventually in the death of the involved nerves. Peripheral, spinal nerves or the brain itself may become involved. Unfortunately, irreparable damage may occur before the cause is recognized.

Hypochlorhydria or achlorhydria are states in which there is a deficiency or total absence of hydrochloric acid in the stomach. When this occurs, the cyanocobalamin bound to proteins in food may not be released in sufficient amounts to combine with R protein and intrinsic factor. This condition eventually results in B$_{12}$ deficiency. In addition, the acid-deficient environment in the stomach allows an overgrowth of gastric bacteria, which in turn produces compounds called analogs that are physically similar but not identical to vitamin B$_{12}$. These vitaminlike compounds compete with the vitamin for absorption, causing a deficiency of the vitamin. The ulcer drug omeprazole (Prilosec) may cause a vitamin B$_{12}$ deficiency because of its effectiveness in reducing the secretion of acid in the stomach.

Smokers were found to have lower levels of B$_{12}$ and folic acid in a study published in the *Journal of the American Medical Association* in 1988. In the study, precancerous changes in bronchial cells of the lungs were noticed in smokers. Supplementation of those vitamins seemed to modify the abnormal cells, suggesting a potential protective effect.

Prolonged exposure to extremely high doses of nitrous oxide, or "laughing gas," may lead to vitamin B$_{12}$ deficiency.

Anemia may result when there is a vast overgrowth of bacteria in the intestines that compete for available vitamin B$_{12}$ with the host. This condition occurs following surgical removal, or resection, of portions of the small intestine.

**TABLE 4 DIETARY CAUSES OF VITAMIN B$_{12}$
DEFICIENCY**

Total vegan (vegetarian) diet
Infants breast-fed by vegan mothers
Rarely alcoholism (folate deficiency is more common)
Dietary faddism, ignorance, religious beliefs, poverty
Inadequate absorption of vitamin B$_{12}$
Deficiency of intrinsic factor secretion in the stomach
  (total or diminished), including pernicious anemia,
  destruction of the gastric mucosa or surgical resection of the stomach
Inhibition of intrinsic factor by immune factors
Disorders of the small intestine, such as celiac disease,
  sprue, bacterial overgrowth, fish tapeworm infestation, malignancy, surgical removal of portions of the
  intestine
Drugs, including para-aminosalicylic acid (PAS),
  colchicine, neomycin, alcohol, possibly oral contraceptives and omeprazol (Prilosec)

**TABLE 5 CONDITIONS THAT MAY REQUIRE
VITAMIN B$_{12}$ SUPPLEMENTATION**

Alcoholism
Anemia, hemolytic (a condition in which anemia is
  caused by destruction of red blood cells)
Cancer of the bowel or pancreas
Fever, prolonged or chronic
Fish tapeworm infestation
Gastrectomy (surgical removal of all or part of the
  stomach)
Gastritis, atrophic with achlorhydria (a condition in
  which the stomach lining wastes away and loses the
  ability to secrete acid)
Metabolic disorders:
  (1) homocystinuria, usually a genetic disorder
      causing failure to thrive, can also be caused by
      inadequate vitamin B$_{12}$ or folate deficiency.
  (2) methylmalonic aciduria, an inherited disorder
      involved in the metabolism of vitamin B$_{12}$
Hyperthyroidism
Infection, prolonged or chronic
Kidney disease
Liver disorders
Malabsorption disorders associated with diarrhea
Stress, prolonged

Dosage

Supplementation of vitamin B$_{12}$ may be necessary
during pregnancy and breast-feeding in vegetarians. For infant formulas 0.15 mcg/kcal (micrograms per kilocalories of B$_{12}$) is required for each
1,000 calories of formula consumed. Multivitamins
with folic acid should also contain vitamin B$_{12}$.

People with pernicious anemia require injections of vitamin B$_{12}$, because the lack of intrinsic
factor in these individuals prevents absorption of
dietary or oral supplements in the intestine.

Toxicity

Although synthetic vitamin B$_{12}$ contains a cyanide
molecule, there is no known toxicity. However,
doses greater than 10,000 times the RDA may
rarely cause allergic reactions with the formation
of antivitamin antibodies. This is more likely to
occur with the hydroxocobalamin form of B$_{12}$.
There may also be acnelike rashes. A suspicion also
exists that extreme excesses (doses exceeding
10,000 mcg per day) of the vitamin enhances the
spread of some cancers.

B$_{15}$, vitamin See PANGAMIC ACID.

B$_{17}$, vitamin See AMYGDALIN.

baeckea An evergreen tree originating in Australia, *Baeckea frutescens,* of the Myrtaceae family,
whose leaves are used by Chinese practitioners to
treat sunstroke and fever.

bala In Ayurvedic medicine, the Sanskrit name
for country mallow (see MALLOW).

balamcanda (black-berry lily, leopard flower)
An herb native to China and Japan, *Belamcanda chinensis,* of the Iridaceae family, whose underground
stem is used by Chinese practitioners to treat ton-
silitis, laryngitis, gonorrhea, breast cancer, dysuria
(painful urination), asthma, cough, swollen liver
and spleen and malaria.

**balm (balm mint, blue balm, melissa, sweet
balm, dropsy plant, garden balm, bee balm)** An
herb common to the Mediterranean area and the

Near East and cultivated in other regions including the United States, *Melissa officinalis*. The herb and leaves, which smell like lemon when bruised, are used by herbalists as a calmative and antispasmodic, and to treat migraine, bronchial cough, toothache, melancholy, cramps, dyspepsia, flatulence, some forms of asthma and female reproductive disorders. Balm tea also has diaphoretic properties.

Balm of Gilead (quaking aspen, white poplar)
The *Populus balsamifera*, or *balsamifera candicans*, and *Populus tremula* trees' buds used in the making of cough syrups and expectorants. Poplar bark is said to relieve fever and aches and pains. Quaking aspen bark is said to reduce fever and headaches and relieve aches and pains.

balmony (snake head, turtle head, salt rheum weed, bitter herb) A perennial herb, *Chelone glabra*, of the Scrophulariaceae family, found in the United States, whose leaves are considered medicinal, especially for improving the appetite. A tea made of the leaves is thought to stimulate the stomach and flow of liver fluids and relieve jaundice, malarial problems and gastrointestinal disturbances. Balmony is also used to expel worms from the body.

balsam fir (Christmas tree) One of the nine species of fir trees in the United States, *Terebinthine canadensis*, of the Coniferae family, whose bark and twigs are considered medicinal for the treatment of rheumatism, kidney dysfunctions, gleet, cystitis, typhoid fever and capillary bronchitis, among other ailments. As a stimulant and expectorant, balsam fir yields products similar in effect to Balm of Gilead (see BALM OF GILEAD).

balsam of Peru (balsam of Tolu, balsam tree) A resin from the bark of the tree native to South and Central America, *Myroxylon balsamum*, which is used as treatment for loosening phlegm in upper respiratory ailments, including bronchitis, colds and cough, as an antipyretic and externally as an antiseptic for wounds and burns, hemorrhoids, pressure sores and frostbite. Balsam of Peru, whose

actual main source is San Salvador, is also used to kill parasites, particularly those causing scabies. Adverse effects may include allergic reaction, increased photosensitivity and skin eruptions.

bamboo See BAMBUSA.

bambusa (giant thorny bamboo) A native Indian plant also cultivated in other regions (*bamboo* is the Malay name), *Bambusa arundinacea*, of the Gramineae family, whose stem, sap and unfolded leaves are used in Chinese medicine to treat fever and rheumatism. Bamboo shavings, known as *zhu ru*, of the *Phyllostachys nigra* species, are used for lung problems. Known as *vamsha rochana* in Ayurvedic medicine, it is used as an expectorant.

baptisia (wild indigo) A leguminous, flowering plant of the genus *Baptisia tinctoria*, of the family Leguminosae, whose name derives from the Greek word *baptisis*, which means dipping. The roots and leaves are used in herbal medicine as a treatment for blood poisoning, ulcerations, typhoid dysentery, typhoid pneumonia, meningitis, diphtheria, sore throat and severe inflammatory disorders. Considered a strong anti-inflammatory and antibiotic, baptisia is also used for swollen glands and infections characterized by putrid discharges. It is also thought to have antiviral properties.

barberry (pipperidge bush) A deciduous shrub of the genus *Berberis* and the family *Berberiaceae*, whose bark is powdered and made into capsules. Homeopaths claim that tincture of the bark of the barberry root promotes the secretion of bile and is effective against bad breath, indigestion, rheumatism, skin conditions, bladder infections, sore throat, menstrual pain, fistula, calculus, herpes, ophthalmia, jaundice and other liver disorders, knee pain, lumbago, tumors and problems of the spleen. Barberry has been called an "old woman's medicine," which refers to its use as a stomach and liver tonic. The Native Americans used barberry-root tea as a blood tonic, cough medicine and remedy for rheumatism, ulcers, heartburn and even tuberculosis. Herbalists also allege barberry's effectiveness against cholera, ringworm and bronchitis.

Barberries and barberry juice are prescribed for fever, diarrhea and other symptoms of typhus.

The official Pharmacopoeia of Russia has cited two barberry species, Amur barberry and Barberry common, as therapeutic treatment for high blood pressure and problems of the female genital organs. Russian folklore has it that barberry treats inflammation, excessive menses and gallbladder problems and has a general ability to stop bleeding.

In Ayurvedic medicine, barberry is known by the Sanskrit name *daruharidra.*

barley (prelate) A cereal grass of the genus *Hordeum,* including *Hordeum vulgare,* whose seed is used in malt beverages, breakfast cereals, animal feed and to make barley water for the treatment of fever, diarrhea and intestinal irritation.

Found in tombs in Asia Minor from about 3500 B.C., barley seeds had been the most favored grain for bread-making in Europe until wheat and rye became more popular. Today, barley is also grown in the United States, especially California, North and South Dakota and Minnesota, and in Canada.

When introduced to Native Americans by early settlers in North America, barley was recognized to be a generally beneficial nutrient. It contains proteins, sugars, starch, fats and B vitamins. Barley is thought to be effective in the treatment of arthritis and rheumatism. Barley water, made by boiling pearl barley in water and strained, is used for fevers, diarrhea in children, bowel and stomach inflammation and as an addition to any diet to promote healthy intestinal bacterial conditions. In Chinese traditional medicine, barley is considered an anti-inflammatory diuretic and a treatment for tumors, gallbladder disorders and jaundice.

basil An annual herb, *Ocimum basilicum,* thought to relieve nausea, headaches, intestinal gas in infants, anxiety, infections and lack of menstruation. Basil, which grows wild in India, parts of Africa, Japan, Iran and Malaysia, among other countries, is also a popular flavoring in European and Mediterranean dishes. There is varied folklore pertaining to basil. To the French, basil is the *herbe royale* (royal herb); Jewish lore holds that basil offers strength during fasting. To the Italians, basil

symbolizes love, and to the Greeks, hate, although the Greek word for king, *basileus,* may be the reason for basil's having been known as the king of herbs. Basil, possibly derived from *basilicus,* meaning serpent, may also have been an ancient antidote for poisonous insect bites. English herbalist Nicholas Culpeper added to basil's folklore by calling it "an herb of Mars and under the Scorpion . . . it is no marvel if it carry a virulent quality with it." Contemporary herbalists believe basil to yield gentle yet reliable therapeutic effects.

In Ayurvedic medicine, *tulsi* is the Sanskrit name meaning "holy basil."

basswood The linden tree, *Tilia americana,* or *Tilia europaea,* native to Europe and the eastern United States, whose flowers are used medicinally for nervousness, indigestion, cramps, insomnia and initial symptoms of a cold. Linden-flower tea is considered by European herbalists to be therapeutic, while linden-flower baths are thought to relieve hyperactivity, insomnia and anxiety. The linden tree also yields linden-flower honey, inner bark that is prepared to treat burns as well as to make rope, and wood especially appealing to wood-carvers.

bay A tree native to Mediterranean shores, *Laurus nobilis,* also known as sweet bay or bay laurel, whose leaves are used chiefly as a flavoring in foods but also as a gastrointestinal tonic and to relieve gas. Cultivated in groves near the healing temples in Ancient Greece, the bay tree was considered sacred to Apollo, Greek god of the sun, and its branches were fashioned into wreaths to be worn by exalted luminaries such as heroes and great artists.

bayberry A shrub of the Myricaceae family, also known as American bayberries, wax myrtle, wax berry, tallow shrub, candle berry and American vegetable wax. Bayberry grows in sandy swamps and other wet woodland areas in the West Indies, along the east coast of the United States from southern New Jersey to Florida, and west to Arkansas and Texas. Besides its berries yielding an aromatic wax used to make candles, bayberry is said to have medicinal properties in its root bark. Herbalists claim that bayberry, or *myrica cerifera,* provides treatment for bronchitis and other bronchopulmonary diseases, cholera, scarlet fever, goiter, typhoid, diseases of the intestinal tract, and uterine, stomach, lung or bowel hemorrhage, among other ailments. The ancient physician Galen noted that bayberries helped relieve colds. Herbalists also prescribe bayberry for sore throats (as a gargle solution) and to improve the circulation of blood throughout the body. Because of the alleged astringent and narcotic properties of the wax, bayberry has also been used as a topical bath for skin irritations including boils and carbuncles.

The Sanskrit name for bayberry in Ayurvedic medicine is *katphala.*

bearberry   See UVA URSI.

bear's foot   A perennial flower, *Polymnia uvedalia,* member of the astor family, shaped like a bear's foot. Also known as leafcup, balsam resin, yellow leafcup and uvedalia, the bear's foot is found in North America. Its root is claimed to have both internal and external therapeutic effects. When boiled in water, the root allegedly provides relief of mammitis (nonmalignant inflammation of the breast), enlarged cervical nodules, enlarged spleen, scrofula, chronic rheumatism and certain malarial conditions. Made into a salve, bear's foot is applied to swollen areas and used as a hair tonic when massaged into the scalp.

beech   A tree, *Fagus grandifolia* and *Fagus sylvatica,* known for its beechnuts and medicinal leaves, that thrives in North America and Europe. According to English herbalist John Gerard, in the 16th century leaves were used in topical treatments of swelling, blisters, excoriations, skin rashes including poison ivy, frostbite and burns. When chewed, the leaves were thought to relieve chapped lips and painful gums. Gerard also claims that beechnuts ease kidney pain, and beechwater (found in the hollow of the tree) washes can cure assorted problems such as scabs on people, horses, sheep and cows.

beechdrop   Cancer root, a parasite of the Orabanchaceae, or broom-rape, family. This wiry plant has a scaly root and bears flowers in late summer.

The tops, stems and root are considered medicinal, having an astringent effect on the body. They are used in the form of tinctures and extracts by homeopaths to treat cancer, asthma, palpitations, gonorrhea, headaches, mouth and stomach ulcers and diarrhea. Externally, beechdrop is said to be effective against all forms of dermatitis.

beef cartilage   See ZYMAIN.

bee pollen   The dusty bloom on the body of the bee. Pollen, a mass of microspores resembling a fine flour found in seed plants, is collected by "pollen baskets" on each hind tibia of the bee. Many nutritionists and herbalists consider bee pollen a 100 percent nutritionally balanced food because it contains enzymes, amino acids, vitamins, hormones and other substances required for healing and rejuvenation of bodily functions. Some of the indications for using bee pollen are aging, allergies, indigestion, prostate disease, sore throat, acne, sexual problems and fatigue, according to some nutritionists, homeopaths and herbalists.

See also BEE PROPOLIS.

bee propolis   A natural antibiotic, antiviral and antifungal substance. Harvested by bees from the resin found under the bark of trees, bee propolis protects beehives against harmful microorganisms. The substance has a strong content of copper, magnesium, silicon, iron, manganese, zinc and other trace minerals, bioflavonoids, amino acids, vitamins C, B and E and beta-carotene. For human use it provides a stimulant for the thymus gland and the immune system. Produced as a soluble concentrate for internal use, as a tincture for topical application and as chewable lozenges, bee propolis is also used to prevent infection, as well as to treat gastric and intestinal ulcers; broken bones; gum, mouth and throat ailments; high blood pressure; arteriosclerosis; pneumonia and viral infections. It is also being tested for use to help heal certain skin cancers and melanoma.

See also BEE POLLEN.

belladonna (poison black cherry, deadly nightshade, dwale)   A perennial plant, *Atropa belladonna,* found in the eastern United States and in

Europe, whose leaves, tops (any growth above the leaves or from leaves) and berries are used as a narcotic, anticholinergic, antispasmodic, calmative, diaphoretic and diuretic. A well-known poison, belladonna (meaning "beautiful lady" in Italian) is the source of various alkaloids, including atropine and scopolamine, used to treat gastrointestinal spasms and diarrhea, according to the United States Pharmacopoeia (USP).

benincasa (dong gua pi, white gourd, wax gourd, Chinese preserving melon)   An annual plant native to southeast Asia, *Benincasa hispida*, of the Cucurbitaceae family, eaten as a vegetable and used for making pickles, whose seeds, rind and fruits are used by Chinese practitioners to treat fever, piles, diabetes, urinary tract diseases, gonorrhea and intestinal inflammation.

benzoin   A balsamic resin derived from the tree *Styrax benzoin* or *Styrax paralleloneuris*, used internally as a stimulant expectorant and an inhalant for the treatment of laryngitis and bronchitis, according to the United States Pharmacopoeia (USP).

bergamot   A mint of the genus *Monarda*, or an essential oil derived from the rind of the orange *Citrus bergamia*, used in the making of perfume. Bergamot is a popular, aromatic flavoring for tea that may offer some of the soothing effects of other mints (see MINT).

beriberi   A disease affecting the neurological, cerebral and cardiovascular systems that is caused by a severe lack of thiamine, or vitamin B_1, in the diet. *Beri* is the Singhalese word meaning weakness, one of the symptoms of beriberi. Other symptoms include abdominal discomfort, poor memory, numbness in the legs, palpitations and increased heart rate, calf-muscle tenderness, sleep disturbances, constipation, anorexia and pain in the heart and chest area.

Symptoms including edema, or swelling, of the legs, face, trunk and serous cavities, high blood pressure, decreased urine output, distended neck veins and muscle tension are characteristic of "wet beriberi."

Symptoms of the form of beriberi known as "dry beriberi" include difficulty walking, loss of memory and disorientation, a staggering gait, jerky eye movements and other signs of the Wernicke-Korsakoff syndrome, which is identified by encephalopathy, or any dysfunction of the brain. Wernicke-Korsakoff syndrome is usually seen in alcoholics, although it can occur in others with malnutrition.

Beriberi, also known as dietetic neuritis, has been endemic in Asia, particularly Burma, Thailand and Vietnam, the Philippines and other Pacific islands, and formerly in regions of the United States in which rice is grown. People who rely on milled rice as their chief food are at risk of developing beriberi. When the grain was hulled and pounded at home, it retained its thiamine content in the bran left on the kernel of rice. But when rice is highly polished during a commercial milling process, it loses its valuable thiamine content. Prevention of beriberi has been implemented by manufacturers of flour and cereals: Thiamine is added to the products (called "enriched") to reduce the incidence of thiamine deficiency.

Secondary conditions may also result from inadequate or impaired absorption or impaired bodily utilization of thiamine. Alcoholics are at risk of a neuritis nearly identical to beriberi, because the consistent consumption of alcoholic beverages suppresses the desire for food and depletes the body of nutrients.

Thiamine may be administered orally or by injection as treatment for the disease. Dietary sources of thiamine include whole and enriched grains, legumes and other vegetables, lean pork, eggs, liver and milk. Infants with beriberi may be treated by administering thiamine to the breast-feeding mother and the infant.

See also ANTITHIAMINE FACTORS; THIAMINE.

beta-carotene   A provitamin, precursor chemical or building block that is converted to vitamin A in humans (see A, VITAMIN).

betaine   Also known as betaine hydrochloride, this alkaloid substance containing 23 percent hydrochloric acid is found in the beet and other plants and used to treat hypochlorhydria, or deficiency of hydrochloric acid as a possible result of carcinoma or anemia.

Betalin S   The trade name for thiamine hydrochloride.
See also THIAMINE.

beth root (birth root, wake robin, Indian balm, American ground lily)   A flowering herb of temperate North America and eastern Asia, *Trillium pendulum,* wild, or *edectum,* of the Liliaceae family, whose root was used by Native Americans as a pain reliever, especially during childbirth. Beth root is also considered a tonic for bleeding and female reproductive disorders including profuse menstruation and leukorrhea. It is also used in the treatment of lung conditions and, in homeopathic medicine, for writer's cramp, fainting, dysentery and diabetes.

bharngi   The Sanskrit name, in Ayurvedic medicine, for the herb *Clerodendrum serratum,* of the family Verbenaceae.

bhringaraj   The Sanskrit name, in Ayurvedic medicine, for the herb *Eclipta,* of the Compositae family, used as tonic alterative, nervine and hemostatic (see ECLIPTA).

bhumyamalaki   The Sanskrit name, in Ayurvedic medicine, for the herb *Phyllanthus nururi.*

bibhitaki   The Sanskrit name for Beleric myrobalan, used in Ayurvedic herbal medicine as a strong laxative and antidote for *kapha,* a *dosha,* or body type, characterized generally by sluggishness. From the species *Terminalia belerica* of the family Combretaceae. Used as tonic, astringent, expectorant and laxative.

bifidus   See PROBIOTICS.

bilberry (huckleberry, whortleberry, hurtleberry)   An herb, *Vaccinium myrtillus,* of the Ericaceae family, that is thought to strengthen capillaries of the eye muscles, thereby reducing eyestrain and increasing night vision.

bilva   An Ayurvedic herbal medicine (*bilva* in Sanskrit, which translates as "bel").

bioflavonoids ("vitamin P")   A group of naturally occurring compounds containing a common structure, widely distributed in plants with biological activity in animals including humans. Citrus bioflavonoids are derived from the rind of green citrus fruits, rose hips and black currants. Although plentiful in the diet, these substances are broken down in the intestine and little if any are absorbed intact. It was theorized in the 1930s that bioflavonoids were useful to treat individuals with fragile or damaged blood vessels. Originally called vitamin P, this substance was renamed when researchers realized they could not prove the group of bioflavonoids to be either essential nutrients or have any value as drugs. Some researchers claim that bioflavonoids boost the effects of vitamin C.

biota (bai zi ren)   A Chinese medicinal herb, *Biota orientalis,* whose seeds are used in the treatment of heart problems.

biotin   A coenzyme manufactured by bacteria normally found in the human intestinal tract and essential in the metabolism of both fats and carbohydrates. Because it is manufactured in humans, it is not a true vitamin (see VITAMIN).
Raw egg white contains the antivitamin substance avidin, which, if ingested in high and prolonged quantity, results in a rash and glossitis (inflammation of the tongue) caused by biotin deficiency. Long-term total parenteral nutrition (TPN), an intravenous method of nourishing people who are extremely ill and/or incapable of eating, may also cause biotin deficiency.
Infants may exhibit the rash seborrheic dermatitis and hair loss due to a lack of biotin, but hair loss only responds to supplementation in a true deficiency of the substance.
There are reports that some individuals may exhibit such Alzheimer-like signs and symptoms as

TABLE 6 FOOD SOURCES OF BIOTIN

Chicken	Yeast	Rice bran
Lamb	Soybeans	Eggs (must be
Pork	Milk	cooked[1])
Beef	Cheese	
Veal	Saltwater fish	
Liver	Whole wheat flour	

[1]Avidin, a substance in raw egg white, antagonizes the action of biotin but is destroyed by cooking.

disorientation, speech disorders, loss of memory, restless legs, tremors and unsteady gait that are actually caused by biotin deficiency. Biotin deficiencies are rare except for some genetically impaired groups of individuals and bodybuilders who eat large quantities of raw eggs (see table). Also, persons treated with antibiotics for a prolonged time might have impaired bacterial synthesis of biotin because of the destruction of normal bacterial flora in the gut.

Although there is no recommended daily allowance (RDA) for biotin, a dosage of 150 to 300 mcg daily promptly improves biotin deficiency.

Biotin is found in many B-complex and multivitamin supplements and is also available as d-biotin tablets. Biotin is thought to be without toxic or other adverse effects.

birch   A tree whose leaves are used in the making of tea that is claimed to help alleviate urinary problems, intestinal worms and rheumatism.

bird's nest (ice plant, ova-ova, fit plant, Indian pipe)   A flowering plant, *Monotropa uniflora*, found in North America from Maine to the Carolinas and in regions toward Missouri, considered an anti-spasmodic, tonic and sedative, especially for use in St. Vitus' dance (chorea, including Huntington's disease, among other types) and seizures in children.

birth control pills and vitamin deficiency   See CONTRACEPTIVES, ORAL.

birth defects and vitamin deficiency   See FOLIC ACID.

bistort (dragonwort, adderwort, snakeweed)   The plant *Polygonum bistorta,* of the family Polygonaceae, whose root is considered by herbalists to be an astringent to treat bleeding and diarrhea. External uses include toothpowder said to be effective against gum disease and a douche to eliminate vaginal discharge.

bitter orange   An oil extract of the citrus fruit used in naturopathic remedies for strep throat and diarrhea.

bitter root (dog bane, milk weed, westernwall)   A perennial, flowering plant of North America, *Apocynum androsaemifolium,* of the family Apocynaceae, whose root is considered medicinal, especially in the treatment of venereal diseases, Bright's disease, rheumatic gout, worms, diabetes, heart diseases, dropsy, facial neuralgia, nausea and vomiting. Used externally, bitter-root milk is said to remove warts.

blackberry   The bush *Rubus fruticosus,* of the family Rosaceae, whose berries are nutritionally beneficial, especially to anemic individuals, and whose leaves and root bark are used as treatment for sore throat, fever, colds, diarrhea, bleeding and dysentery. Blackberries contain sugars, vitamins C and A and other nutrients, and, in Chinese traditional medicine, are thought to provide a cooling "Yin tonic" for nourishing the blood.

black cohosh (bugbane, black snakeroot, rattleroot)   An herb containing natural estrogen with none of the carcinogenic properties found in synthetic estrogen. Black cohosh is claimed to be effective for the treatment of menstrual cramps and to regulate menses.

black haw (stagbush, American sloe)   The *Viburnum prunifolium,* of the family Caprifoliaceae, whose stem and root bark are used in herbal medicine as a uterine tonic to prevent miscarriage, relieve menstrual pain and help relieve menopausal distress such as hot flashes and night sweats, and as an antispasmodic for treating diarrhea, asthma, palpitations and other cardiac problems, nervousness and mood swings.

black mustard (brown mustard, red mustard) The oil (also known as allylisothiocyanate) of mustard seeds from the plant *Brassica nigra.* It is used topically, particularly as a plaster, in the treatment of bronchial pneumonia and pleurisy and in homeopathic medicine for sore throat, runny nose and hay fever symptoms. Internal use of mustard oil may cause stomach and kidney irritation, and it is not recommended for individuals with vascular disorders, ulcers or renal disease. An overdose of black mustard may cause problems, including vomiting and diarrhea, stomach pain, cardiac and respiratory distress, sleepiness, coma or death.

black pepper (*maricha,* in Sanskrit) A pungent, hot spice used throughout the world mainly to improve the taste of foods, from the East Indian plant of the Piperaceae family. Pepper is used in Ayurvedic medicine to relieve swelling, hives (external use), intestinal worms, dry hemorrhoids, constipation, flatulence and loss of appetite.

black root (Beaumont root, oxadaddy, physic root, tall Veronica, Bowman's root, Culver's root, whorlywort, tall speedwell) The perennial herb chiefly of the eastern United States, *Leptandra virginica,* is used for the treatment of constipation and liver and gallbladder ailments.

black teas Beverages made by adding boiling water to dried and fermented leaves from the evergreen shrub *Thea sinensis* grown throughout the world. Black teas contain natural fluoride, caffeine and polyphenols, which serve as antioxidants that do not impede iron or protein absorption and combat free radicals and degenerative diseases.

See also GREEN TEAS; TEA.

blackthorn (sloe, wild plum) A flowering bush, *Prunus spinosa,* of Europe and regions of Asia whose fruit is an ingredient in sloe gin and whose flower is made into remedies for oral and pharyngeal inflammation. Blackthorn is also used as a laxative and to relieve cramps and indigestion. In homeopathic medicine, it is considered a remedy for neuralgia, tension headaches and urinary problems and as a cardiac tonic.

black walnut (butternut, lemon walnut, oilnut, white walnut) Remedy made from the bark and root of the American tree *Juglans nigra.* It is used to treat hemorrhoids, liver and gallbladder problems and, in homeopathic medicine, for headache, hepatitis and various skin disorders. Black walnut also yields Juglone, a compound that is a mild laxative and also is antibacterial, is antihelminthic and has antitumor properties.

bladderwrack See SEAWRACK.

blessed thistle (holy thistle, St. Benedict thistle) An annual plant native to southern Europe or western Asia and cultivated elsewhere, thought to be a tonic to stimulate circulation to the heart, stomach and liver. Many herbalists believe blessed thistle, *Cnicus benedictus* of the family Compositae, increases the flow of oxygen to the brain and boosts memory capabilities. It is also said to reduce fever, stop bleeding and resolve blood clots and treat hepatitis. Artichoke leaves, a member of the thistle family and usually eaten as a vegetable, are also used for a tea thought to restore normal liver functioning. Milk thistle is considered a healing and protective liver tonic (see ARTICHOKE).

bletilla A ground orchid of China and Japan, *Bletilla striata,* of the Orchidaceae family, whose stem is used in Chinese medicine to treat tuberculosis, chest pain, bloody sputum or vomitus, coughs, abscesses and swellings.

blindness and vitamin deficiency See EYE DISEASES.

blood coagulation See K, VITAMIN.

blood levels of vitamins Laboratory tests available to determine adequacy or deficiencies of vitamins or minerals. Only a few tests are frequently used, including vitamin B_{12}, folic acid and iron levels to assist in the diagnosis of anemia. Minerals can be measured also, but most often these tests are run to detect toxicity.

bloodroot (redroot, red Indian paint, tetterwort)

An herb, *Sanguinaria canadensis,* of the Papaveraceae family, thought to be a treatment for coughs and colds and a stimulant to the heart and digestive system. In herbal medicine, bloodroot is used as an expectorant for asthma, productive coughing, croup, sinus congestion and laryngitis. External uses include tinctures or powders to treat athlete's foot, skin rashes and cancer and gum disease.

blue cohosh (papooseroot, squawroot)

An herb, *Caulophyllum thalictroides,* of the Berberidaceae family, similar in effect to black cohosh. The rhizome, or root stem, is used in herbal medicine to relive labor pain and various difficulties related to menses, such as lack of menses, irregularities and pain. It is also used for the treatment of worms and genitourinary disorders (see BLACK COHOSH).

blue flag (flag lily, poison flag, liver lily, fleur-de-lis, wild iris)

An herb, *Iris versicolor,* of the family Iridaceae, whose rhizome, or root stem, is used in extract form, thought to be effective in the treatment of cancer, skin diseases, blood dyscrasias, constipation, rheumatism and liver ailments. In herbal

---

TABLE 7 TESTS AVAILABLE

Test	Use
Calcium (blood)	Elevated calcium levels occur in hyperparathyroidism, some kidney disorders, some cancers, especially tumors of lung, kidney, pancreas and ovary or metastatic cancer. Also hypervitaminosis A or D, myeloma, sarcoidosis, milk-alkali syndrome (excessive use of calcium-containing drugs), hyperthyroidism, acromegaly, Addison's disease, drugs including diuretics and estrogens. Causes of low calcium levels: low levels of albumin and total protein, hyperparathyroidism, osteomalacia, vitamin D deficiency, rickets, kidney disorders, malabsorption or malnutrition, neonatal tetany, Milkman's syndrome, pancratitis, high phosphorus, IV fluids, drugs including anticonvulsants and barbiturates
Calcium (urine)	Elevated in some bone disorders, kidney stones and other kidney disorders, rickets, vitamin D toxicity, hyperparathyroidism. Decreased when taking oral contraceptives, vitamin deficiency, some kidney disorders, vitamin D–resistant rickets, hypoparathyroidism
Carotene (blood)	Elevated in pregnancy and excessive intake of carrots. Depressed in malabsorption, some metabolic disorders, heat stroke and liver necrosis.
Ferritin (blood)	Evaluation of microcytic anemia, iron storage disorders, iron metabolism
Folates (folic acid) (blood)	Anemia evaluation
Iron (blood)	Anemia evaluation
Vitamin A	Hypervitaminosis A. Vitamin A deficiency
Vitamin B_1	Deficiency
Vitamin B_2	Deficiency
Vitamin B_6	Deficiency
Vitamin B_{12}	Deficiency, anemia evaluation
Vitamin C	Evaluation of scurvy
Vitamin D	Evaluation of parathyroid and kidney disorders
Vitamin E	Deficiency in hemolytic disease in premature infants, neuromuscular disease in infants and adults with cholestasis

medicine, blue flag is also used as an appetite suppressant for obese individuals.

blue vervain The herb *Verbena officinalis*, of the family Verbenaceae, whose aerial portions, or tops, are used in herbal medicine in the treatment of liver disorders, menstrual pain, nervousness, ascites, mastitis, influenza, colds and fever. Vervain is also thought to increase the flow of breast milk.

blue violet A flowering herb claimed to relieve headache, head congestion and internal ulcers.

bog bean (bog myrtle, moonflower, water shamrock, water or bean trefoil, buck bean, marsh clover) An aquatic bean plant of the northern hemisphere, *Menyanthes trifoliata*, that yields remedies for loss of appetite and indigestion and, in homeopathic medicine, treats urinary problems, diabetes and headaches. Once considered a treatment for scurvy, bog bean is not recommended for individuals with colitis or diarrhea.

boldo *Peumus boldo*, an aromatic evergreen shrub found on the west coast of South America, whose leaves serve as a remedy for indigestion, intestinal cramping, appetite loss and liver and gallbladder disorders. Boldo, which increases digestive juices and bile and relieves digestive-tract spasms, is not recommended for individuals with gallstones, bile duct obstruction or liver disease.

bone growth and structure See CALCIUM; OSTEOPOROSIS; RICKETS.

bone meal Ground or crushed bone used as fertilizer and a source of easily absorbed calcium. Bone meal is also high in phosphorus.

boneset (feverwort, thoroughwort) An herb, *Eupatorium perfoliatum*, of the family Compositae, prepared as an infusion to treat colds, influenza and constipation. Boneset it also thought to relax muscles, stomach, intestines, uterus and gall ducts.

borage (burrage) A flowering European herb, *Borago officinalis*, of the family Boraginaceae, thought to reduce fever and irritation of skin and mucous membranes, including the mucous membranes of the lung. Borage, whose seeds are a rich source of gamma linolenic oil, is also said to increase breast milk.

boron A nonmetallic element found as a compound in such substances as boric acid or borax and in plant and animal tissues. Along with arsenic and aluminum, boron, or bromine, is considered a nonessential trace element of no known function or need in the human diet. There is some evidence that postmenopausal women on low-boron diets may be at increased risk for osteoporosis, and a diet high in fruits and vegetables may prevent calcium loss and bone demineralization.

boswellic acid One of four triterpene acids found in the herb *Boswellia serrata* that has been standardized in amount and used in Ayurvedic herbal treatments for various problems, including arthritis. Boswellia and vitamin E are combined in a topical preparation for arthritic pain relief.

bovine cartilage A nutritional supplement used for the treatment of degenerated cartilage, or osteoarthritis, along with other supplements, such as shark cartilage, EPA (eicosapentaenoic acid), coenzyme Q10, yucca root, devil's claw, cat's claw, vitamins C and E and N-acetyl-glucosamine (glucosamine). Both cartilage and connective tissue require glucosamine sulfate and glucosamine HCL in order to maintain strength and flexibility.

brahmi In Ayurvedic medicine, Sanskrit for gotu kola.
See also GOTU KOLA.

bran The cracked outer coating of the seed of a cereal grain such as oats or wheat that has been separated from the milled product, i.e., flour or meal, through the process of sifting (bolting). Added to the diet, bran is used to prevent and treat constipation because of its indigestible cellulose content, which introduces bulk into the intestines. Any edible product containing digestion-resistant cellulose, hemicellulose, lignin, gums, mucilages and pectin is considered helpful to the elimination function of the body. Studies have been made on the effectiveness of added fiber to the diets of individuals with high blood pressure, diabetes, colon cancer, gallstones, irritable bowel syndrome, colon polyps and other problems. Oat bran became extremely fashionable during the early 1990s, when some researchers proclaimed it a cancer-preventing agent. The studies have not yet proven all the claims, but it is accepted that foods rich in fiber, including whole-grain products, bran flakes, beans, fruits, leafy vegetables, nuts, root vegetables and prunes, are beneficial in the prevention of constipation.

brand name products   See GENERIC PRODUCTS.

brassica (mustard)   The cabbage plant, *Brassica juncea, cernua, napiformis, oleracea* or *gongylodes,* of the Cruciferae family, whose seeds and leaves are used by Chinese herbalists to treat various disorders, including colds, lumbago, rheumatism, ulcers, cystitis, stomach problems, diabetes, pneumonia, arthritis and neuralgia.

breast disease and vitamins   The controversial results from several studies designed to determine if antioxidant vitamins protect against breast or other cancers. In 1984, British investigators measured frozen blood from more than 5,000 women and determined that those with breast cancer had significantly lower beta-carotene than healthy women. The same observers found that those with low vitamin E levels were five times more likely to develop breast cancer.

In 1990, researchers at the University of Toronto analyzed data from a number of studies and concluded that large amounts of vitamin C seemed to protect women against breast cancer. However, participants in the Harvard Medical School's Nurses Health Study, who consumed more than 1,300 mg vitamin C or 600 I.U. of vitamin E daily, had no apparent protection against breast cancer when compared to those not taking the antioxidants.

brewer's yeast   A yeast (of the fungus family), resulting from the brewing process of beer, that may be dried and used as a source of proteins and B-complex vitamins. Brewer's yeast, usually sold as a powder in health food stores, can be an ingredient in breads, pancakes, milkshakes and a wide variety of foods.

brindal berry   The English name of *amlavetasa,* the Sanskrit name of an Ayurvedic herb.

bromelain   A proteolytic enzyme with the trade name Ananase, found in the pineapple plant and known to be a meat tenderizer and a substance that clots milk, and having anti-inflammatory properties that may benefit muscle injuries, sinusitis, post-operative swelling, and arthritis. Pineapple juice, which contains bromelain, helps reduce oral swelling after a tooth extraction.

brucea   A shrub native to the Malay Archipelago, East Indies and China, *Brucea javanica,* of the Simaroubaceae family, whose seeds are used by Chinese herbalists to treat both constipation and diarrhea, amoebic and chronic dysentery and hemorrhoids.

buchu   A plant, *Agathosma betulina,* of the family Rutaceae, whose leaves have been touted for their effectiveness as a diuretic, an agent that helps rid the body of excess water, and urinary pain-reliever. Buchu leaves were used by the Khoikhoi of South Africa.

buckthorn   A tree, *Rhamnus cathartica,* whose bark is said to promote regular bowels and alleviate appendicitis, worms and warts. Buckthorn berries are made into a syrup with honey, allspice and ginger that is used as a laxative for children.

buddleia (butterfly bush)   A flowering shrub of China, *Buddleia officinialis,* of the family Loganiaceae, named for English botanist Adam Buddle (1660–1715). The shrub's flower buds contain buddlein, an alkaloid, and the flowers and leaves are used in Chinese medicine to treat night blindness, eyestrain and cataracts. The roots of the poisonous *Buddleia lindleyana* are used for stunning fish, killing insects and treating asthma and bloody, productive cough.

buffered vitamins Modification of vitamins that are acidic, such as ascorbic acid (vitamin C), so that megadoses can be taken without irritating the stomach. Sodium ascorbate, a buffered form of vitamin C, should be avoided by people with hypertension and others on low-sodium diets.

bugleweed (gypsywort, water or sweet bugle, Virginia water horehound) A North American perennial plant, *Lycopus virginicus*, was first discovered along the banks of streams in Virginia. Its fresh or dried aboveground parts are harvested during flowering season and used in remedies for tension, breast pain, mildly overactive thyroid, insomnia, nervousness and premenstrual syndrome. Bugleweed inhibits thyroid activity and levels of prolactin, a hormone that helps the production of breast milk. It is not recommended for individuals with thyroid insufficiency, those on thyroid medications or those who anticipate undergoing tests that involve radioactive isotopes. Bugleweed may cause enlargement of the thyroid.

bupleurum (ch'ai hu) An herb, *Bupleurum chinese*, of the family Umbelliferae, whose root is considered in Chinese herbal medicine to be a liver detoxicant and an agent against nausea, anxiety, dizziness, pain and fever. Bupleurum is also thought to strengthen the eyes and limbs.

burdock (lappa, beggar's buttons, bardane) An herb, *Arctium lappa*, of the family Compositae, whose root, seeds, and leaves are claimed to purify the blood by removing toxins and treat severe skin problems and arthritis. In Japan, burdock root, called *gobo*, is eaten like carrots.

burns and nutrition Burns cause a loss of fluids and electrolytes, which may be life-threatening. Since burn patients may require total bed rest, serum calcium may fall to levels that precipitate bone loss. This condition can be minimized by calcium supplementation and starting exercise as soon as possible. In addition, zinc levels fall, impairing wound healing and causing loss of appetite.

butcher's-broom (kneeholy, sweet broom, pettier) The herb *Ruscus aculeatus*, of the family Liliaceae, used in herbal medicine as a vascular anti-inflammatory and a pain reliever in arthritis and rheumatism. Hemorrhoid pain and swelling are treated with an ointment made from butcher's-broom.

butternut An American oily-nut tree, *Juglans cinerea*, of the walnut family, whose bark is thought to strengthen the intestines and relieve constipation, fever and colds.

C, vitamin   See ASCORBIC ACID.

cabbage   A common leafy vegetable originating in Europe, *Brassica oleracea,* that was given high praise by the ancient Greeks and Romans, particularly Hippocrates, Pythagorus and Cato the Elder, as a medicinal plant. In *Herbal,* a 17th-century writing by Nicholas Culpeper, cabbage (earlier known as colewort) was credited with healing all manner of ills, including kidney stones and shortness of breath. Dubbed "the poor man's medicine" in Europe, cabbage is considered effective in cleansing the liver (because of its sulfur content) and keeping the intestines healthy (because of its vitamin C, bulk, water and fermentation bacteria). Cabbage has also been used in the treatment of worms, anxiety and depression.

See also BRASSICA.

cadmium   A metal similar in appearance and properties to tin. Elemental cadmium and its salts are toxic. It is unknown if traces of this mineral are essential in human nutrition. If required, it is sufficiently plentiful in food, water and air to satisfy human needs.

caesalpinia (sappan tree, brazilwood)   A tree, *Caesalpinia sappan,* of the Leguminosae family, native to the Malay Peninsula and India, that yields heartwood, from which synthetic aniline dyes are made. In Chinese medicine, heartwood also can be made into a decoction for the treatment of bleeding during and after childbirth, excessive menstrual flow, coughing blood and bruises, among other similar uses.

cajunput (cajeput, white tea tree, tea tree)   The tree *Melaleuca leucadendron,* of the family Myrtaceae,

whose oil is distilled and used in herbal medicine preparations to treat colds, flu and yeast (*Candida albicans*) infections. Internal use of cajunput is restricted, however. External uses include treatment of arthritis pain, fungal infections, pimples, cradle cap, plantar warts, cuts, bruises and various topical injuries, itching and scalp irritation. Inhalation of the oil vapors may be effective for congested sinuses.

calamus (sweet flag, haulm, sweet sedge)   The plant *Acorus calamus,* of the family Aracae, named from the Greek word *kalamos,* meaning reed, whose aromatic rhizome, or root stem, contains a carcinogenic essential oil, B-asarone. (The American, as opposed to the European, calamus is reported to lack this oil.) In herbal medicine, calamus has been used for treating liver, stomach and intestinal ailments. It is also said to help overcome the desire for tobacco. Native Americans chew the calamus root to boost their stamina and endurance. The Chinese consider the calamus root therapeutic for hypertension, coughs, constricted veins, irregular heart rhythms, lung congestion and bacterial infection. Asian Indians use calamus root as a cooking spice and for nervousness, particularly in Ayurvedic medicine, which maintains that calamus root increases concentration. Ayurvedic practitioners also believe that calamus root's anti-anxiety properties aid in helping individuals with a marijuana habit. Both in marijuana and tobacco cessation therapies, calamus is said to create a slight nausea when taken in conjunction with either substance.

calciferol   See D, VITAMIN.

calcium   The most abundant mineral and the fifth most plentiful substance in the body. The average adult contains from 2 to 3 pounds of calcium, of which 99 percent is found in the bones and teeth. The remaining 1 percent is found in the circulatory system and aids in regulating various body functions. The newborn's skeleton contains about 30 grams of calcium, most of which is deposited during the third trimester of pregnancy.

Calcium, which is absorbed from the small intestine, requires the presence of vitamin D.

Uses

Essential for healthy bone composition, calcium alone cannot increase bone mass after the age of 20. Although calcium supplements probably do little to reduce the incidence of hip fractures in the elderly, there is little downside to supplements. A French study in elderly women given 800 International Units of vitamin D₃ (see D, VITAMIN) and 1.2 grams of calcium daily demonstrated more than a 40-percent reduction in hip fractures.

Results have been mixed in studies designed to see if high calcium intake lowers blood pressure. While animal studies seem to indicate that high calcium intake may protect against colon cancer, proof in humans is lacking.

Deficiency

Osteoporosis is the most common and serious complication of inadequate calcium intake or absorption. As calcium intake diminishes, calcium is resorbed from bones, especially the spine and jaw, the first bones to show evidence of osteoporosis. Vitamin D is essential for the utilization of calcium, and it may be prudent for women at highest risk, such as those older than 65 who are housebound, reside in nursing homes or live in areas where winters are long with minimal sun exposure, to take 200–400 I.U. of vitamin D daily.

It has been found in several studies that women taking thiazide diuretics for the treatment of hypertension had a reduction in the number of hip fractures as high as 30 percent. It is known that these drugs interfere with the excretion of calcium by the kidneys, and that the increased blood levels may result. However, other studies dispute the findings and report only a modest 10 percent increase in bone density for women who have been on up to 10 years of thiazide therapy.

Regular weight-bearing, vigorous exercise seems to protect against osteoporosis because stressed bone stimulates new bone production via osteoblast cells. But any benefit is lost within one year of ceasing the exercise.

Low blood-calcium levels cause increased muscle sensitivity, resulting in muscle spasms, or tetany. Muscle cramps occur when blood-calcium levels are very low and are particularly more common during pregnancy. Infants fed undiluted cow's milk are at increased risk for tetany.

Recommended Dietary Allowances

In 1994 The National Institutes of Health Consensus Development Panel made recommendations for calcium intake (see Table 8). This expert group recommends a modest increase in calcium for most individuals that should not exceed 2,000 mg per day. Higher levels should be monitored carefully and may cause adverse effects. Peak bone mass is probably attained from ages 11 to 24 years. Women older than 50 who are on estrogen have a lower requirement equivalent to premenopausal women. Since calcium absorption from cow's milk

---

TABLE 8 1994 RECOMMENDATIONS BY THE NATIONAL INSTITUTES OF HEALTH CONSENSUS DEVELOPMENT PANEL ON CALCIUM REQUIREMENTS

Infants up to 6 months	400 mg/day
Infants 6 to 12 months	600 mg/day
Children 1 to 5 years	800 mg/day
Children 6 to 10 years	800–1,200 mg/day
Adolescents and young adults (11 to 24 years)	1,200–1,500 mg/day
Men 25 to 65 years	1,000 mg/day
Men older than 65 years	1,500 mg/day
Women 25 to 50 years	1,000 mg/day
Women older than 50 years	1,000 mg/day with estrogen therapy* 1,500 mg/day if not on estrogens
Pregnant or nursing women	1,200–1,500 mg/day*

*Although estrogen is known to slow down bone loss and prevent osteoporosis, estrogen replacement therapy in some individuals has been known to cause various problems, including hypoglycemia, blood clotting, salt and fluid retention, and the development of tumors, fibroids, and endometriosis.

is less efficient than from human milk, formulafed infants have an increased requirement.

Supplements Available

Calcium supplements, generic or brand-name, are readily absorbed and work best when taken with meals. Dietary sources such as cheese, milk and yogurt are much more expensive. Care must be taken to assure that sources of calcium used do not contain toxic amounts of lead. Seventy brands of calcium supplements were analyzed for lead content. Five categories of the supplements were identified: dolomite, bone meal, refined- and natural-source calcium carbonate and calcium chelates. Lead levels ranged from 0.03 mcg/gram to 8.83 mcg/gram. Twenty-five percent of the products supplied daily lead quantities exceeding the federal Food and Drug Administration's "provisional" total tolerable daily intake of lead for infants and children through age six. Therefore, caution must be used to assure that calcium supplements, especially those given to children with milk intolerance, have lead contents as low or lower than the levels found in milk products.

In addition to the possibility of lead contamination, calcium in dolomite is very poorly absorbed. Although bone meal is easily absorbed, it also contains large amounts of phosphorus, which may be undesirable (see PHOSPHORUS).

Toxicity

Most adults can tolerate a calcium intake of up to 2,500 mg per day, but constipation and possibly increased incidence of kidney stones may occur with persistence of high ingestion. Very high levels of calcium may interfere with the absorption of iron, zinc and other minerals from the intestine. Renal function may deteriorate in the presence of continued excessive calcium intake. In any case of hypercalcemia (high calcium), hypomagnesemia (low magnesium) and hypokalemia (low potassium) should also be considered.

See also Appendix V.

calcium-channel blocking drugs Drugs used in the treatment of high blood pressure and heart disorders. They play no role in blood-calcium levels and do not interact with calcium supplements.

See also CALCIUM.

TABLE 9 CALCIUM MYTHS

- Myth: The body can utilize only small quantities of calcium.
- Truth: Most adults can tolerate up to 2,500 mg of calcium per day.
- Myth: All foods containing calcium are absorbed equally.
- Truth: Soybeans, kale, bread and dairy products contain readily absorbable calcium, whereas calcium-rich spinach provides almost no available calcium.
- Myth: High fiber interferes with the absorption of calcium.
- Truth: While bran, spinach and rhubarb do inhibit calcium absorption, psyllium (Metamucil) does not.
- Myth: All calcium supplements are the same.
- Truth: Calcium citrate is the most easily absorbed but contains a lower concentration of calcium (24 percent) than calcium carbonate (40 percent). Calcium lactate contains only 13 percent and calcium gluconate 9 percent of calcium per tablet.
- Myth: Calcium intake must be reduced in persons with kidney stones.
- Truth: A low-calcium diet may actually increase the risk of calcium kidney stones.
- Myth: Calcium must be in the form of a soluble salt to be absorbed.
- Truth: With rare exceptions, taking supplements with meals is the key to calcium absorption.
- Myth: Persons with achlorhydria (inadequate secretion of hydrochloric acid in the stomach) are unable to absorb calcium carbonate and require calcium citrate, a more expensive form of supplement.
- Truth: These individuals can absorb calcium carbonate if it is taken with meals.
- Myth: Persons taking calcium-channel blocking drugs such as verapamil (Calan, Isoptin, Veralan); diltiazem (Cardiazem, Dilacor); nifedipine (Procardia, Adalat) and others used to treat hypertension, angina pectoris and heart arrhythmia (irregularities) should avoid calcium supplements.
- Truth: Calcium supplements can be taken by those individuals.
- Myth: All calcium supplements are equally safe.
- Truth: Dolomite and bone meal have high concentrations of calcium, but may be contaminated by lead or other toxins.

calcium pantothenate   A form of pantothenic acid contained in supplements of the B-complex vitamin.

See also PANTOTHENIC ACID.

calendula (pot marigold)   A flowering herb, *Calendula officinalis*, whose flower petals have been used as topical treatment of wounds, sores and wasp and bee stings. Infusions, or teas, made from the flowers have been used to treat toothache, conjunctivitis (inflammation of the lining membrane of the eye), ulcers and fever. Calendula petals also have the culinary advantage of being less expensive than saffron, an important spice in Asian Indian and Spanish cuisine.

calico (sheep laurel, spoonwood, mountain laurel, lambkill)   The flowering, evergreen bush *Kalmia latifolia*, of the Ericaceae family, found in hilly, rocky regions of the United States, whose leaves have been used in folk medicine as an anti-syphilitic, astringent and sedative. While herbalists claim that large doses of calico may be poisonous, they also use it in the treatment of fevers, jaundice, inflammation and neuralgia. In homeopathic practice, a tincture of calico leaves is thought to relieve angina pectoris (chest pain), Bright's disease, dropsy, painful menstruation, gout, headache, sun headaches, syphilitic sore throat, ill effects of tobacco, ringing in the ears, dizziness, vomiting, lumbago and other problems.

Californian poppy   The poppy plant *Eschscholtzia california*, originally found in California, may be used as a dried herb or liquid extract for the treatment of depression, anxiety, migraines, insomnia and other sleep disorders, bed-wetting, nervous disorders, chronic fatigue syndrome, liver and bladder disorders and weather sensitivity, among other ailments.

calorie-dense foods   Foods that contain minimal amounts of vitamins or minerals but relatively large amounts of calories. Calorie-dense foods include those high in fat and sugar such as bacon, hot dogs and cookies.

camellia   Flowering shrubs and small trees of the Theaceae family, named for the Moravian Jesuit George Joseph Camellus of the 17th century. The flowers of *Camellia japonica*, indigenous to China and Japan, are used by Chinese practitioners to treat bleeding of the uterus and nose and coughing of blood. The tea plant, *Camellia sinensis*, yields caffeinated green tea and black tea from its leaves and is used as a tonic for the central nervous system, heart and flow of urine.

See also GREEN DRINKS AND SUPERFOODS; GREEN TEAS.

camomile (chamomile, Hungarian camomile, single camomile)   A common European herb of the genus *Anthemis*, especially *A. nobilis*, and the related genus *Matricaria*, including *M. chamomilla* and *M. recutita*, of the Compositae family, whose leaves and flower heads contain medicinal properties. With its high calcium content, camomile tea is a popular remedy for indigestion, colds, flu, teething pain, back pain, diarrhea, menstrual cramps, anxiety and insomnia. German camomile is considered the most potent anti-inflammatory of all other varieties of camomile, which may account for its effectiveness against the pain of sciatica, gout and herniated vertebral disc.

camphor (cemphire)   Distilled from the wood of the evergreen camphor tree, *Cinnamomum camphora*, originally found in Japan and Taiwan, camphor is a remedy for hypertension, respiratory problems, such as cough and bronchitis, cardiac arrhythmia, rheumatism and cardiac weakness.

See also CINNAMOMUM.

campsis (Chinese trumpet creeper, Chinese trumpet flower)   A flowering vine, *Campsis grandiflora*, of the family Bignoniaceae, whose flowers and roots are considered medicinal by Chinese practitioners. The Greek word for curve, *campsis* has curved stamens. The flowers are used to treat diabetes, itching, fever, rectal bleeding, painful menses, skin allergy and other problems. The roots are said to relieve rheumatoid arthritis and muscle paralysis.

canarium (kenari-nut tree)   The tree *Canarium album*, of the family Burseraceae, native to

Indochina and South China, that yields a fruit resembling an olive and containing an oily kernel used for candies and cooking. The fruit is also used in Chinese medicine for sore throat and diarrhea, and as an antidote for poisoning by contaminated or poisonous fish. The seeds are powdered and used as an anti-inflammatory.

cancer prevention Relatively risk-free measures that may prevent or delay the onset of cancer, or malignancy. Cancer is a disease in which cells lose their normal structure, exhibit unlimited growth and spread, by invasion of surrounding tissues or by the circulatory system in a process called metastasis, to distant sites. The cancerous, or abnormal, cells interfere with the tissues' ability to function. Initially healthy cells or their genetic code is altered by exposure to a substance called a mutagen or carcinogen. A second phase called the promotion stage is necessary for cancer to occur. This phase may take many years to develop and may not be apparent for 20 to 30 years. For cancer to develop, the abnormal cell must be in contact with something that will stimulate its growth.

The National Academy of Sciences believes that up to 60 percent of cancer is caused by nutritional factors. Diets high in vitamin A and beta-carotene, the plant form of vitamin A that the body converts to vitamin A, appear to have cancer-protective properties. Those who have diets low in vitamin A and beta-carotene seem to have an increased risk of developing cancer. Both smokers and chewers of tobacco have low levels of vitamin A and increased precancerous cells in the tissues of the mouth, throat and lungs. Smokers may also have low levels of vitamin B_{12} and folate. Vitamin A may also offer protection to persons exposed to "second-hand" smoke and pollution.

The antioxidant vitamin E has been promoted as a cancer preventive because of its apparent ability to stabilize cell membranes and reduce free radicals. So far, study results have been mixed and inconclusive.

Experiments with vitamin K suggest that it may block the growth of cancerous cells in some tumors.

Folic-acid deficiency may predispose some women to cervical cancer. Folate supplements appear to prevent damage to cervical cells. Vitamin

C seems to block the conversion of nitrites in processed foods to nitrosamines, which are thought to be carcinogenic to the stomach, colon and bladder. Its antioxidant properties also may have protective properties similar to vitamin E. Individuals with colon cancer may consume diets low in calcium and vitamin D.

Selenium is another antioxidant. People who live in areas where the selenium content of soil is high have lower incidence of cancers. Similarly, patients with malignancies including Hodgkin's disease, breast, colon and bladder cancer and leukemia have low blood levels of selenium.

While diets rich in vitamins and minerals may be protective against malignancy, the safety of large doses, or megadoses, of vitamins is questionable. Some studies suggest that excessive amounts of vitamin C, iron and zinc may inhibit the immune response, thus increasing the risk for cancer, infections or other diseases.

See also AMERICAN CANCER SOCIETY GUIDELINES ON DIET AND NUTRITION; ANTIOXIDANTS.

cancer treatment with vitamins Alternative and highly controversial nutrient therapy for malignant disorders. Traditional treatment for cancer is often frustrating because it frequently fails to prevent pain and death, and nausea may be unbearable. Therefore, anything that promises to prevent, cure or at least slow the process of cancer is welcome. Unfortunately, some practitioners offer alternative cancer therapies that rely on unproven vitamin or mineral regimens that may be toxic as well as ineffective. Additionally, they may be substituted for traditional or experimental drug protocols that may be effective.

Even well-meaning scientists, such as Nobel Prize recipient Dr. Linus Pauling, have been caught up in promoting vitamins, especially vitamin C, as a cancer treatment. A study published in the *Proceedings of the National Academy of Sciences* in 1976 by Linus Pauling and Scottish researcher Ewan Cameron reported that 100 terminally ill cancer patients who received large doses of vitamin C lived up to 20 times longer than those who did not receive supplements. However, the article sparked great contovery among scientists who doubted the validity of the study. Examination of study methods show that there may have been bias, intentional or not, in favor of the group that received vitamin C. Other studies have also produced contradictory results. A properly controlled "double-blind" study at the Mayo Clinic found that those cancer patients receiving 10 grams of vitamin C daily appeared to do no better than the group receiving a placebo.

Pauling objected vigorously to the fact that patients in the Mayo study had previously received chemotherapy, thus influencing the outcome.

Multiple vitamin-mineral supplements that supply at least the recommended daily allowances (RDA) are frequently given to patients as part of their therapeutic regimen. Occasionally the use of other supplements appears to be beneficial. For instance, zinc improves the sensation of taste in some cancer patients, which therefore may improve appetite and nutritional status. Interestingly, the basis for the anticancer drug methotrexate's effect comes from its ability to fool cancer cells into thinking the drug is folic acid. Since folic acid stimulates the reproductive processes of cells, methotrexate effectively blocks the spread of cancer cells. Thus, folic acid supplementation may actually stimulate a tumor.

cannabis See HEMP SEED.

canthaxanthin A carotenoid, similar to beta-carotene, but, unlike beta-carotene, it is not converted to vitamin A in the body. Early research indicated this substance might have some cancer-protective properties.

capsicum (cayenne, red pepper, bird pepper, African pepper, chili pepper) The plants *Capsicum minimum (Roxb), frutescens* and *annuum,* of the family Solanaceae, grown in America (mainly south of Tennessee), Asia and Africa, whose fruit is eaten as a vegetable and used in the making of the hot, pungent spice. Chinese and other herbalists use the fruit as a tonic to stimulate the heart and circulation and stomach activity; unfortunately it is also linked to stomach distress and intestinal gas. Cayenne, however, is thought to be effective against bleeding in the lungs, toothache (the leaves

are the medicinal part for this), cramps and other ailments. Homeopathic medicine uses dried cayenne pods as a treatment for mouth ulcers, diarrhea, delirium tremens, asthma, headache, motion sickness, obesity, gout, sciatica, sore throat and a number of other problems.

The Russians commonly use red pepper in vodka as a home remedy for colds, stomach problems, rheumatism and lack of appetite.

See also CAYENNE.

capsule A hard or soft enclosure suitable as a container for drugs. Capsules are usually made from gelatin and animal by-products. "Vegicaps" are available from one manufacturer, Solgar, for vegetarians and those who adhere to a kosher diet.

See also GELATIN.

caraway A flowering biennial or perennial plant, *Carum carvi,* of the Umbellifer family, whose aromatic seeds are used as seasoning in various ethnic cuisines and by Chinese practitioners and other herbalists to aid digestion; expel gas; calm the nerves; counteract spasms, colic in infants and uterine cramps; and promote the onset of menstruation and lactation. When cooked and eaten, the roots are thought to tonify the intestines. Caraway grows wild in the northern United States, Europe and Asia, and is cultivated in most parts of the world, particularly in England, the Netherlands and Morocco.

carbohydrate A major class of chemical substances composed of carbon, hydrogen and oxygen, including sugars, dextrins, glycogen, starches and celluloses. As a fundamental source of energy, carbohydrates are stored in all the body's tissues as glycogen and are especially plentiful in the liver and muscles. Carbohydrates are dispatched from their storage sites when necessary.

The abundance of glucose and its polymers surpasses the quantity of all other organic chemical compounds found on earth, including fuel hydrocarbons just below the earth's crust.

Carbohydrates are absorbed by the body in the form of glucose, galactose and fructose—three sugars. Among the sources of carbohydrates are legumes, whose grains, vegetables, potatoes, fruits, honey and sugars. Because the calories obtained from sugars and candy lack essential amino acids, vitamins and minerals, they are considered "empty calories."

cardamom (sha ren, bastard cardamom, Malabar cardamom, ela) A perennial native to southern and eastern India, *Elettaria cardamomum,* of the ginger family, used as a spice and in folk and Ayurvedic medicine as an appetite stimulant, antiflatulent (carminative) and stomachic (an agent that invigorates stomach function).

cardiomyopathy A disease of the heart muscle in which the heart may become enlarged and lose its pumping efficiency, resulting in congestive heart failure. Selenium deficiency predisposes some individuals, primarily children, to a form of cardiomyopathy called Keshan's disease.

See also SELENIUM.

cardiovascular disease prevention and antioxidant vitamins The presence of oxidized low-density, or LDL, cholesterol is thought to clog arteries by stimulating macrophages, cells in the immune system, to ingest LDL particles, converting them to "foam cells." The oxidized LDL also damages the arterial walls, accumulating fats, cellular debris, platelets and the mineral calcium in the process. When the buildup becomes sufficient, the coronary arteries (blood vessels that supply life-sustaining blood to the heart muscle) become clogged, leading to angina pectoris (the pain of heart disease) and myocardial infarctions (heart attacks). Atherosclerosis also can occur in the carotid arteries and the extremities, often leading to strokes. Supplements of the antioxidant vitamin E seem to lower the risk of heart attacks by up to 37 percent, according to one of two Harvard University studies involving 39,910 male pharmacists and other health-care professionals followed for four years. Doses from 100 to 249 International Units (I.U.) of vitamin E daily were adequate with no extra benefit from higher doses. Since vitamin E also seems to reduce blood clotting (similar to the effects of aspirin), the question remains of which mechanism, the influence of the vitamin on blood clotting or the antioxidant effects on LDL, is responsible for this risk reduction.

The second of the two Harvard studies followed 87,245 healthy female nurses for eight years and found that those taking 100 I.U. of vitamin E daily were 34 percent less likely to suffer a heart attack.

A comparison of a small group of men taking 800 I.U. of vitamin E daily suggests protection against the oxidation of LDL more effective than beta-carotene, vitamin C or placebo. The study, conducted at the University of Texas, was reported in 1993.

Conclusion

Studies suggest, but do not prove, that approximately 100 I.U. of vitamin E daily reduces the risk of heart disease. It is impossible to get 100 I.U. of vitamin E from a balanced diet, but there does not seem to be any harmful effect from taking that quantity of vitamin E in a supplement.

See also ANTIOXIDANTS; E, VITAMIN.

carica (papay, pawpaw) The plant *Carica papaya,* of the Caricaceae family, thought to have originated in Mexico and Costa Rica, whose dried fruit pulp, leaves and latex are used by Chinese practitioners. The pulp reduces foot distress, including swelling. The leaves are for the treatment of ulcerations, boils, wounds and swellings. The latex, a meat tenderizer and ingredient in the manufacture of chewing gum and cosmetic products, is dried and used to expel intestinal worms and treat splenomegaly (enlarged spleen), skin blemishes, warts and corns.

carnitine A nonessential amino acid that helps regulate fat metabolism, carnitene potentiates fat oxidation, reduces excess triglycerides, decreases ketone levels and aids the metabolism of prostaglandin.

See also AMINO ACIDS.

carotenoids A group of yellow to deep red pigments, synthesized by plants, that concentrate in animal fat when ingested. An example is beta-carotene, which is converted to vitamin A in the body.

See also A, VITAMIN.

carrot   An herb, *Daucus carota,* of the family Umbelliferae, whose orange-colored root is edible. An average carrot is about 7 inches in length and provides roughly four times the Recommended Daily Allowance (RDA) of beta-carotene, which the human body converts to vitamin A. Although it contains only about 30 calories, a carrot will also provide fiber, vitamin C and potassium. Canned and frozen carrots lose about half their vitamin C but retain most of the beta-carotene and other nutrients. Excessive intake of carrots will result in a deep yellow or orange skin discoloration that can be reversed by eliminating carrots from the diet.

carthamus (hong hua, false saffron, bastard saffron, safflower)   A flowering herb, *Carthamus tinctorius,* of the Compositae family, that may have originated in Eurasia and whose flowers are used in Chinese medicine to treat internal bleeding, painful menses and the coughing of blood. Other uses include inducing menstruation and stimulating the circulation. It is also prescribed for women after giving birth or carrying a dead fetus.

cascara sagrada (Persian bark, sacred bark, chittem bark)   A flowering tree of the West Coast of the United States and in South America, *Rhamnus purshiana,* of the Rhamnaceae family, whose aged, dried bark extract is used as a cathartic, listed in the United States Pharmacopoeia (USP). Cascara was recognized by Native Americans as an effective laxative. In Russia, cascara sagrada is called Krushina or Joster, and is also used in homeopathic medicine for the treatment of rheumatism.

cassava   The perennial herb *Manihot esculenta,* from which root (or rootstock) tapioca and other puddings are made. Grown in the tropics, cassava is a rich source of starch and is an effective catalyst in the conversion of solar energy into carbohydrates. It is also used as a thickening agent in pie fillings and other foods.

cassia (sicklepod, sickle senna)   A flowering herb of the Philippines, Indonesia, India, Japan and China, *Cassia tora,* of the Leguminosae family, whose seeds are used in Chinese medicine to treat herpes, eye ailments such as conjunctivitis, vertigo, earache, constipation and skin diseases.

castor bean (castor-oil plant, Palma Christi)   The plant *Ricinus communis,* of the Euphorbiaceae family, whose bean or seed yields an oil when pressed that is used internally as a cathartic (castor oil) and externally as an emollient. The oil contains glycerides of ricinoleic, isoricinoleic, stearic, linoleic and dihydroxystearic acids, which act as laxatives in the digestive tract. After the beans have been pressed to extract the oil, the poisonous substance ricin is left. In the past, castor oil was routinely given to children to keep their bowels regular. Its terrible taste often created indelible memories of childhood. Herbalists also prescribe castor oil as a treatment for food poisoning, and, administered along with anti-worm medications, to expel worms. Castor oil is recognized in the United States Pharmacopoeia (USP).

catalase   An enzyme that catalyzes the breakdown of hydrogen peroxide into water and oxygen. Catalase, found in most cells, works with superoxide dismutase (SOD) to inhibit the production of free radicals.

catalysis   A process in which a velocity of a chemical reaction is increased by the presence of a substance that is not consumed by the reaction. Enzymes, synthesized from amino acids, act in conjunction with B-complex vitamins as catalysts in the body.

A catalyst is a substance, such as an enzyme, that enables a chemical reaction in other substances, particularly a reaction that may be faster or otherwise unusual without the help of the catalyst. The catalyst itself remains unchanged.

See also CATALASE; CHYMOTRYPSIN; COENZYME Q10.

catalyst   See CATALYSIS.

cataracts and vitamins   See EYE DISEASES.

catechu (cutch)   An extract from the heartwood of the Indian tree *Acacia catechu,* used in Asian medicine as a remedy for oral disorders, such as gingivitis and toothaches, diabetes and skin conditions. Catechu may be prepared as a mouthwash or as a tincture to be taken internally.

catnip (catmint) A highly aromatic mint, *Nepeta cataria*, of the Labiatae family, commonly known for its attractiveness to cats. But a tea made from the leaves, according to herbalists, is used for relieving the accumulated effects of stress, including nervousness and insomnia. Catnip is also prescribed as a treatment for diarrhea, fevers and colds, and hyperactivity in children. Catnip may be combined with camomile, spearmint and lemon balm as a remedy for insomnia.

cat's claw A South American herb, *Uncaria tormentosa*, used as a treatment for strengthening immunocompromised individuals, such as those with AIDS, cancer and viral infections. Cat's claw also has anti-inflammatory properties and is used in South American medicine as a treatment for arthritis, intestinal inflammation and ulcers. It has been considered a remedy for various ailments, including asthma, menstrual disorders, depression, wounds and hemorrhoids.

cat's foot (cudweed, Life Everlasting) The flowering plant *Antennaria dioica* grows in Europe, Asia, and America. Its flowers may be prepared as a tea and taken as a remedy for muscle spasms and intestinal problems. It is called "Life Everlasting" because its flowers do not wilt for about a year after being cut.

cayenne (paprika, chili pepper, red pepper) A pepper plant, *Capsicum annuum*, native to Mexico and Central America, from which capsaicin is extracted as a pain reliever. Used in topical creams and as a liquid taken internally, capsaicin is said to relieve pain caused by shingles, bursitis, diabetic neuropathy, muscle spasms and tension, rheumatism, alcoholism, motion sickness, malaria, yellow fever, indigestion, arteriosclerosis, stroke, gas and cardiac problems. Internal use of cayenne may cause diarrhea and cramps, and use over an extended period of time may result in chronic gas-

tric disorders and kidney, liver or nerve damage. An overdose may be life-threatening.

See also CAPSICUM.

celandine (tetterwort, chelidonium) An evergreen perennial of the United States and Europe, *Chelidonium majus*, of the Papaveraceae family, whose herb and root are used in herbal medicine as a diuretic, an expectorant and a laxative. Early use of celandine included the treatment of jaundice. In Russian folk medicine, celandine preparations are used for spasmatic conditions of the liver, kidney, bladder and gallbladder, stomach problems and swellings. Among the homeopathic applications of celandine are liver, spleen and skin disorders, cancer, chorea, gonorrhea, hemorrhoids, headache, nosebleed, whooping cough, jaundice, stomachache, diarrhea, pneumonia, rheumatism, gallstones and influenza. External uses include the treatment of metastatic skin conditions, warts and cuts. The celandine plant is poisonous to animals.

celery (smallage) A biennial or annual herb, *Apium graveolens*, of the Umbelliferae family, that originated in southern Europe, Asia and Africa, whose root and seeds are considered of medicinal use by herbalists as a tonic, nerve sedative and carminative. In India and Pakistan, celery (*ajmoda*) is used to treat numerous problems, such as bronchitis, asthma, liver and spleen ailments, rheumatism, hiccoughs, intestinal gas, hives, urinary retention and discharges, lack of menses, fever and cough. Homeopathic medicine uses celery-seed tincture for tension headache, heartburn, toothache, vomiting, hives and the retention of urine.

celiac disease See MALABSORPTION.

cellulose A fiber found in cotton, trees and other plants, as well as in foods such as bran, broccoli, oranges, parsnips, cabbage, turnips, wheat and other whole grains, spinach, apples, celery, apricots, asparagus, onions, beans, oatmeal, prunes and beets. A polysaccharide, cellulose contains a large number of glucose units and stimulates the digestive and elimination process, but, as a fibrous form of carbohydrate, it provides no nutrients to humans.

celosia (wood flower) A weed of Asian origin, *Celosia argentea* and *cristata* (cockscomb), of the Amarantaceae family, named from the Greek word *kelos,* meaning burned, used in Chinese medicine for dysentery, various menstrual difficulties, bleeding in the intestines and lungs, cough, eye inflammations and abnormal sensitivity, headache and worms.

The plant was eaten by prisoners of war in Thailand during World War II to prevent nutritionally related diseases such as beriberi and pellagra, and it has been known also as an aphrodisiac and anticancer agent.

See also BERIBERI; PELLAGRA.

centaury (bitter clover, rose pink) A flowering plant, *Sabbatia angularis,* of the family Gentianaceae, grown in Europe and the United States, used in herbal medicine as a tonic, fever reducer and diaphoretic, and for the treatment of dyspepsia, rheumatic and other joint pain, diarrhea, eye inflammations and homesickness (which may be a form of depression in this context). In Russian folk medicine, centaury tea with vodka is given for parasitic tapeworm, hypertension and liver and gallbladder maladies.

centella (Asian pennywort, Indian pennywort) A tropical weed, *Centella asiatica,* of the Umbelliferae family, sometimes eaten as a vegetable and, in Chinese medicine, used to stimulate the appetite, promote digestion and treat ulcers, skin problems and bowel complaints.

chaenomeles (Japanese quince) Deciduous shrub native to China and cultivated in Japan and elsewhere, *Chaenomeles speciosa,* of the family Rosaceae, named from the Greek words *chaino* (split) and *meles* (apple), whose fruit is used in Chinese medicine for the relief of sunstroke, indigestion, colic, joint pain, cholera, muscle spasms and diarrhea.

chaga (birch mushroom) A North American tree, *Inonotus obliquus,* of the family Polyporaceae, whose internal granulated parts (from the middle layer of a fungus, or mushroom-type growth sawn off the tree, as if removing a blackened wart) are used by Native Americans for medicinal purposes. In herbal folk medicine, chaga was given great credit for effectiveness against stomach pain, cancer, tuberculosis of the bone and other disorders. The Medical Academy of Science in Moscow touts the use of chaga for malignancies and inoperable conditions, for purifying the blood and regenerating (or rejuvenating) organs.

chamomile See CAMOMILE.

chaparral (chaparro, greasewood, creosote bush, gobonadora, dwarf evergreen oak) The plant *Larrea divaricata,* of the family Zygophyllaceae, and plants of more than 100 botanical types of desert Artimesia, whose leaves and stems are considered in Native American medicine to be antiseptic, tonic and diuretic. Chaparral tea is an old Native American remedy for melanoma. Chaparral contains nordihydroguariaetic acid (NDGA), thought to be the substance that inhibits cancerous growth. It is also used by herbalists for the treatment of chronic backache, leukemia, prostate disorders, pulmonary ailments, kidney infection and arthritis, among others. It is considered an expectorant and weight reducer.

chelated mineral supplements Minerals in which a natural or synthetic substance called the chelator is chemically combined and which some advocate as being better absorbed and therefore more available for utilization by the body. However, this claim may not be true, since the acidic nature of stomach juices breaks down the chelated product into its individual components. Therefore, there is probably no difference in absorption of chelated or nonchelated minerals. There are a few instances when chelated compounds such as iron or zinc may be less irritating to the stomach and therefore better tolerated. Chromium picolinate, another chelated mineral, may also be better absorbed.

See also AMINO ACID CHELATES.

chelation A process in which metal complexes are formed. Chelating agents are used as treatments for metal poisoning. Although promoted by some as "better" supplements, there is no scientific basis for this.

See also CHELATED MINERAL SUPPLEMENTS.

cherry bark (choke cherry, wild black cherry bark) A large North American fruit tree, *Prunus virginiana*, of the Rosaceae family, whose bark is used as a vehicle and flavoring in cough medicines. Homeopaths and Native American herbal-medicine practitioners use cherry bark, which contains hydrocyanic acid and malic acid, to prepare remedies for diarrhea (in children), bronchitis and dyspepsia.

chestnut (Spanish chestnut, horse chestnut) A North American, Asian and southern European tree, *Castanea dentata*, of the family Fagacaea, that produces nuts containing carbohydrates; minerals including phosphate of potash, magnesia, sodium, and iron; and some protein. The leaves and inner bark are considered medicinal as a tonic, sedative and astringent. Herbalists use a tea of chestnut leaves for chronic cough, hiccoughs, fever and diarrhea. The horse chestnut is cultivated in Russia as Konsky cashtan, and, in folk medicine, is used to treat arthritis, rheumatism, intestinal inflammation, gynecological problems and hemorrhoids.

chewable vitamins Supplements that can be chewed to make them more palatable for children or those who have difficulty swallowing tablets or capsules. Young children must be observed for overdoses because these products may taste like candy. Chewable vitamin C may cause tooth decay because the acidic nature of the vitamin may wear away tooth enamel.

chickweed (starwort, adder's mouth, tonguegrass, satin flower, stitchwort, starweed, winterweed) An annual or biennial weed, *Stellaria media*, of the Caryophyllaceae family, found throughout the world and used in Native American and herbal medicine as a carminative, demulcent, expectorant and laxative. Also a vegetable, chickweed resembles spinach and can be eaten in salad. Homeopathic uses of chickweed include treatment of gout, inflammation of the liver, psoriasis and rheumatism.

chicory (succory, endive) An American and European perennial, *Cichorium intybus*, of the Compositae family, whose rootstock and flowering herb are used in folk, Native American and homeopathic medicine. Chicory tea is said to remove phlegm from the stomach, purify the liver and spleen and counteract gout, arthritis and stiff joints. A tincture made of the dried root is used for amblyopia, constipation and headache. Chicory (*Tzicory*, in Russian folk medicine) is also used as a sedative of the heart and central nervous system.

children, herbs for Herbs meant for adults may be more potent when used by children. The usual child dosage is one-eighth to one-half the adult dose, according to the child's body weight. Many ailments affecting children may be treated with herbal remedies, particularly those prepared with the intention of strengthening the child's body and immune system and preventing illnesses. For example, for diarrhea, a child may take peppermint tea, slippery elm mixed with skim milk, brown rice, apples or carob powder mixed in apple juice. For constipation, a child can have raisins soaked in senna tea, molasses in water or a teaspoon of psyllium husk in aloe juice. A child with indigestion may benefit from chamomile or fennel tea, soy milk instead of cow's or goat's milk or ground cinnamon or ginger in water. Acidophilus liquid or powder in juice promotes good digestion. Licorice tea or sticks or zinc lozenges may be offered to a child with a sore throat. Chest congestion in children may be relieved with peppermint or raspberry tea and with herbal steam inhalation preparations, such as eucalyptus oil or tea tree oil. For prevention of illness, children may benefit from protein drinks, sugar-free multivitamin and mineral supplements, chewable vitamin C, bifidobacteria, certain raw foods and other nutritional and supplemental foods and preparations.

On the other hand, some herbal or home remedies should *not* be given to very young children. For example, honey, which may be contaminated with botulism or other toxic microorganism, should not be given until the child is at least two years old.

See also C, VITAMIN; CHAMOMILE; FENNEL; LICORICE; MULTIVITAMIN AND MINERAL SUPPLEMENTS.

chimonanthus (wintersweet) A Chinese flowering deciduous shrub, *Chimonanthus praecox,* of the Calycanthaceae family, whose flowers are used in Chinese medicine to treat sore throat and burns. *Chimonanthus* is the Greek word for winter flower.

China orange (citrus dulcis, sweet orange)
Originally an Asian citrus tree, *Citrus sinensis,* that yielded fruits whose outer peel was prepared as a remedy for loss of appetite and indigestion.
See also ORANGE PEEL.

Chinese foxglove root From the herb *Rehmannia glutinosa,* a preparation used as a remedy in traditional Chinese medicine for digestive disorders, menstrual irregularities, heart palpitations, constipation, stiffness in joints, hearing and visual problems, low back pain, menopausal symptoms, insomnia and chronic fever. When the root is cooked in wine, it is used as an antiaging tonic. Side effects may include diarrhea, distended abdomen and gas.
See also REHMANNIA.

chitrak (plumbago) An Ayurvedic herb thought to reduce hyperacidity and promote digestion.

chlerodendron (glory-bower, tubeflower, Kashmir-bouquet) Tropical shrubs or trees of the Verbenaceae family, named from the Greek words for chance and tree, whose leaves are used by Chinese practitioners to treat hypertension, beriberi, nosebleed, gonorrhea, intestinal bleeding, rheumatism and dermatitis.

Chlorella The genus name of unicellular green algae.
See also ALGAE.

chloride A salt of hydrochloric acid and principal inorganic anion in the extracellular fluid necessary to maintain a normal fluid and electrolyte balance in the body. Normal chloride occurs in concentrations of 96 to 106 milliequivalents per liter of plasma. Higher concentrations are present in the gastric juices and cerebrospinal fluid.

Chloride deficiency occurs only when there is also a loss of sodium caused by excessive sweating, chronic diarrhea or vomiting or some kidney disorders. These losses may result in metabolic alkalosis, a disorder of the body's pH, or acid-base balance, which may lead to coma or death.

Dietary intake is generally as sodium chloride (common table salt). Small amounts are available when potassium chloride supplements are used for the treatment of potassium deficiencies associated with diuretic use.

Toxicity
Only in the presence of severe dehydration is excessive dietary intake of chloride, as salt, of any significance. Hyperchloremia may cause high blood pressure.
See also POTASSIUM; SODIUM.

chlorophyll The green color in plants in which photosynthesis takes place.
See also ALGAE.

cholesterol See CARDIOVASCULAR DISEASE PREVENTION AND ANTIOXIDANT VITAMINS.

choline A substance found throughout animal and plant tissues or made synthetically. Choline is not a vitamin, despite claims by some that it is part of the B-complex. It was first discovered in hog bile in 1862. The amino acid methionine and folic acid are essential for choline's synthesis in humans.

Choline is important for the structure of all cell membranes, lipoproteins and surfactant for normal lung function. Choline may be vital in the production and transportation of fats from the liver and may prevent fatty liver. Researchers are trying to determine if alcoholic cirrhosis is caused by the toxic effects of alcohol alone or of that toxicity aggravated by nutritional deficiencies including choline.

Choline may also have important functions in the central nervous system as a component of sphinogomyelin in membranes and the neurotransmitter acetylcholine. Acetylcholine may be deficient in some neurological disorders of the elderly, and large dietary intake of choline was thought by some researchers to be of some possible benefit for memory loss. Unfortunately, this benefit has proved elusive in conditions such as Alzheimer's disease. There have been claims that chronic headache sufferers benefit from choline supplements.

Dietary Sources

The average diet contains 400 to 900 mg of choline, found principally as lecithin in eggs, liver and other organ meats, lean meats, brewer's yeast, wheat germ, soybeans, peanuts and green peas. Lecithins are used as an emulsifier in chocolate and margarine, whereas vegetables such as cauliflower and lettuce contain free choline.

The American Academy of Pediatrics recommends that infant formula contain 7 mg of choline per 100 kilocalories, equivalent to the amount found in human milk, to assure adequate growth and development in newborns.

Toxicity

While large doses of choline produce liver and spleen damage and possibly alter the immune system in laboratory animals, this finding has not been demonstrated in humans. But an abnormal accumulation of sphinogomyelins in the nervous system results in the hereditary Niemann-Pick disease, characterized by enlargement of the liver and spleen, anemia and progressive physical and mental deterioration. With an onset in infancy, Niemann-Pick usually results in death before a child is three.

chondroitin   A complex carbohydrate present in the connective tissue of mammals, including the cornea and cartilage, prepared in chondroitin sulfate capsules and in chondroitin sulfate/glucosamine combination capsules and tablets as a remedy for osteoarthritis, torn ligaments and tendons, gout pain, inflammation of or damaged cartilage of the joints, headaches, respiratory and allergy problems, wounds and antiaging. Chondroitin draws fluid into the tissues, which results in nutrients flowing to the damaged area and more resilient cartilage consistency and thus better shock absorption. It is also said that chondroitin prevents certain enzymes from weakening connective tissues; in some cases, because of its sugar molecules called glycoaminoglycans, it can

help rebuild cartilage that has been injured. In addition, use of chondroitin is reported to reduce the need for nonsteroidal anti-inflammatory drugs (NSAIDS) and other painkillers for individuals with osteoarthritis. Chondroitin and combinations thereof are still under investigation for actions and effectiveness.

See also ARTHRITIS.

chromium   A trace mineral thought by some to be deficient in people with diabetes and having an influence on insulin and carbohydrate metabolism. Chromium, in association with insulin, may also play an important role in the synthesis of protein. Studies have not been completed to determine the validity of these claims.

See also CHROMIUM PICOLINATE; DIABETES MELLITUS.

chromium picolinate   An essential trace mineral necessary for normal glucose metabolism and regulation of sugar in the body. Chromium, which was discovered in the 1950s, curbs the appetite by suppressing hunger pains, controls blood cholesterol levels, helps prevent infection, helps control and produce insulin and promotes the synthesis of proteins. Food sources of chromium and chromium picolinate include brewer's yeast, honey, whole grains, meats, liver, cheese, corn oil, grapes, raisins, eggs, black pepper, thyme, potatoes and clams and other seafood. Some experts claim that the combination of chromium, niacin and glutathione is most effective in the treatment of diabetes, because of its ability to potentiate the production of insulin.

See also BREWER'S YEAST; CHROMIUM; GLUTATHIONE.

chronic fatigue syndrome (CFS) (chronic mononucleosis, chronic Epstein-Barr virus infection, post-viral fatigue syndrome, myalgic encephalomyelitis)   A disorder characterized by overwhelming fatigue associated with a prolonged recovery period. Tasks that were formerly routine become difficult or impossible. The fatigue is accompanied by poor concentration and memory, depression, headaches, sleep disturbances, aches and pains.

The condition may begin insidiously without apparent cause, or following an acute infection, described as early as 1869 as "neurasthenia . . . a physical not a mental state" by the American neurologist George Beard. Clusters of cases have been blamed on mass hysteria since clinical findings are usually nonexistent.

Recently, several viruses have been proposed as causes, but so far this has not been scientifically documented. Epstein-Barr virus, enteroviruses, retroviruses, herpesvirus type 6 and the T-cell lymphotropic virus type II have all been implicated as possible causes of CFS.

Alternative therapies including megavitamin formulas; royal jelly, a substance obtained from bees; and diets restricting yeasts and sugar have been prescribed for CFS. However, the Chronic Fatigue Syndrome Research Group at the Center for Disease Control in Atlanta warns that no dietary or vitamin therapy has proven effective in treating the condition.

An Australian study has demonstrated improvements in physical, psychological and functional symptoms following therapy with intravenous gamma globulin, suggesting that chronic fatigue syndrome, by whatever name, is an organic disease process and not a psychosomatic disorder.

See also FATIGUE.

chrysanthemum, Chinese (chu hua, ju hua) A flowering plant of the Compositae family, named from the Greek words *chyros* (golden) and *anthos* (flower). *Chrysanthemum morifolium* flowers are used in Chinese medicine as a tea in order to stimulate circulation and vision and treat menstrual, digestive, liver and potency problems, night blindness and nervous disorders. The flowers and stem of *Chrysanthemum indicum* are used to treat hypertension and skin infections.

chymopapain One of the proteolytic food enzymes found in unripe papaya that aids the digestion of proteins.

chymotrypsin A digestive enzyme that helps convert food into chyme (from the Greek word *chymos,* meaning juice), which is a thick liquid mixture of partially digested food and fluids secreted by the stomach and small intestine during digestion.

cibotium (Scythian lamb) A Chinese and Malaysian forest fern, *Cibotium barometz,* of the Dicksoniaceae family, whose stem is used by Chinese practitioners as a liver and kidney tonic, and to treat infertility, lumbago, rheumatism and bone diseases.

cigarette smoking's effects on absorption of vitamins and minerals Smokers have lower bone density than nonsmokers, and calcium supplements may be helpful. Vitamin C is metabolized, or broken down, more quickly in smokers, who may require more than twice as much of the vitamin. The National Research Council recommends at least 100 mg of vitamin C daily. Vitamin E deficiency may also be more likely in smokers.

cimicifuga (bugbane) An herb, *Cimicifuga foetida,* of the Ranunculaceae family, of Europe, Siberia and China, named from the Latin words *cimicis* (bug) and *fugio* (to flee), and thought to have insecticidal properties. In Chinese medicine, bugbane root is used as a sedative, painkiller and treatment for measles, headache and diarrhea.

cinchona (Jesuit's bark, Peruvian bark) Parts, including the dried bark, of the cinchona evergreen tree native to tropical American mountain regions that constitute the main source of the drug quinine, for the treatment of malaria and cardiac and other ailments. It is named after the countess of Cinchon, who introduced the substance's medicinal properties to Europe. Cinchona (*Cinchona pubescens*) is also used as a remedy for anorexia, indigestion, bacterial infections, fever, chronic dysentery, gout, nephritis, gas, muscle cramps, splenomegaly, leg ulcers and cancer. Potential side effects include allergic reaction to quinine and quinine-based medications and exacerbation of any bleeding problem, such as hemophilia. Cinchona is usually prepared as a liquid extract or as tea. Overdose of quinine (roughly, 10 to 15 grams) may lead to heart failure and asphyxiation.

cinnamomum (cinnamon, rou gui, gui zhi, twak)
Evergreen trees and shrubs of the Lauraceae family, found from Southeast Asia to Australia. *Cinnamomum camphora* (camphor tree) of China, Taiwan and Japan yields wood and oil used externally to relieve pain and congestion. *Cinnamomum zeylanicum*, of India, Sri Lanka and the Malay Peninsula, is the source of cinnamon, the spice known throughout the world, as well as cinnamon oil, which, according to Chinese medicine, may be a narcotic poison when taken internally and a treatment for nausea and vomiting. The *zeylonicum* bark is used to treat rheumatism, tuberculosis and headache, and as a respiratory and circulatory stimulant.

The *Cinnamomum cassia* native to Burma yields cassia oil used in the making of chocolate and, from its bark, twigs and branches, medicinal preparations that relieve menstrual problems, indigestion, headache, fever, colds and joint and abdominal pain.

citronella (lemongrass)　From the *Cymbopogon* species, citronella is an Asian medicine made from the grass used as a remedy for indigestion, gas, worms and disorders of the throat. It is also a popular insect repellant and fragrance in household products. Citronella may cause lung damage if its oil is inhaled.

See LEMONGRASS.

citrus (chen pi, orange or tangerine peel)
Fruit-bearing, evergreen shrubs and trees of the Rutaceae family, originally of South and Southeast Asia and now cultivated throughout the world if the climate permits, whose leaves, roots, fruit and fruit peels are generally recognized as medicinal by most conventional practices of medicine and nutrition, including allopathic, Chinese traditional, Ayurvedic and Native American. Some of the fruits of the citrus shrubs and trees are oranges, lemons and grapefruits, rich in vitamin C.

In Chinese medicine, the leaves, root and fruit peel of citron, or *Citrus medica*, native to India, are used to treat lumbago. Any citrus fruit offers vitamin C, which wards off scurvy. To prevent scurvy, English sailors sucked limes to obtain the nutrient, thus becoming known as "limeys." Chinese practitioners also use both ripe and unripe fruits to relieve diarrhea, cramps, chest congestion and spleen and stomach problems.

See also ASCORBIC ACID.

cleavers (goose grass, bedstraw, catchstraw, clivers)　A flowering herb, *Galium aparine*, of the Rubiaceae family, commonly found in Europe and the United States, especially along river banks, and used in Native American medicine as a tonic, diuretic and as a remedy for the occurrence of stones in bodily organs.

clematis　A climbing vine (in Greek, *klematis* means climbing plant) of the Ranunculaceae family. *Clematis chinensis* roots are used in Chinese medicine as a treatment for jaundice, constipation, irregular menses, lumbago, arthritis, backache, alcohol poisoning and scanty urine. The stem of *Clematis montana*, of the Himalayas, provides a remedy for excessive or painful urination and insomnia.

clove (ding xiang, lavanga)　A tropical evergreen tree, *Caryophyllus aromaticus*, *Eugenia caryophyllus* or *Syzygium aromaticum* of the myrtle family, used as a spice and a source of oil. Native to the Spice Islands and the Philippines, though cultivated in South America, Sumatra and the West Indies, clove oil relieves toothaches and nausea. The oil is distilled from the dried flower buds.

cnidium (chuanxiong, Chinese lovage)　A Chinese, Siberian and eastern European herb, *Cnidium monnieri*, of the Umbelliferae family, whose seeds are used in Chinese medicine and are thought to be a stimulant (particularly for menstrual flow), aphrodisiac and sedative.

cobalamins　See B_{12}, VITAMIN.

cobalt　A metallic element that is an essential constituent of vitamin B_{12}. There is no evidence of human deficiency, and therefore no Recommended Dietary Allowance (RDA) has been established.

See also B_{12}, VITAMIN.

cocaine abuse See TYROSINE.

cocoa (cacao, chocolate) Cocoa is the main ingredient in chocolate products. It is sometimes used as a remedy for diarrhea, though it may also cause constipation, as well as for intestinal and urinary tract disturbances and other disorders. Certain compounds in cocoa expand respiratory passages, dilate blood vessels, act as a cardiac tonic and relax muscles. Despite recent enthusiasm that chocolate (whose Latin name, *Theobroma cacao*, means "food of the gods") is beneficial, in addition to being a popular food, it remains in significant amounts a possible trigger for migraine, tachycardia, sleep disorders and allergic reactions.

cod liver oil A supplement rich in omega-3 fatty acids and fat-soluble vitamins A and D. Excessive amounts can cause toxic accumulation of A and D.

See also A, VITAMIN; D, VITAMIN; OMEGA-3 FATTY ACIDS.

codonopsis (bonnet bellflower, dang shen) A flowering, twining herb with heart-shaped aromatic leaves, *Codonopsis pilosula,* of the Campanulaceae family, originally found in Northeast Asia. The plant's name is the Greek word for "bell-like," which describes the bell-shaped flowers. The roots are used in Chinese medicine to prevent gonorrhea and relieve heart palpitations, diabetes, hypertension, breast cancer, diminished sexual desire, amnesia, asthma, insomnia and menstrual difficulties. Some believe codonopsis root may offer a substitute for the widely known stimulant ginseng.

coenzyme A nonprotein compound that binds with a protein (apoenzyme) to form an active enzyme. Some B-complex vitamins, such as pantothenic acid, are converted in the body to coenzymes.

See also COENZYME A.

coenzyme A A compound derived from the B-complex vitamin pantothenic acid required to convert carbohydrates, fats and some proteins to energy.

See also COENZYME; PANTOTHENIC ACID.

coenzyme B_{12} (adenosylcobalamin) One of two active forms of vitamin B_{12} synthesized after the ingestion of the vitamin.

See also B_{12}, VITAMIN; COENZYME.

coenzyme Q-10 An enzyme activator found in rice bran, wheat germ, fish, eggs, beans and nuts. Synthesized in the liver, this coenzyme catalyzes cellular energy throughout the body and converts nutrients into adenosine triphosphate (ATP), or "fuel" for every cell. Some experts claim that a deficiency of coenzyme Q-10 contributes to congestive heart failure and other cardiac conditions. As the body ages, synthesis from food intake decreases, and the enzyme may be taken as a supplement. Coenzyme Q-10 is said to inhibit the aging process, promote weight loss and cardiac health, boost the immune system and treat hypertension and periodontal disease.

See also UBIQUINONE.

coenzyme R The former name for biotin.

See also BIOTIN.

coffee charcoal From the Latin *Coffea arabica.* Roasted, blackened, and powdered coffee beans used as a remedy for diarrhea and sore throat. Coffee, whose main active ingredient is caffeine, is used as a homeopathic remedy for nervousness and neuralgia and as a component in conventional headache medications. Originally derived from the beverage coffee in Caffa, part of Ethiopia, and produced in Arab countries in the early 15th century before reaching Europe, coffee charcoal does not rely on its caffeine content for the therapeutic effect. Instead, it works as an astringent for body tissues and therefore may have the adverse effect of interfering with other medications. An overdose of coffee charcoal powder may lead to anorexia, diarrhea, vomiting, insomnia, restlessness, cardiac irregularities, muscle spasms and general poisoning.

See also KOLA NUT; TEA.

Cohen, Kenneth (1952–) Health educator, traditional healer and author of books including *The Way of Qigong: The Art and Science of Chinese Energy Healing* (Random House, New York, 1999) and *Hon-*

oring the Medicine: The Essential Guide to Native American Healing (Ballantine Books, New York, 2003). Cohen, who holds M.A. and M.S.Th. degrees, has written extensively about Eastern and Western herbalism, including on the use of plant extracts and preparations now in widespread use as both dietary supplements and remedies for illness.

coix (Job's tears, yi yi ren)   A flowering, southeast Asian grass named *Coix lacryma-jobi,* or tears of Job, by the Swedish botanist Carl Linnaeus, who created the system of naming and classifying plants. Of the family Gramineae, coix kernels (in Greek, *koix* means palm) are used in Chinese, Japanese, Indian and Filipino medicine to treat fever, rheumatism, gonorrhea and other ailments.

colombo (kalumb, calumbo)   A southeast African climbing perennial, *Cocculus palmatus,* whose rootstock is used in herbal medicine to treat diarrhea, nausea and vomiting, fever, dyspepsia and colon disorders.

coltsfoot (kuan dong hua, British tobacco, foal's foot, flower velure, butterbur)   A flowering, perennial plant, *Tussilago farfara,* of the United States, Europe and the East Indies, whose leaves and flowers are used in herbal medicine for diarrhea and numerous respiratory problems, including pleurisy, bronchial asthma and hoarseness.

comfrey (knitbone, bruisewort, healing herb, gum plant, salsify, blackwort, wallwort)   An American and European flowering perennial plant, *Symphytum officinale,* of the family Boraginaceae, whose rootstock is made into a decoction and used as a gargle for sore throat and bleeding gums. When drunk, this decoction is considered by herbalists to remedy various symptoms of indigestion. Comfrey contains calcium, phosphorus, potassium, and vitamins A and C, and when powdered, its rootstock may be applied to minor cuts and burns to promote healing.

Comfrey tea, however, which has been popular for hundreds of years as a therapeutic agent, is now the subject of much controversy because of its pyrrolidine content, a substance that may cause liver dysfunction and cancer. While pyrrolidine and other alkaloids found in comfrey have not been proven to be carcinogenic, herbalists recommend cautious use of comfrey. Comfrey's chief reputation as a healing herb for external use on wounds and broken bones is largely attributable to the plant's allantoin content. Allantoin, a white crystalline substance found in amniotic fluid, is thought to stimulate cell growth.

condurango (eagle vine)   The bark of an asclepiadaceous vine, about 30 feet long and two feet wide, beaten, separated from the stem and sun-dried, is used as a diuretic, stomachic and alterative remedy in the treatment of early stage cancer. Reportedly condurango has no effect in inhibiting or halting the progress of the disease. There are many varieties of the plant, and the species experimented with in cancer is the *Condurango blanco,* used in South America as an alterative in chronic syphilis. While it increases the circulation, an overdose may produce convulsions, paralysis, vertigo and visual disturbances.

contraceptives, oral, and vitamin deficiency   Drugs that inhibit ovulation and effectively prevent pregnancy also depress serum folic acid levels. Therefore they may increase the risk of birth defects related to folate deficiency if pregnancy occurs in women who have recently used these products, also known as birth control pills.

cooking methods' effect on nutrients   While many people believe that eating vegetables raw is the best way to obtain the nutrients they offer, experts now believe that minimal cooking, which involves the use of heat, may yield optimal results in terms of the food's digestibility and making the nutrients available to the body.

For example, raw carrots are low in fat, but carrots cooked lightly in a microwave oven make the beta-carotene more available. Dr. John W. Erdman, Jr., director of the University of Illinois division of nutritional sciences at Champaign-Urbana, explained in an article that, because chunks of raw carrot may not be broken down by digestive enzymes, a person may not be able to absorb more than 1 percent of the carrot's beta-carotene. A cooked carrot preserves the beta-carotene and also offers more available protein and fiber, even though some water-soluble, heat-labile vitamin C is sacrificed. Juicing, which does not involve heating but does serve to pulverize food, is another effective way to create bioavailability of nutrients.

In addition, the cooking of vegetables creates a greater availability of starches. A potato eaten raw offers about 30 percent of its starch, but a cooked potato offers 95 percent. Raw cauliflower and broccoli are among other vegetables with high amounts of starch.

If vegetables are boiled, about 50 percent of their vitamins C and B and minerals will be destroyed. Vegetables should be cooked in as little water as possible only long enough to soften them slightly (this result is often called al dente), whether steaming or microwaving. Of boiling, steaming and microwaving, the last is considered the method that preserves the most nutrients of foods, especially vegetables.

According to Dr. Paul Lachance, chairman of the Food Science Department of Rutgers University, New Brunswick, New Jersey, Chinese wok cooking (also called "stir-frying") and pressure-cooking methods are also recommended. Stir-frying requires no water, and the small amount of oil that is used helps foods retain their nutrients. Beta-carotene, for example, is absorbed best when the vegetable containing it is cooked in oil. A pressure-cooker heats foods quickly, allowing them little or no contact with water. Foods boiled while enclosed in a plastic bag also maintain their nutrients because the nutrients cannot leach into the water.

copper   A metallic element essential in human nutrition. The average adult has stores of about 100 to 150 mg of copper in the liver, brain, heart, kidney and hair. Copper plays an essential role in the utilization of iron in the synthesis of hemoglobin. Copper is also involved in the metabolism of vitamin C, the sense of taste and collagen elastin, bone and myelin (the covering for nerves) development. Copper is involved in a number of enzymatic reactions for the production of energy, oxidation of fatty acids and formation of the skin pigment melanin.

Ceruloplasmin is a substance in the blood containing six atoms of copper that appears to serve as a transport vehicle for the mineral to tissues where it is needed.

Deficiency

Although human deficiencies are rare, malnourished South American children were shown to have anemia, low white blood cell counts, poor bone formation and growth impairment from diets lacking in copper. In adults, deficiencies have been found in patients on total parenteral nutrition (TPN), the intravenous provision of the total caloric needs of a patient who cannot take food orally. A rare inherited disorder, Menkes' steely hair disease, involves impairment of copper utilization. Spue, a malabsorption disease, and the kidney disorder nephrotic syndrome cause inadequate protein and therefore the body may fail to produce sufficient ceruloplasmin necessary for the metabolism of copper. The evidence for an increase in cholesterol, glucose and heart disease in persons whose copper intake is very low has been inconsistent. However, there may be an increased incidence in heart disease for those individuals whose zinc-to-copper dietary intake was elevated. Copper supplementation has experimentally raised HDL ("good" cholesterol) and lowered total cholesterol in copper deficient animals and humans.

Dietary Sources

Liver and other organ meats, shellfish, nuts, legumes, whole-grain cereals and raisins provide the highest dietary levels of copper. Copper intake may be increased by the influence of acidity in the water supply from contact with copper pipes. The federal Food and Drug Administration (FDA) in the Total Diet Study between 1982 and 1986 showed a daily copper intake of 1.2 mg for adult males and 0.9 mg for females. Infant ingestion was 0.45 mg and 0.57 mg daily for infants and toddlers, respectively.

Recommended Dietary Requirement

The National Research Council's Food and Nutrition Subcommittee recommends 1.5 to 3 mg per day as a safe and adequate level for copper ingestion for adults, although there has been insufficient data to establish a Recommended Daily Requirement (RDA). There may be an increased need for copper during pregnancy, since birth defects have been shown in experimental animals deficient in this mineral. Copper is stored in the liver by the human fetus. For infants 0.6 mg per day is recommended (0.7 mg for babies six to 12 months). Premature infants and infants exclusively breast-fed may need supplementation of copper. The American Academy of Pediatrics recently recommended that infant formulas provide 60 mcg of copper per 100 kilocalories, therefore providing an average 0.4 mg of copper daily. For seven-to-10-year-old children, 1.0 to 2.0 mg per day are recommended; for preadolescent and adolescent girls, 1 to 1.3 mg per day is recommended.

Supplements

Copper is generally included in multivitamin-mineral supplements. Copper gluconate is preferred over copper sulfate because it is easier to digest.

Toxicity

Wilson's disease is an inherited disorder that causes hepatitis (inflammation of the liver), kidney and neurological dysfunction and degeneration of the lens of the eye from copper excess. Vitamin C may interfere with the absorption of copper, while being of some benefit in Wilson's disease.

Acute poisoning, which may be fatal, is characterized by nausea, vomiting, abdominal pain, diarrhea, headache, dizziness and a metallic taste.

Typical American diets contain less than 5 mg of copper per day. Levels up to 10 mg per day are probably safe for adults. Toxicity is extremely rare in the United States. Elevated copper levels are sometimes found in individuals with the following conditions: viral infections, rheumatoid arthritis, rheumatic fever, systemic lupus erythematosus (SLE), leukemia, some cancers and post-heart attack. It is not known what role copper plays in the presence of disease. It is not clear if copper helps fight these conditions or if it is part of the disease process. Interestingly, drugs containing copper are often helpful in fighting some of these diseases. It has been theorized that copper-containing drugs help repair tissues damaged by many diseases.

coptis (goldthread, huang lian) A Chinese herb, *Coptis chinensis,* of the Ranunculaceae family, whose underground stem is used in Chinese medicine to promote lactation and to treat nausea and vomiting, fever, conjunctivitis and bleeding.

coriander (dhanyaka) An annual plant, *Coriandrum sativum,* of the carrot family, with aromatic fruits, grown in Europe, North and South America and the Mediterranean region, whose seeds are used as a spice in (Asian) Indian cuisine and, in herbal and Ayurvedic medicine, as an antispasmodic, carminative and stomachic. Coriander, once considered an aphrodisiac, may also be prepared as a topical treatment for rheumatism.

corn (maize, yu shu shu) The plant originating in America and recognized as valuable by Native Americans, *Zea mays,* a cereal grass, whose grain is used to make cornmeal and whose kernels are eaten as a vegetable and used in animal feed. Now cultivated in China and many other parts of the world, corn is also thought to have medicinal properties. Tea made from corn silk (*yu mi xu,* in Chinese) was used as a diuretic by Native Americans to ease bladder and kidney infections. Invalids were routinely fed corn porridge because it is easy to digest.

cornflower (cyani, bluebonnet, bachelor's button) An annual European herb, *Centaurea cyanus,* whose blue flowers are used by herbalists as a remedy for stomachache or indigestion.

corn poppy (corn rose, flores rhoeados) Dried petals of the poppy flower (*Papaver rhoeas,* [Fam. Papaveraceae]), indigenous to Eastern Europe, North Africa and Asia, are used traditionally in remedies for aches, colds and respiratory disorders, insomnia, minor pain and anxiety and as a natural coloring and flavoring (from poppy seeds). Syrup made of red poppy was listed in the British Pharmacopoeia as early as 1885 and again in 1898. One study found that an ethanolic aqueous extract of *Papaver rhoeas* petals, which contain anthocyanins, produced a sedative or lethal effect in mice, which corresponds to a dosage much larger than that recommended for poppy flowers used traditionally by humans. Poppy flowers contain mucilage, anthocyanin glycosides and approximately 12 percent isoquinoline alkaloids, of which up to 50 percent is rhoeadine. Urticaria has been reported from contact with the fresh flowers, and the use of gloves during harvesting is recommended. Traditionally prepared as a tea, poppies are known for their potential to cause poisoning (stomach pain and vomiting) in children. When taken in large doses, poppy flowers cause convulsions and coma in cattle, cramps in rats and stimulates respiration in rabbits. The toxicological effect of the alcoholic and aqueous plant extract administered intraperitoneally was determined in mice, and the large dosages required to illicit toxicity indicated that the plant is safe when consumed in recommended dosage for humans.

cornus (shan zhu yu, Japanese cornel, Japanese cornelian cherry) A Chinese, Korean and Japanese tree or shrub, *Cornus officinalis,* of the Cornaceae family, that bears flowers and fruit. The plant contains a guinol glycoside, perhaps responsible for the use of cornus in Chinese medicine as a remedy for excessive urine discharge. The fruit is also used to treat intestinal worms, vertigo, backache, night sweats, excessive menses and fever.

cottonroot A biennial or triennial herb, *Gossypium herbaceum,* of the Malvaceae family, native to Asia and cultivated in the United States, among other regions, whose inner root bark is considered in homeopathic medicine to be a treatment for lack of menses, sterility, painful menstruation, ovarian pain, vomiting related to pregnancy and labial abscess.

couch grass (dog grass, twitch grass, agropyrum) The plant *Triticum* or *Agropyrum repens,* of the Gramineae family, found in North America and Europe, whose rootstock and rhizome are used in Native American medicine for the treatment of bladder irritation and infection, catarrh, gout, jaundice and enlarged prostate. Couch grass contains vitamin C, carotene, glucose and other nutrients.

cowslip (palsywort, herb peter, paigles) A North American and Arctic flowering perennial, *Primula officinalis,* of the Primulaceae family, known to the Greeks as "Paralysis." Cowslip flowers and leaves are used in Native American medicine as an antispasmodic and sedative, particularly cowslip tea for vertigo, seizures, anxiety, bladder and back pain and palsy. Homeopathic medicine prescribes cowslip tincture for fevers, migraine,

neuralgia, eczema and dizziness. In folk medicine, cowslip is also considered an expectorant, diuretic and diaphoretic. The root and rhizome are given as an extract or powder combined with other herbs as a laxative and digestive tonic.

cramp bark (guelder rose, high cranberry, snowball tree, squaw bush) A North American flowering, fruit-bearing shrub, *Viburnum opulus,* of the Caprofoliaceae family, with acidic berries high in vitamins C and K. Viburnine, the substance considered medicinal in the plant, is in the dried bark of the stem. Cramp bark and the related *Viburnum prunifolium* (black haw) are prescribed in Native American and herbal medicine for uterine and menstrual problems, including premenstrual syndrome (PMS) and cramps and other gynecological complaints. Cramp bark is also used as an antispasmodic and to treat rheumatism and heart palpitations.

cranberry A small evergreen shrub, *Vaccinium macrocarpon,* characterized by dark pink flowers and cranberries. Native to bogs and mountain forests from Tennessee to Alaska, the shrub blooms from late spring until the end of the summer, producing its fruit in the fall. Cranberry was first documented in North America in 1621 when the Pilgrims were rumored to have eaten its berries on Thanksgiving. New England sailors ate them, thereby preventing scurvy, a disease resulting from vitamin-C deficiency. In the mid-1800s, German chemists discovered that the urine of those who ate cranberries contained a bacteriostatic compound. Cranberry juice is a common and effective remedy, mainly to prevent and inhibit bacterial urinary tract infections (UTI).

cranesbill (wild geranium, dovesfoot, storksbill) An American flowering plant, *Geranium maculatum,* of the Geraniaceae family, whose dried root is used in Native American and herbal medicine as an astringent, especially useful in the treatment of diarrhea, dysentery and infantile cholera, as a styptic, to check hemorrhage, leukorrhea, diabetes, nosebleed, Bright's disease and excessive discharge of mucus.

crataegus (hawthorn, Chinese hill haw) Deciduous trees or shrubs of the north temperate regions, *Crataegus cuneata* and *pinnatifida*, whose ripe fruits are used in Chinese medicine in the treatment of diarrhea, dysentery and stomachache.

crawley (chickentoe, coral root) A flowering North American plant, *Corallorhiza odontorhiza*, whose powdered root in warm water is a remedy for fevers, especially because of its diaphoretic and sedative properties, according to herbalists and Native American medicine.

C-reactive protein (CRP) An abnormal blood chemical, or globulin, that when detected in the blood indicates the active phase of acute illnesses, such as rheumatic fever. It also appears in the event of inflammation in heart vessels. According to the January 12, 2003, issue of *Time* magazine, "New studies have provided the strongest evidence yet that inflammation is a better predictor than cholesterol levels of your risk of heart disease. What won't change is your doctor's advice. CRP levels are lowered in the same ways by which cholesterol is reduced: diet, exercise and statins."

crocus (saffron) A flowering plant, *Crocus sativus*, of the Iridaceae family, originally from Asia Minor and named from the Greek word *krokos*, meaning saffron, a popular coloring and food-flavoring agent. In Chinese medicine, the stigmas of the flowers are dried and prepared as a remedy for lack of or irregular menses, asthma, seizures and whooping cough. Crocus is also thought to be a blood and circulation tonic. In Ayurvedic medicine, the herb called *nagakshar* in Sanskrit is known as cobra's saffron.

croton A Chinese, Burmese, Laotian, Vietnamese and Malaysian evergreen, *Croton tiglium*, of the Euphorbiaceae family, cultivated for its seeds, used in Chinese medicine as a powerful purgative. Croton oil, obtained from the seeds, is poisonous.

crowfoot (buttercup) A perennial flowering herb, *Ranunculus bulbosus*, of the Ranunculaceae family, that grows in colder regions of North America and Europe. Crowfoot parts cause mouth ulcerations when chewed. Once used by beggars to incite pity, crowfoot is prepared as a tincture in homeopathic medicine for the treatment of alcoholism, chilblains, delirium tremens, epilepsy, jaundice and liver pain, rheumatism, hay fever and other ailments.

cubeb (Java pepper, tailed pepper) A flowering, fruit-bearing perennial, *Piper cubeba*, that grows in regions near New Guinea and Sumatra, whose unripe berries resembling black pepper are used in herbal medicine to treat intestinal gas, respiratory congestion and indigestion. Cubeb oil is prescribed for gonorrhea and urinary tract problems.

cumin *Cuminum cyminum*, a plant of the carrot family, has been used since ancient times as a spice and for medicinal purposes. Now cultivated throughout the world, cumin has aromatic seeds and oil that are used as a remedy for indigestion, worms and inflammation, to encourage lactation and, in certain cultures, to induce abortion. Cumin may interact with barbiturates, phenobarbital, prolonging their effect in the body. Some reports claim that cumin also has anti-infective properties and may interfere with blood clotting.

curculigo (xian mao) A tropical flowering herb, *Curculigo orchioides*, of the Hypoxidaceae family, whose underground stem is used in Chinese medicine as a remedy for impotence, lumbago and joint pain, and as a tonic and aphrodisiac.

curcuma (turmeric, jiang huang, haridra) An Indian and tropical, aromatic herb, *Curcuma domestica*, of the Zingiberaceae family. A flavoring and coloring agent, turmeric means yellow in Sanskrit, and had many uses in Hindu traditions. The underground stem is used by Chinese practitioners to promote the manufacture of hemoglobin, dissolve clots and stop bleeding. It is also prescribed for dysentery, stomach disorders and abdominal and chest pain. Native to India, wild turmeric, or *Curcuma aromatica*, treats excessive gas, seizures, liver ailments and other problems.

cuscuta (tu si zi, devil's guts, dodder, lady's laces, bride's laces) The plant *Cuscuta japonica*, of the Convolvulaceae family, of both China and

Japan, whose seeds are prescribed by Chinese practitioners to treat prostatic inflammation, impotence, premature ejaculation, vertigo, lumbago and nervous disorders.

cyanocobalamin   See B₁₂, VITAMIN.

cyathula (hookweed)   A flowering plant, of the Amarantaceae family, used in Chinese medicine as a laxative and antiarthritic.

cycas (sago palm, Japanese fern palm)   A type of palm tree, *Cycas revoluta,* of the Cycadaceae family, grown in Japan and southern China, whose seeds are considered by Chinese herbalists to be a tonic, expectorant and antirheumatic.

cymbopogon (lemon grass, rohisha)   A grass native to India and Sri Lanka and cultivated in the tropics, *Cymbopogon citratus,* of the Gramineae family, used as a food flavoring and an oil for soap and perfume. Chinese and Ayurvedic herbalists prescribe the plant for coughs, colds and bloody sputum, and as a diaphoretic.

cynanchum   Various species of a northern Chinese and Japanese herb of the Asclepiadaceae family, with a fragrant root and flowers. Cynanchum is prescribed in Chinese medicine to treat urethral problems, fever, cough, pneumonia, difficult breathing and other ailments.

cyperus (nut grass, sedge root, xiang fu)   A flowering, weedlike plant, *Cyperus rotundus,* of the Cyperaceae family, whose tubers are used in Chinese medicine to ease various menstrual problems, chest pain, dysentery, headache and indigestion.

cypress (gopher wood)   Originally a Mediterranean tree or shrub, *Cupressus,* of the Coniferous Cupressaceae family, whose cones or nuts are used in Native American medicine and by herbalists to arrest bleeding. Homeopaths prescribe a tincture of cypress berries and leaves for tumors, warts and other ailments.

cysteine   An amino acid containing a crystalline sulfur that oxidizes into cystine, found in many proteins and known to be a major source of metabolic sulfur. Cysteine works as an antioxidant along with vitamins C and E and selenium and stimulates white blood cell functioning in the immune system. When used in conjunction with evening primrose oil, cysteine inhibits the effects of tobacco and alcohol and may relieve or prevent hangover. It is also said to relieve bronchial asthma, psoriasis and other skin disorders and alopecia, and to help prevent dental plaque.

See also AMINO ACIDS; C, VITAMIN; EVENING PRIMROSE; E, VITAMIN; SELENIUM.

D, vitamin (vitamin D$_1$ or calciferol, cholecalciferol [vitamin D$_3$], ergocalciferol [vitamin D$_2$])
An essential vitamin manufactured in the skin during exposure to the sun. Dietary supplements may be necessary for those lacking sunlight exposure. Vitamin D is a generic term for a family of compounds known as vitamins D$_1$, D$_2$ and D$_3$. Chemically these substances are called sterols, and their metabolic products have the ability to prevent rickets in children or osteomalacia in adults. Vitamin D is fat-soluble and requires dietary fat that absorbs the vitamin from food sources or supplements in the digestive tract.

Vitamin D$_2$ is derived from plants and can substitute for vitamin D$_3$ in the human body. Calcium balance is regulated by the interaction of three hormones, vitamin D, parathormone (PTH) and calcitonin. PTH is secreted by the parathyroid gland and calcitonin, which antagonizes or blocks the effects of PTH, by special cells in the thyroid gland.

Functions of Vitamin D

Considered a hormone, vitamin D is responsible chiefly for regulating the absorption and use of calcium and phosphorous and facilitating the formation of normal bones, cartilage and teeth. Other important functions of vitamin D include maintaining normal nerve conduction and muscle contractions, especially those of the heart muscle. Vitamin D regulates the supply of calcium in the blood and plays a role in the utilization of magnesium.

Some researchers theorize that vitamin D might aid in the prevention or treatment of cancer and assist in regulating the immune system. Vitamin D was formerly advocated as a treatment for lupus vulgaris (tuberculosis of the skin) that is now considered unacceptable. Vitamin D has been reported to lessen the severity of psoriasis.

Vitamin D Deficiency

Rickets is caused by inadequate exposure to sunlight or dietary lack of vitamin D and occurs in childhood. It is characterized by malformed and weak bones because of poor calcium and phosphorous deposition. Defective mineralization of both bones and cartilaginous material in the epiphyseal growth plate becomes apparent as the child grows. Weight-bearing bones buckle, the head becomes malformed, wrists and ankles become enlarged and the sternum bows to resemble a pigeon breast. The severity of the changes varies with the degree of vitamin D deficiency. Early recognition may escape even trained health professionals but should be considered in an infant who is restless, sleeps poorly, sweats profusely, repeatedly turns its head from side to side and has delayed dentition (formation of teeth). The infant will have reduced mineralization of the skull, or craniotabes, and bossing of the skull and delayed closure of the fontanelle. Sitting and crawling skills may be delayed beyond the normal stage of development in which they are usually demonstrated. Costochondral beading, known as rachitic rosary, occurs. Rickets is readily recognized when the toddler develops the typical bowed legs, knock knees and kyphoscoliosis (lateral curvature of the spine with an anteroposterior hump) shortly after starting to walk.

Deficiencies of vitamins C, D and other nutrients often coexist, and symptoms of vitamin D deficiency may mask or modify important symptoms and X-ray findings of scurvy.

With widespread availability of vitamin D–fortified milk, rickets is rarely seen except in northern climates with limited sunlight. The production of vitamin D is blocked or inhibited by other factors, such as the pigmentation of the skin.

The darker the skin, the less readily the vitamin is formed. Malnourished black infants are more prone to rickets than Caucasian or other light-skinned infants. Substances or situations that block the sun's ultraviolet rays include smoke, fog, smog, clothing and windows.

Children with celiac disease or other disorders of fat absorption, and those taking anticonvulsants for seizure disorders, are at risk of vitamin D deficiency and rickets. Although vitamin D supplementation corrects the bone structure, it may be too late to correct deformed bones.

The hallmarks of osteomalacia—softening and deformities of the bones of the arms, legs, spine, thorax and pelvis—result from a deficiency of calcium or vitamin D. Osteomalacia occurs after the epiphyseal growth plates fuse, thus the term "adult rickets." Although bone fractures are uncommon, chronic pain and muscle weakness add to the symptoms of the disorder.

Osteomalacia is commonly confused with osteoporosis, in which bone fractures are common. In the later stage of osteoporosis, muscle weakness is rare, and pain is only present when brittle bones become fractured. Osteomalacia most commonly occurs in women who have had multiple pregnancies and are also vitamin D or calcium deficient.

Aging reduces the ability of the body to manufacture vitamin D. Hearing loss may be related to malformation of the bones in the middle ear or changes that occur to these bones in the elderly. Elderly invalids are also more likely to have inadequate sunlight exposure or have poor dietary intake of required nutrients.

Studies in the United States suggest that 30 to 40 percent of hip-fracture victims have vitamin D deficiencies. Those at risk for vitamin D deficiency are infants, pregnant women and individuals with little or no sunlight exposure, especially the disabled.

Calcitrol, a vitamin D derivative, vitamin D_3, is used in the treatment of osteoporosis in Japan, where estrogen therapy is not well accepted. Calcitrol is also used in Australia and New Zealand. There is a considerable risk of vitamin D toxicity with the use of calcitrol.

"The Mediterranean Osteoporosis Study" (in the *British Medical Journal*) failed to show that vitamin D, fluorides or anabolic steroids reduced the incidence of hip fractures in postmenopausal women at increased risk. However, estrogen, calcium or calcitonin were protective, reducing risk by 55, 25 and 31 percent, respectively, in a group of more than 5,500 women.

A contradictory account of 138 women studied at Cambridge University similarly reported in the *British Medical Journal* confirmed that increasing vitamin D intake to 400 International Units daily or exposing the skin to sunlight for 30 minutes daily would increase bone density by 5 to 10 percent and reduce the occurrence of bone fractures by an estimated 20 percent.

Vitamin D may be especially important during winter in northern latitudes such as Sweden, where calcium alone increases bone density in the summer, but density is lost during the winter unless 400 units of vitamin D are added to the diet.

Sun-blocking agents with a skin-protection rating of 8 or greater prevent the formation of vitamin D in the skin. It is unlikely that children or most adults would use sunscreens often enough to develop vitamin D deficiency, but some elderly persons concerned about skin cancer may become deficient.

Causes of Vitamin D Deficiency

Dietary deficiencies of vitamin D are rare in the United States and other developed countries. Intestinal disorders that interfere with dietary absorption usually only are associated with vitamin D deficiency if the afflicted individuals lack sufficient exposure to the sun or have rare disorders of the metabolism. Vitamin D deficiency causes hypocalcemia and hypophosphatemia, or diminished blood levels of calcium and phosphorus. The deficiency in turn causes stimulation of the parathyroid gland. The hormone secreted by the gland pulls calcium out of bones to restore the calcium in the blood to adequate levels. This process causes rickets in infants and children and osteomalacia in adults.

Drugs such as the anticonvulsant drug phenytoin (Dilantin) may impair the effectiveness of vitamin D.

Dosage

Dosages of vitamin D are usually expressed as International Units (I.U.) of cholecalciferol, with

TABLE 10 COMPARISON OF OSTEOMALACIA AND OSTEOPOROSIS

	Signs and Symptoms	Prevention	Treatment*
Osteoporosis	pain from fractures muscle weakness is rare fractures are common skeletal deformities only related to fractures widespread loss of bone density normal blood levels of calcium, phosphorus and alkaline phosphatase normal or high levels of calcium in the urine	adequate calcium intake (1,000 mg in premenopausal women and 1,500 mg after menopause) + estrogen therapy + regular weight-bearing exercise	calcitonin, calcium, estrogens, fluoride (controversial) vitamin D (used in Japan) is controversial and can be toxic
Osteomalacia	chronic bone pain muscle weakness (may result in a gait disturbance) fractures are rare skeletal deformities are common bone density loss is usually limited to the spine low calcium and phosphorus blood levels high alkaline phosphatase blood levels low calcium levels in the urine	adequate sunlight and/or vitamin D in the diet or supplements	vitamin D supplements

*Author's note: The treatments currently available for osteoporosis are either expensive, not very effective, toxic or all of these.

400 I.U. being equivalent to 10 mcg of the vitamin. Five to 7.5 mcg (200 to 300 I.U.) should be given only to those infants who are fed unfortified formulas. However, the rare infant with a malabsorption disorder or who is the offspring of a mother with a vitamin D deficiency may require up to 750 mcg or 30,000 I.U. daily for a short period.

Ten mcg (400 I.U.) are recommended during pregnancy and lactation if there is inadequate dietary vitamin D or sunlight. The same amount is generally advisable in the elderly.

When Vitamin D supplements are given to treat deficiency, the dose should be reduced to the Recommended Dietary Allowance (RDA) as soon as symptoms are improved and before bone healing is complete, because the effects of vitamin D persist for prolonged periods and may result in elevated calcium levels and kidney damage. If doses larger than 10 mcg per day of vitamin D are taken for extended periods, blood-calcium levels and 24-hour urine specimens should be monitored frequently. Vitamin D supplements are available in 400 and 1,000 I.U. strengths over-the-counter and 25,000 and 50,000 I.U. by prescription.

A fair-skinned person can probably manufacture 10,000 I.U. of vitamin D in one day. In temperate climates, 10 minutes of sunbathing daily throughout the summer months will provide adequate stores of the vitamin for the colder months. Infants and children who must remain on a milk-free diet can obtain an adequate supply of calcium, vitamin D and other essential nutrients from vegetables, including broccoli, kale, turnip greens or tofu.

Drug Interactions

The cholesterol-lowering drug cholysteramine and mineral oil both interfere with the intestinal absorption of vitamin D. Phenytoin and phenobarbital, drugs used in the treatment of seizures, speed up the metabolism of vitamin D.

Most problems with the use of vitamin D interacting with other drugs occur in the presence of hypercalcemia (elevated blood-calcium levels) and heart or kidney disease. Heart irregularities may occur with the use of digoxin and other digitalis derivatives or verapamil. In the presence of elevated calcium levels associated with the vitamin's use, arrhythmias (heart irregularities) may occur. Thiazide diuretics in the presence of vitamin D may cause hypercalcemia in the presence of hypoparathyroid disease. Persons with kidney failure should avoid taking magnesium-containing antacids with vitamin D.

Toxicity

Vitamin D is highly toxic, especially in infants and children who have developed hypercalcemia. Sensitive infants may develop high calcium levels with as little as 10 mcg or 400 I.U. daily. Prolonged exposure to excessive doses that may be slightly above 25 mcg (1,000 I.U.) per day for infants may result in mental retardation, lagging physical growth, elfin facies (resembling the facial features of an elf), kidney failure and death. Older children and adults may develop weakness, loss of appetite, vomiting, diarrhea, excessive thirst and urination as well as mental changes associated with elevated blood-calcium levels from doses of vitamin D exceeding 1.25 mg or 50,000 I.U. daily. Prolonged used of megadoses may also result in kidney failure and death. In the absence of severe kidney damage, hypervitaminosis D is usually reversible with cessation of vitamin D.

See also ASCORBIC ACID.

daidzein (daidzin)   A substance reported to inhibit desire for alcohol.

See also KUDZU.

daikon radish   A vegetable rich in vitamin C, daikon contains active enzymes that aid digestion, particularly of starchy foods.

daily minimal requirements   See RECOMMENDED DIETARY ALLOWANCES.

d-alpha-tocopherol (natural vitamin E)   See E, VITAMIN.

damiana   The plant *Turnera diffusa*, of the family Turneraceae, native to Texas, southern California, Mexico, South America and the West Indies, whose leaves are made into a tea and used in the treatment of depression, coughing and congestion and as a mild aphrodisiac in the case of decreased sexual desire.

dandelion (pu gong ying, lion's tooth, blow ball, cankerwort)   The biennial or perennial plant *Taraxacum officinale*, of the family Compositae, originally from Greece. Dandelion may be eaten as a vegetable, made into wine and tea and, in herbal medicine, used for the treatment of bladder, kidney, gallbladder, pancreas and spleen obstructions, stomachaches, hepatitis, high blood pressure, anemia, fluid retention, weight loss and breast cancer.

Dandelion leaves contain vitamins A, B, C and G, sodium, protein, iron, calcium, phosphorus and inulin. Tea, coffee or a vodka beverage made from dandelion root was once dubbed the "life elixir" by advocates of home remedies and was considered a blood purifier; liver, gallbladder, spleen and female organ tonic; and treatment for rheumatism, urinary tract problems and skin diseases. Homeopathic medicine also prescribes dandelion tincture for diabetes, jaundice, neuralgia, night sweats, typhoid fever and mapped tongue.

daruharidra   See BARBERRY.

datura (downy thorn apple, horn-of-plenty)   A flowering plant, *Datura metel*, of the Solanaceae family, originally thought to be from eastern India or southwestern China, whose leaves, seeds and fruit contain poisonous tropane alkaloids, and whose leaves and seeds are the source of scopolamine, a sedative and motion-sickness drug.

Datura has a strange history of uses, including as a trance-inducer by ancient priests of Apollo in Greece, as a preoperative sedative of the Incas, as a way for robbers in Indian, Malaysian and other cultures to debilitate their victims and as an intoxicant of African boys during rite-of-passage ceremonies. However, to Chinese Buddhists, datura is considered sacred because they believe rain from heaven fell on the datura plant when Buddha spoke.

In Chinese medicine, the flowers are used for the treatment of nervous disorders, muscle pain, asthma and colds.

decoction The method of extracting the essences or medicinal properties from hard or coarse herb stems, barks and roots. The herb part or parts may be simmered in water until one-third of the water has evaporated. The herbs are then strained and the liquid retained for use.

dendrobium (shi hu) The plants *Dendrobium nobile, monile* and *hancockii,* of the Orchidaceae family, named from the Greek words *dendron* (tree) and *bios* (life). Chinese practitioners use mainly the stem, but also the whole plant, in the treatment of arthritis, fever, impotence, pain and cough.

dentes The Latin word for teeth. Nutritionally, normal dentition (the number and arrangement of teeth) and healthy teeth and gums depend on calcium, which gives the teeth their rigidity, and other nutrients, including vitamin C, for healthy collagen matrix and optimal strength and integrity of teeth and mouth. A lack of protein may result in small, irregularly shaped teeth, a delay in the appearance of teeth and susceptibility to cavities. A lack of vitamin A may contribute to poorly formed teeth and possibly the delayed eruption of teeth, as well as problems involving the keratin matrix of enamel. Magnesium is important for the development of tooth enamel. Phosphorus deficiency may result in poor mineralization, and iron, zinc and fluoride deficiencies may cause susceptibility to cavities.

Dental health requires that individuals:

a) restrict the ingestion of sweets, especially at bedtime,

b) drink fluorinated water and provide infants with fluoride supplements if fluorinated water is not available,

c) restrict the ingestion of sticky foods (such as caramel, nougat, fruits that stick to the teeth longer than required by the normal eating time, etc.),

d) brush the teeth and floss regularly, after every meal and snacks if possible, or rinse the mouth with water,

e) eat foods containing calcium and phosphorus,

f) eat high-fiber foods that inhibit dental cavities and stimulate the flow of saliva, such as raw vegetables, and,

g) when appropriate, substitute low-fat cheese for sweet dessert, because cheese is high in calcium and promotes the formation of acid and saliva that inhibit cavity development. Chocolate, tea, coffee and beer, all of which contain the acid tannin, help prevent cavities. (Children without dietary restrictions may eat regular cheeses.)

denutrition An alternate term for malnutrition, or a deficiency of nutrients that causes debilitation, weakness, disease processes and other problems. Malnutrition exists in individuals as well as populations throughout the world.

depression See STRESS.

dermatitis Skin inflammation characterized by itchiness, redness and various types of eruptions or lesions. Nutrition-related dermatitis may involve desquamating changes of the skin, or abnormally pigmented areas, usually on the legs, thighs, buttocks and extremities, that resemble flaking paint or "crazy pavement." Desquamation on the trunk is associated with kwashiorkor, a severe, life-threatening protein deficiency common to children in many Third World countries.

Dermatitis has many causes, including allergic, hereditary, infectious and psychological. Depending upon the type of dermatitis, vitamins E, A and D salves or creams, mineral ointments and other topical applications, along with alterations in diet and nutrient supplementation, especially in the case of a vitamin or mineral deficiency, may be recommended as treatment.

desmodium The climbing plants, *Desmodium triquetrum, pulchellum, triflorum* and *styracifolium,* of the Leguminosae family, named from the Greek word *desmos* (chain). In Chinese medicine, desmodium preparations are prescribed for numerous ailments, including intestinal worms, infantile convulsion, indigestion, internal blood clots, dysentery and colic.

dessicated liver Dried, powdered beef liver available in tablet form in health food stores as an iron and multinutrient supplement.

devil's claw (grapple plant, wood spider) *Harpagophytum procumbens,* an herb used as a remedy for appetite loss, indigestion, liver and gallbladder problems, rheumatism, skin disorders, pain and problems of pregnancy. Native to south and central Africa, its medicinal value is found in its freshly chopped or pulverized roots. Devil's claw stimulates digestive juices, bile production and appetite, and it also fights inflammation and relieves minor pain. The herb may not be recommended for individuals with peptic or duodenal ulcers.

dhanyaka See CORIANDER.

diabetes mellitus A chronic disorder of the body's ability to metabolize carbohydrates. Beta cells in the pancreas fail to secrete an adequate amount of insulin, a hormone essential for maintaining a normal blood-sugar level and the utilization of glucose. Symptoms include hyperglycemia (elevated blood sugar), sugar in the urine, excessive urination, extreme thirst, increase of food intake and genital itching.

It has been speculated that micronutrients, especially zinc and chromium, play a role in the development of carbohydrate intolerance leading to diabetes mellitus, both Type I, insulin-dependent, and type II, non-insulin-dependent. Supplementation with micronutrient minerals is considered experimental, and there may be some as-yet-undetermined risk.

Standardized diets, exercise regimes and insulin therapy for people with diabetes are geared toward balancing carbohydrates, proteins and fats and improving glucose utilization. In addition, many nutritionists, homeopaths, naturopaths, herbalists and others offer alternative treatments, especially with herbs that affect blood-sugar levels. Untreated diabetes may lead to coma, acetone (sweet) breath odor, nausea, headache, vomiting, difficulty in breathing, a sense of drunkenness, delirium, weakness or deep coma and subsequent death.

dicalcium phosphate The substance containing two atoms of calcium used in dietary calcium supplements.

diets, fad Weight-reduction regimes that become a sensation or popular through the media that may or may not be nutritionally sound. They include liquid formulas, calorie restrictions, fasting techniques and diets emphasizing one type of food or another in the diet over a certain period of time. No one diet is a panacea for people who wish to lose weight, and a healthy nutritional status depends upon biopsychosocial aspects of the individual. Some diets cause a state of ketosis in dieters, which may reduce the desire for food and increase the rate of weight loss. Ketosis is an accumulation of ketones—acetone, betahydroxybutric acid and acetoacetic acid—as a result of inadequate metabolism of fatty acids and carbohydrate deficiency. High-fat diets, starvation, poorly monitored diabetes mellitus, pregnancy and postoperative ether anesthesia are often linked with ketosis.

Other problems frequently exist alongside fad diets. Milkshake-type preparations become boring, weight lost quickly may be as quickly replaced, psychological and other individual factors may not be taken into account and nutrient deficiencies may emerge.

digestion The body's process of breaking down ingested foods into forms that are most readily absorbed by the gastrointestinal tract and the nutrients distributed throughout body tissues. While salt, glucose and other simple sugars, water and crystalloids can be absorbed intact, fats, starches and protein require considerable breakdown into smaller molecules. Digestion begins with the enzyme ptyalin, in the saliva, that splits starch. The partially digested starch then proceeds to the stomach and the intestines for further breakdowns by other enzymes such as pepsin, lipase, trypsin, invertase, and other enzymatic substances in the pancreatic juices and the epithelial cells of the small intestine. Fats are mostly digested in the small intestine. Proteins go through several digestive stages before they are converted into amino acids. Whatever remaining materials the body has not converted into valuable nutrients become waste material and are eliminated at the end of the digestive tract, through the rectum.

dill weed The herb *Anethum graveolens,* of the family Umbelliferae, used primarily as a flavoring spice. Dill weed is also an herbal medicine for treating colic, stomachaches, indigestion, abdominal cramps, colds, influenza and coughs. It is also said to increase breast milk.

dioscorea (yam, shan yao) The vines *Dioscorea opposita, nipponica, bulbifera, tokoro, japonica* and *hispida,* of the Dioscoreaceae family, found in Korea, Japan and China, whose tubers are edible and also used in Chinese medicine. The Chinese yam, which contains the anti-inflammatory agent diosgenin, provides preparations for the treatment of numerous ailments, including diarrhea, dysentery, arthritis, rheumatism, rheumatoid arthritis, sore throat, poisonous snakebite, cough and premature ejaculation.

diospyros (Japanese persimmon) A Japanese and Chinese deciduous tree, *Diospyros kaki,* of the Ebenaceae family, with edible fruit often made into jam and cosmetic products. In Chinese medicine, diospyros fruit, fruit juice and fruit stalk are used to treat high blood pressure, cough, hiccough and diarrhea.

dipsacus (Venus' basin, teasel, xu duan) European, western Asian and North African herbs, *Dipsacus asper* and *japonicus,* of the Dipsacaceae family, named from the Greek word *dipsakos* (thirst). Dipsacus roots are used in Chinese medicine to treat pain, lumbago and excessive menses.

dl-alpha-tocopherol (synthetic vitamin E) See E, VITAMIN.

dogbane (catchfly, bitterroot, honeybloom, milk ipecac, western wallflower) An American flowering perennial, *Apocynum androsaemifolium,* whose rootstock is used in herbal medicine as an emetic (to induce vomiting), expectorant, stimulant and cathartic. While the leaves appear to be poisonous to animals, the plant with its milky juice is thought to be effective against gallstones, stomachache, constipation and dropsy.

dog poison (fool's parsley, small hemlock, fool's cicely) A North American and European annual plant, *Aesthusa cynapium,* whose herb is used in homeopathic medicine to treat nervous stomach and spasms. The leaves and roots, which resemble parsley, are poisonous.

dogwood (Virginia dogwood, flowering cornel, green ozier, Florida cornel, cornelian tree, budwood, borwood) Shrubs, trees and herbs of the Cornaceae family, found in Canada and the United States. The *Cornus florida* flowers, according to Native American herbal medicine, have a soothing property similar to camomile (see CAMOMILE) and the bark is used to make a healing ointment. Homeopathic medicine uses tincture of dogwood bark for dyspepsia, fever and pneumonia.

dolichos (Egyptian bean, hyacinth bean, lablab bean, seim bean) A tropical bean plant thought to be of Asian origin, *Dolichos lablab,* of the Leguminosae family, whose bean is eaten as a vegetable in India and whose flowers and seeds are used in Chinese medicine to treat poisoning from fish and vegetables, sunstroke, colic, infectious dysentery, cholera and rheumatism.

dolomite The mineral CaMg $(CO_3)_2$, a calcium magnesium carbonate originating in limestone and crystals. Although in wide use as a calcium supplement, it is not only poorly absorbed, but is often contaminated with lead, which may be toxic.

See also CALCIUM.

dong quai (tang kwei) The plant *Angelica sinensis,* of the Umbelliferae family, well known in Chinese traditional medicine as a "female" treatment. The root of the plant is prescribed for menstrual cramps and other menstrual discomfort, menopausal symptoms, hypertension, insomnia, anemia, constipation and other problems.

See also ANGELICA.

don sen (tang shen) The *Codonopsis pilosula* plant, of the Campanulaceae family, whose root, similar in action to ginseng, is prescribed in Chinese traditional medicine for strengthening the *chi,* or vital energy, throughout the body. Don sen is also used for indigestion caused by excessive gastric acid and as treatment of infections, inflammation and diabetes.

See also GINSENG.

double-blind study Also known as an open-label study, a technique for the purpose of scientific experimentation and study in which neither the researchers nor the subjects know which treatment (nutrient, drug, placebo, etc.) the subjects are receiving or participating in. A double-blind study seeks to eliminate any bias on the part of researchers and subjects that may skew the results. When the experiment is over, the treatments and subjects are revealed and the data analyzed.

dragon root (jack-in-the-pulpit, wake robin) A North and South American flowering plant, *Arum triphyllum,* of the Araceae family, whose dry root is used in Native American medicine as a stimulant and expectorant, especially in the treatment of asthma, whooping cough, colic, chest pain and other ailments. Homeopathic medicine uses tincture of the plant's fresh tuber or corn for headache, diphtheria, swollen glands, hoarseness, pain in the jaw and numerous other problems.

drynaria (oak-leaf fern) The tree *Drynaria fortunei,* of the Polypodiaceae family, whose stem is used in Chinese medicine to treat bleeding, gangrene, kidney weakness and other ailments.

dryobalanops (Bornean camphor-tree, kapur) The Malaysian, Javan and Bornean tropical tree *Dryobalanops aromatica,* of the Dipterocarpaceae family, that yields camphor. In Chinese medicine, camphor preparations treat chicken pox and sore throat and tonify the body.

dyer's broom (furze, greenweed, waxen woad, dyer's whin) A northeastern American and European perennial shrub, *Genista tinctoria,* that bears fruit. The shrub's flowering twigs are used in herbal medicine to make tea, considered effective against gallstones, gravel and hypotension. Dyer's broom tea is also a vasoconstrictor with properties similar to those of nicotine.

E, vitamin (d-alpha-tocopherol, or natural vitamin E; dl-alpha-tocopherol, or synthetic vitamin E)
Alpha-tocopherol, the most active of the eight forms of vitamin E found naturally. This fat-soluble vitamin was named from the Greek *tokos,* meaning offspring, and *pherein,* meaning to bear. Vitamin E is absorbed into the lymphatic circulation from the gastrointestinal tract and has been shown to have antioxidant, or protective, actions in the cells. The vitamin is stored in all tissues, and vitamin E deficiency is rare. Approximately three-fourths of the vitamin are excreted in the bile, while the balance becomes a metabolite or altered form in the urine.

Naturally obtained d-alpha-tocopherol is more potent than synthetic dl-alpha-tocopherol, a racemic (optically inactive) mixture. Vitamin E may be the only vitamin in which the natural form is superior to the synthetic.

There have been many unproven claims supporting the supplementation of this vitamin by "megavitamin" promotors for many years. Until recently, medical investigators could find no proven human requirement. Vitamin E is known to be essential for laboratory-animal, but not human, fertility. The results of two Harvard University studies published in 1992 show promising results for the reduction of heart-attack risk in men and women through moderate doses of vitamin E.

History
In 1922, Evans and Bishop reported failed pregnancies in rats fed diets thought to contain all required nutrients. In 1924, Sure discovered a missing nutrient required for rat reproduction: He named it vitamin E. By 1931, Pappenheimer and Goettsch demonstrated that chicks deficient in vitamin E had abnormal brain development, while rabbits and guinea pigs developed muscular dys-

trophy. The same year, Olcott and Mattill found a high concentration of vitamin E in the lipids of lettuce. These investigators also demonstrated the antioxidant properties of vitamin E. In 1936, Evans derived the vitamin from wheat-germ oil. By 1938, Fernholz established its chemical structure, and Evans and Calhoun named it tocopherol.

Deficiency
Vitamin E rarely may cause hemolysis (destruction of red blood cells), resulting in anemia in humans with malabsorption problems. It may also cause degeneration of axons of the spinal cord and peripheral nerves. Vitamin E has many other proven deficiencies in animals.

Dosage
The estimated adult daily requirement is 10 to 30 mg per day. The daily requirement is increased by the dietary intake of polyunsaturated fat. Dosages from 100 to 250 I.U. daily, used in the Harvard studies cited above, seemed adequate to reduce heart-attack risk.

Recommended Dietary Allowances
The Food and Nutrition Board Subcommittee on the Tenth Edition of the Recommended Dietary Allowances arbitrarily established a value based on customary American dietary intake of 10 mg for adult men and 8 mg for women, who are generally smaller. The daily requirement is diminished or increased by the amount of dietary intake of polyunsaturated fatty acids (PUFA) varying from 5 to 20 mg per day.

Vitamin E requirements may be increased in persons taking large doses of iron. The daily requirement for vitamin E may be diminished in the presence of diets high in selenium or other antioxidants.

Toxicity

Most individuals can tolerate prolonged ingestion of large amounts of vitamin E, and many authors of vitamin books state there are no proven cases of vitamin E toxicity in doses up to 1,200 units per day. However, doses of 800 to 1,500 International Units or more may depress prothrombin levels, interfere with the action of vitamin K and the clotting of blood. This is especially risky in patients taking oral anticoagulants such as warfarin sodium (Coumadin) to prevent blood clots. Premature infants given vitamin E may develop various adverse effects, including jaundice and thrombocytoopenia (low platelet counts), which may cause bleeding.

The *New England Journal of Medicine* reported an increased risk of hemorrhagic strokes in a study of 29,000 Finnish men taking vitamin E in a cancer-prevention study. There was not an increase in total deaths in the group taking alpha-tocopherol. The authors of this study attributed their finding to the vitamin's effects on platelet function. In the same study, there was a diminished incidence of prostate cancer.

In addition, high doses of vitamin E may cause nausea, flatulence or diarrhea and an allergic contact dermatitis. There are rare reports of heart palpitations that led to fainting. Individuals known to be hypertensive (having high blood pressure) may have a slight rise in their pressure at the onset of vitamin E therapy and should begin with a dose of no more than 100 I.U. and be monitored as they increase the dose.

TABLE 11 RECOMMENDED DIETARY ALLOWANCES FOR VITAMIN E

Age	Milligrams of d-alpha-tocopherol
Birth to 6 months	3
6 to 12 months	4
1 to 3 years	5
4 to 6 years	6
7 to 10 years	7
11 to 14 years	8
Males over 14	10
Females over 14	8
Pregnancy	10
Lactation	11

TABLE 12 POTENCIES OF VITAMIN E SUPPLEMENTS

1 mg of product	International Units (IU)
d-alpha-tocopherol	1.49*
d-alpha-tocopheryl acetate	1.36**
d-alpha-tocopheryl acid succinate	1.21**
dl-alpha-tocopheryl	1.10*
dl-alpha-tocopheryl acetate	1.00**
dl-alpha-tocopheryl acid succinate	0.89**

*Unstable because of oxidation in the presence of light
**Light stable

Dr. H. J. Roberts, of the Palm Beach Institute for Medical Research, an authority on vitamin E, differs in his opinion of the safety of this vitamin. Although premature infants may exhibit low platelet counts, adults may have thrombocytosis (increased platelets). Dr. Roberts attributes cases of thrombophlebitis (blood clots in the deep veins of the legs) that may lead to life-threatening pulmonary emboli (blood clots in the lungs) and gynecomastia (enlarged breasts) to as little as 300 International Units (I.U.) of vitamin E. The Vitamin Nutrition Information Service estimates that in 1990, up to 7.3 million adults took vitamin E supplements, and the majority of those individuals took 400 units daily. Ten percent of the population took 800 units, and about 3 percent took 1,200 units, although the adult requirement has been calculated at only 8 to 10 mg.

Chronic excess doses of vitamin E may also increase the levels of androgenic and estrogenic hormones and cholesterol, impair wound-healing, cause hypoglycemi (low blood sugar), lower levels of thyroid and increase vitamin D requirements.

Vitamin E has been implicated in the deaths of 38 infants given the vitamin intravenously for reasons not fully understood.

See also CARDIOVASCULAR DISEASE PREVENTION AND ANTIOXIDANT VITAMINS.

echinacea (purple cornflower, black sampson)

A flowering perennial plant, *Echinacea angustifolia,* of the Compositae family, native to western American prairies, whose root is used by Sioux Indians to treat rabies, snakebites and systemic poisoning. Echinacea is sometimes considered a natural anti-

**TABLE 13 ADVERSE OR TOXIC EFFECTS OF
VITAMIN E**

Blood clots—deep vein thrombophlebitis, pulmonary
  embolism
Decreased blood clotting for individuals taking oral
  anticoagulants
Increased risk of hemorrhagic stroke
High blood pressure
Impaired wound-healing
Allergic contact rash
Gastric distress—nausea, flatulence and diarrhea

toxin. Homeopathic medicine prescribes a tincture
made of the entire plant for appendicitis, pus in the
blood, gangrene and various types of poisoning,
and Russian folk medicine uses echinacea as both
an internal and external antiseptic.

eclipta (han lian cao, bhringaraj [Sanskrit]) A
flowering weed, *Eclipta prostrata,* of the Compositae
family, of India, Japan, China, Taiwan, Indochina,
the Philippines and elsewhere, used by Chinese
and Ayurvedic practitioners as a remedy for vertigo, bloody vomitus and urine and lumbago.

elder (elderberry, sambucus) A North American shrub, *Sambucus canadensis, nigra, racemosa* and
ebulus, of the Caprifoliaceae family, whose root and
rootstock, bark, leaf buds, leaves, flowers, young
shoots and berries are considered medicinal by
herbalists. In the form of tea, wine, infusion,
decoction and tincture, elder is used as a remedy
for a wide range of ailments, including urinary and
kidney problems, edema, rheumatism, constipation, neuralgia, sciatica, diarrhea, cholera and
headaches attributable to colds. In the *canadensis*
species of elder, internal use of fresh plant parts can
cause poisoning. In the *nigra,* berries must be
cooked before eating or making juice. The berry
seeds of the *racemosa* are poisonous, and the berries
of the *ebulus* are poisonous.

**elecampane (deviat sil [Russian], pushkaramula
[Sanskrit], elf dock, scabwort, aunee, horseheal)**
A perennial herb, *Inula helenium,* of the Compositae family, that resembles horseradish and grows in
northern Asia, Europe and eastern North America.
The use of elecampane root in Ayurvedic and
Native American medicine includes treatment for
respiratory, breast and liver diseases, dyspepsia and
malignant fever. Homeopathic tinctures are prescribed for erysipelas, sciatica, cough, back ache,
toothache and cramps.

electrolytes See CHLORIDE; POTASSIUM; SODIUM.

elettaria See CARDAMOM.

**eleuthero (touch-me-not, devil's shrub, wild
pepper, euleutherococc)** *Eleutherococcus senticosus,* of the Araliaceae family, is a deciduous perennial shrub that thrives in Asia, and is used in
traditional Chinese medicine as a general tonic and
in the treatment of stress, low back pain, kidney
and lung ailments, rheumatoid arthritis, high
blood pressure, hypercholesterolemia, impotence,
decreased appetite and impotence. Eleuthero
extracts have also been used to promote the sense of
well-being in individuals suffering from depression,
insomnia, hypochondria, angina, cancer, acute
craniocerebral trauma, rheumatic heart disease, and
hypotension. According to Dennis J. McKenna, et
al., in *Botanical Medicines: The Desk Reference for Major
Herbal Supplements,* Second Edition, clinical studies
conducted in Russia on more than 2,000 healthy
subjects indicate that eleuthero "can increase (1)
human ability to withstand adverse physical conditions, (2) increase mental alertness and work output
and (3) improve the quality of work output and athletic performance. Eleuthero also appears to have
some adaptogenic properties in the treatment of
various mental disturbances."

elsholtzia An aromatic Chinese herb, *Elsholtzia
splendens,* of the Labiatae family, named for the
German botanist and physician John Sigismund
Elsholtz (1623–1688). The seeds are used in Chinese medicine as a remedy for typhoid, stomachache and colds.

emilia (Cupid's shaving brush) A tropical herb,
Emilia sonchifolia, of the Compositae family, eaten
in salad in Indochina, whose leaves are used by

Chinese practitioners to reduce fever and as a remedy for dysentery.

enriched foods   See THIAMINE.

enzymes   Complex proteins in living cells that are catalysts for temperature-sensitive biochemical reactions. Several hundred enzymes are recognized to date, although it is believed that nearly 1,000 exist in mammals. An example of an enzyme is ptyalin. Ptyalin, a component in saliva, splits starch and begins the process of digestion. Other digestive enzymes are amylases, pepsins, lipase, trypsin, chymotrypsin, carboxypeptidase, enteropeptidase, maltase, lactase, sucrase and nucleosidases.

epazote (Mexican wormseed)   The plant *Chenopodium ambrosioicles,* of the Chenopodiaceae family, that grows in Central America (and is also cultivated in China), whose aerial portions and seeds are used in herbal medicine to treat flatulence and worms.

ephedra   See MA HUANG.

epilepsy   See ANTICONVULSANT DRUGS AND VITAMIN INTERACTIONS.

epimedium (lusty goatherb)   A North American and Chinese herb, *Epimedium pimedium grandiflorum* and *sagittatum,* of the Berberidaceae family, that contains vitamin E, oleic and linolenic acids and other biochemicals. Epimedium is used in Chinese and western herbal medicine to stimulate the production of androgen and is therefore considered effective against male problems such as impotence and prostate and testicular ailments. Other medicinal uses of epimedium include treatment for hypertension, bronchial asthma and weakness in kidney function.

ergocalciferol   See D, VITAMIN.

ergot (mother of rye, cockspur rye, hornseed, smut rye)   A fungus, *Claviceps purpurea,* that is a source of LSD and ergotamine tartrate, which is listed in the United States Pharmacopoeia (USP) and used to treat migraine and cluster headaches

and, after childbirth, to induce vasoconstriction and uterine contraction. Trade names for this drug are Ergostat, Ergomar and Gynergen.

In Western herbal medicine, the dried sclerotia of ergot is also used to treat headaches and prevent hemorrhage after childbirth and menstrual problems. Ergot poisoning may be caused by overdose of the drug or by ingesting rye bread contaminated by the *Claviceps purpurea* fungus. Symptoms of ergot poisoning include vomiting and abdominal cramps, excessive thirst, diarrhea, dilated pupils, marked weakness, twitching of the extremities, absence of urination, seizures (sometimes); as a secondary condition, gangrene may develop in the extremities. Treatment may include gastric lavage, a saline cathartic, anticonvulsants and inhaled amyl nitrate, though ergot poisoning may be fatal.

eryngo (rattlesnake master)   The flowering plant *Eryngium aquaticum,* of the Umbelliferae family, that grows in the New Jersey Pine Barrens and in southern and western locations, with a tuberous, parsnip-like root, considered in Native American and homeopathic medicine the useful part of the plant. Tincture of eryngo root provides a treatment for influenza, gleet, gonorrhea, constipation or diarrhea, cough, conjunctivitis, urinary incontinence and sexual weakness, among other ailments. It is also used for jaundice and sluggishness of the liver.

essential fatty acids (linoleic, linolenic, arachidonic acids)   See FATTY ACIDS.

eucalyptus (blue gum, fever tree)   The aromatic evergreen tree, and sometimes shrub, native to Australia and cultivated in numerous other regions, *Eucalyptus globulus,* of the myrtle family. The oil from the *globulus species'* mature leaves is a popular ingredient in over-the-counter preparations such as cough drops for respiratory distress. Tea made from the leaves should not be ingested, but rather inhaled to open and soothe mucus-laden nasal and bronchial passages. There are about 600 species of the myrtle (Myrtaceae) family. Certain species attract bees that yield eucalyptus honey. The eucalyptus has a peppermint-lemon fragrance.

Native American medicine prescribes eucalyptus oil, leaves and bark preparations for bronchitis, asthma, diphtheria, malaria and neuralgia. Home-opathic medicine uses the essential oil and fresh leaves for bladder infections, dysentery, strychnine poisoning, syphilis, worms, kidney diseases, aneurism, gout and many other ailments.

eucommia (du zhong) A Chinese deciduous tree, *Eucommia ulmoides,* of the Eucommiaceae family, whose bark is used in Chinese medicine to treat hypertension, back ache, impotence and off-set the threat of miscarriage.

evening primrose (sundrops) One of many flowering, perennial herbs, *Oenothera biennis,* of the *Onagraceae* family, that grows in the United States, whose leaves and bark provide Native American and homeopathic preparations to treat nervous-ness, gastrointestinal disorders, nervous or spas-modic cough, diarrhea, hydrocephaloid and gynecological complaints.

exercise and supplements The degree of one's physical activity determines the required quantity of some nutrients, especially sodium, potassium, thiamin, riboflavin and niacin. An ideal diet designed to meet the increased needs of an athlete should provide the requirements without the need for supplements. However, because few people eat all the foods necessary to provide the ideal balance of nutrients, vitamin and mineral supplements can satisfy dietary gaps. Adequate hydration (water) is also essential because of extra losses that occur during vigorous exercise.

Sodium and potassium help maintain normal body water balance. Though these minerals are lost in sweat, the losses are usually quite small and are easily replaced by normal diet. Salt tablets should not be used.

In some situations, well-balanced diets are abandoned. For example, wrestlers may be on low-calorie diets for weight-class maintenance but con-tinue to expend high amounts of energy. Many athletes mistakenly believe that vitamins are a direct source of energy. They are not. Vitamin sup-plements in excess of the recommended dietary allowances (RDAs) will not enhance performance, increase strength or endurance, prevent injury or illness, provide energy, or build muscles.

There are instances where taking supplements may make sense. Athletes who are at highest risk for iron deficiency and who may need supple-mentation include females who lose iron through menstrual bleeding, males and females who eat no red meat, marathon runners who may damage red blood cells by pounding their feet on the ground during training, endurance athletes who may lose significant amounts of iron through heavy sweating and teenagers who are growing rapidly. Iron should always be used under a physician's supervision because of the possible increased risk of toxicity (see IRON). There are reports of athletes taking up to 10,000 milligrams of vitamin C daily. Not only has no benefit to tak-ing such massive doses of vitamin C or any other vitamin been proven, there also may be consider-able risks from taking megadoses. Clearly, research on both physical and psychological effects of vitamin C is needed.

Some women who exercise strenuously stop menstruating. This condition, called "athletic amenorrhea," is caused by diminished estrogen production. Since estrogen deficiency is a major risk factor for developing osteoporosis, these women may be at increased risk for the early onset of osteoporosis. Therefore, calcium supplements become beneficial to those women.

Athletes are more prone to zinc deficiency because of losses through sweat and urine. Most individuals generally do not get the RDA of this important mineral; however, meat, eggs, and seafood are excellent sources of zinc and may help offset a deficiency. In some cases supplements may be necessary.

Chromium is important for the utilization of glucose and supplements seem to be safe. How-ever, whole wheat, peanuts, prunes, apples, mush-rooms and wine are good sources of this mineral.

(Adapted with permission from a lecture by Laura Tedesco, R.D., C.D.E., nutritionist at the Joslin Center for Diabetes at Saint Barnabas, Toms River, New Jersey.)

eyebright The herb *Euphrasia officinalis,* of the Scrophulariaceae family, whose aerial portions are used in western herbal medicine to treat inflamma-tions, sinus congestion and conjunctivitis. Eyebright may be taken internally or used externally, primarily as an eyewash.

eye diseases Dysfunction and other detrimental conditions of the eye. Night blindness, inadequate night vision, has long been recognized as being related to vitamin A deficiency. Vitamin E deficiency in premature babies is a suspected cause of retinal damage that may lead to blindness. Cataracts and macular degeneration are causes of diminished vision and blindness that may be prevented or delayed by improved nutrition, including adequate amounts of the antioxidant vitamins.

Two studies on vitamins and cancer were conducted by the National Eye Institute and the Chinese Academy of Medical Sciences in Beijing, China. In the first study, 2,141 45- to 74-year-olds were given two brand-name multivitamins plus 25,000 International Units (I.U.) of beta-carotene or a placebo for five years. The older individuals, aged 65 to 74, had a 43-percent reduction in vision-limiting nuclear cataracts, a type of cataract that clouds the center of the lens of the eye. In the second study group, 3,249 Chinese were given 2.3 mg of riboflavin (vitamin B_2) and 40 mg of niacin daily for five years. These are approximately twice the United States Recommended Daily Allowances (RDA). Those individuals had about a 50 percent reduction in the nuclear cataracts (see also RIBOFLAVIN). Interestingly, persons taking other antioxidants, 25,000 I.U. of beta-carotene, 30 I.U. of vitamin E and 50 mcg of selenium, showed no reduction in their chances of developing the cataracts, but they did have a reduced risk of stomach cancer. It must be recognized, however, that the Chinese population studied were undernourished, which may have increased their chances of having eye problems.

See also A, VITAMIN; E, VITAMIN; GOLDEN RICE; NIGHT BLINDNESS.

false unicorn (helonias) The plant *Chamaelirium luteum,* of the Liliaceae family, whose root is considered by herbalists to be a uterine tonic, diuretic and antiworm remedy. Not to be confused with *Helonias bullata,* an endangered species according to the federal government, false unicorn is also prescribed for "morning sickness" during pregnancy, stomach-aches, anorexia, lumbosacral pain, intestinal parasites, lack of menses and menstrual pain.

fast foods Meals consisting mainly of hamburgers, fried chicken, french fried potatoes and soft drinks produced extremely quickly and provided "over the counter." The highly successful industry has created much concern over the nutritive quality of the food, most of which is fried and garnished with cheese, bacon, mayonnaise and other substances of questionable nutritive value. Nutritionists believe that the intake of such fast foods, as well as pizza, submarine sandwiches and hot dogs, should be limited and the intake of healthier choices of foods emphasized.

fat Vital dietary macronutrients including grease, oil, lipids (fat or fatlike substances) that are not water-soluble. Chemically esters of glycerol with fatty acids, triglycerides or neutral fat. Fats, which yield 9 kilocalories of energy per gram, should compose 20 to 30 percent of a normal diet. Most fats ingested in the diet are in the form of triglycerides. Triglycerides contain both saturated and unsaturated fatty acids. Saturated fats, such as palmitic and stearic, are usually solid at room temperature. Monosaturated fats are liquid at room temperature and harden or thicken when refrigerated. Polyunsaturated fats, including oleic and linoleic, are liquid at room temperature.

Deficiency

Insufficient dietary fat can lead to deficiencies in vitamins A, D, E and K, the fat-soluble vitamins. These vitamins require fat for absorption from the gastrointestinal tract and utilization by cells. Deficiencies can cause problems with bone development, night blindness and skin disorders.

Excess or Toxicity

Although fats are a vital component of the diet, excessive intake of dietary fat has been linked to breast and colon cancer. Excessive dietary fats may bind to calcium and interfere with calcium absorption.

See also A, VITAMIN; D, VITAMIN; E, VITAMIN; K, VITAMIN.

fatigue Tiredness attributable to long periods of work or other activity, stress or the effect of a psychotropic drug. Profound tiredness and weakness may also be the result of malnutrition, the general deficiency of proteins, carbohydrates, minerals and vitamins; a disease process such as anemia, cardiac damage and oxygen and endocrine insufficiency; and psychogenic, environmental or physical challenges. Nutritionists may be consulted as part of the health-care team for individuals suffering any form of fatigue, including chronic fatigue syndrome, in order to determine if dietary factors are involved and whether the diet should be altered and supplements administered.

See also CHRONIC FATIGUE SYNDROME.

fat-soluble vitamins Vitamins A, D, E and K stored in fat, or lipid, tissue as well as some organs, especially the liver. These vitamins are insoluble in water and require dietary fats and bile acids to be absorbed through the intestinal tract membranes. Excess intake of these vitamins may cause toxicity because of their ability to be stored.

See also A, VITAMIN; D, VITAMIN; E, VITAMIN; K, VITAMIN.

fatty acids Straight chain monocarboxylic acids, many of which occur naturally in fats. Essential fatty acids for the synthesis of prostaglandins (potent biochemicals important for a variety of physiologic processes) and membrane structure, include polyunsaturated arachidonic, linoleic and linolenic acids. These essential nutrients must be supplied by the diet, although arachidonic acid can be made in the body from linoleic acid. Requirements of essential fatty acids are 1 to 2 percent of dietary calories in adults and 3 percent for infants. Pyridoxine, vitamin B_6, is required for the metabolism of essential fatty acids.

Deficiency

Essential fatty-acid deficiency, characterized by failure of growth and skin rashes, is found in formula-fed infants on a skim-milk formula low in linoleic acid.

See also LORENZO'S OIL.

FDA See Appendix V; Appendix VII.

Fen-phen A combination of the drugs Pondimin (fenfluramine), Redux (dexfenfluramine), and phentermine. Concurrent use of phentermine and fenfluramine has been reported to help obese individuals lose weight. Phentermine decreases appetite, while fenfluramine allows for an increased sensation of gratification. The two drugs are anorectic drugs, which permits reducing the dose of both agents and reduces adverse side effects.

However, a major controversy emerged concerning the use of Pondimin and Redux, which have been associated with heart valve, pulmonary, cardiovascular and neuropsychological damage. Generally, three types of injuries can occur: heart-valve damage ("valvulopathy"), primary pulmonary hypertension and endocardial fibrosis. Phentermine and fenfluamine, marketed separately since the 1970s, were combined as Phen-Fen for weight loss and approved by the Federal Food

and Drug Administration in the early 1990s. Gradually thereafter, evidence linking the combination drug to toxicity and, in particular, primary pulmonary hypertension—and subsequent lawsuits by consumers—loomed so large that the pharmaceutical manufacturer of Phen-fen removed it from the market in order to begin further investigation.

See also DIETS, FAD; QUICK WEIGHT-LOSS PROGRAMS.

fennel (hui xiang, finocchio, shatapushpa [Sanskrit]) A perennial European herb, *Foeniculum vulgare,* of the carrot family, similar to celery but with an anise-like taste and aromatic seeds. Italians eat fennel cooked or raw, especially in salad, in the tradition of the ancient Romans, who believed fennel was dietetic. The ancient Greeks thought eating fennel gave them courage and longevity. Northern Indian cuisine uses fennel seeds mixed with tiny hard candies and shreds of coconut as an after-dinner "digestive." In herbal medicine, fennel is known to promote digestion, relieve intestinal gas, freshen the breath and promote lactation in nursing mothers. The seeds may be eaten or made into a tea, which is also considered a calmative. In addition, fennel is used as an expectorant and antispasmodic.

fenugreek (methi [Sanskrit]) A flowering annual plant, *Trigonella foenum-graecum,* of the Leguminosae family, whose name in Latin means "Greek hay." Native to Asia, fenugreek seed was used as medicine by the ancient Egyptians and Hippocrates. Modern herbal medicine prescribes fenugreek preparations for tuberculosis, bronchitis, fever, gout, neuralgia, sciatica, fistula, swollen gland and other sufferers. Some believe fenugreek to be an aphrodisiac.

fern, female (brake fern, stone brake, rock polypod) An American perennial, *Polypodium vulgare,* whose rootstock is used in herbal medicine to expel worms (particularly tenia worms) and treat respiratory problems, jaundice, fever, diminished appetite and hoarseness. The medicinal use of the rootstock of male fern, or *Dryopteris filixmas,* was documented by the ancient Greeks and Romans as an anthelmintic, though a prolonged male fern content in the body may cause poisoning, blindness and death.

Osmunda regalis, known by many names, including buckhorn brake, water fern or king's fern, is a European and African perennial used to treat internal obstruction, coughs and jaundice. The cinnamon fern, or *Osmunda cinnamomea,* native to North America, is used in similar ways as, but is somewhat less effective than, buckhorn brake, and when boiled in milk, it yields a mucilage that can counteract diarrhea.

fertility and vitamins Research in the 1920s identified vitamin E as essential to reproduction in animals. Despite intense scrutiny since, this finding has remained unproved in humans.

ferula See ASAFOETIDA.

feverfew (featherfew, pyrethrum, febrifuge) A European and American flowering plant, *Pyrethrum parthenium,* of the Compositae family, used in Native American and homeopathic medicine as a remedy for tension, poor circulation, dizziness, ill effects of opium, colic, flatulence, indigestion, colds, worms, menstrual problems, rheumatism, convulsions, delirium and St. Vitus' dance (chorea).

fiber, dietary Parts of food not readily absorbed that resist chemical digestion enzymes in the gastrointestinal tract and promote healthful bowel elimination. Dietary fibers are principally complex carbohydrates including cellulose, hemicellulose and lignin, polysaccharides, gums, mucilages and pectin. These substances are obtained from wheat, oats or algae. Lignin is a noncarbohydrate constituent in plant cell walls. Intestinal microorganisms can convert small quantities of dietary fibers to fatty acids that can be absorbed.

Some food labels may still list fiber content as "crude fiber," but this term is nutritionally obsolete. There is no accurate relationship between dietary and crude fiber.

Benefits
Dietary fibers are hygroscopic, or absorb water, adding moisture and bulk to the stool, thereby improving bowel function.

Sources
The average American consumes an average of 15 to 25 grams of fiber daily. The National Research Council recommends that adequate fiber be obtained from consumption of natural foods rather than by taking proprietary supplements. Fiber-rich foods include oat bran, whole-wheat and whole-grain breads and cereals, fruits containing pectin, especially apples, and legumes. There is evidence that diets rich in plant fiber reduce the incidence of heart disease, gallstones, diverticulosis, colon cancer and diabetes. Questions remain whether fiber alone or other related dietary changes are responsible for these protective effects. It is theorized that adequate fiber promotes rapid passage of suspected carcinogens through the digestive tract, reducing the opportunity for toxins to come in contact with mucosal surfaces in the bowel. Softer stools with increased mass may also dilute the concentration of carcinogens.

Excess
More than 50 grams of fiber daily may cause intestinal distress. Although rare in the United States, excessive fiber intake may bind with calcium and trace minerals reducing absorption of iron and zinc.

fibrocystic breast disease See BREAST DISEASE AND VITAMINS.

ficus Old World trees, shrubs and plants of the Moraceae family, with edible fruits. The stems, leaves, roots and fig of the *Ficus pumila,* or creeping fig, grown in East Asia, are used by Chinese practitioners for the treatment of hernia, rheumatism, fever, sore throat, dysentery and inflammation of the bladder. The *Ficus retusa,* also known as Indian laurel and Malayan banyan, an evergreen tree that grows between India and New Guinea, is used for toothache, swollen feet, rheumatism and pain.

fig See FICUS.

fillers Lactose, starch, sugar and other substances added to foods, drugs and supplements to increase bulk, strength, viscosity, opacity and weight.

firmiana (phoenix tree, Chinese parasol tree)
An East Asian deciduous tree, *Firmiana simplex*, of the Sterculiaceae family, whose seeds, fruits and roots are used in Chinese medicine to treat swellings, mouth abscesses in children and skin disorders.

fish oil   See OMEGA-3 POLYUNSATURATED FATTY ACIDS.

flavonoids   A group of antioxidants, including quercetin, kaempferol, myricetin, apigenin and luteolin, found in vegetables, fruits, tea and wine. Dutch researchers found a reduction in coronary artery risk among a group of 805 high-risk men aged 65 to 84, as reported in the British medical journal *Lancet*. There was no significant reduction in cardiac problems in a control group of 693 with no previous cardiac history. It is postulated that flavonoids reduce or prevent oxidation of low-density cholesterol (LDL), inhibiting the buildup of atherosclerotic plaque.

See also BIOFLAVONOIDS.

flax (linseed, lint bells, winterlien)   A North American and European flowering annual, *Linum usitatissimum*, of the Linaceae family, cultivated for its bast fiber and seed. In herbal medicine, a decoction of ripe seeds (immature seed pods may cause poisoning) is used as a remedy for cough, digestive and urinary disorders and other problems. Linseed oil, commonly known as an oil-paint thinner, is used to help eliminate gallstones. When eaten, the seeds work as a laxative by swelling in the intestines, thus promoting elimination of feces.

In Ayurvedic medicine, flax tea may be taken as a laxative, expectorant and decongestant, and flax seeds are thought to be energizing and of therapeutic value in relieving asthma and chronic cough.

fluid balance   See ELECTROLYTES.

fluoride   A binary compound of the nonmetallic, gaseous element fluorine. Fluoride ions combine with bones and teeth to strengthen them. Fluoridation of community water supplies to a level of 1

TABLE 14 ESTIMATED SAFE AND ADEQUATE DIETARY INTAKE OF FLUORIDE*

Birth to 6 months	0.1–.5 mg
6 to 12 months	0.2–1.0 mg
1 to 3 years	0.5–1.5 mg
4 to 6 years	1.0–2.5 mg
7 to 11 years	1.5–2.5 mg
Adults	1.5–4.0 mg

*Because there is insufficient information on which to base Recommended Dietary Allowances (RDA) for fluoride, a range is given.

part per million have achieved a 50 to 75 percent reduction in dental caries (cavities). In nonfluoridated areas, infants and children are usually given daily vitamin supplements containing fluoride, or fluoride alone.

Fluoride used experimentally to treat osteoporosis has been disappointing. Although fluoride stimulates bone growth, the resulting bone formation may be poorly mineralized and may be structurally unsound. However, when fluoride is combined with calcium supplements and vitamin D, there may be decreased fractures. The addition of estrogen therapy to the above regimen may be even more effective.

Toxicity
Fluorosis, or fluoride toxicity, results from excess doses of supplements, or accidental ingestion of fluoride-containing insecticides and rodenticides or chronic inhalation of industrial gases or dusts. Fluorine and fluorides are cellular poisons that inhibit the breakdown of glucose. They react with calcium to form insoluble compounds and cause hypocalcemia (decreased calcium). Characteristic findings indicate osteosclerosis and osteomalacia resulting in skeletal changes, such as dense bones, neurologic complications due to bony overgrowth and calcification of ligaments. Anemia, weight loss and weakness may also occur. Mottling of teeth may result if excessive fluoride is ingested during the formation of enamel.

Acute poisoning causes severe abdominal pain, nausea, vomiting and diarrhea. Calcium loss causes tetany, convulsions and eventually death from cardiac or respiratory arrest.

fluorine See FLUORIDE.

folacin See FOLIC ACID.

folate See FOLIC ACID.

folic acid (folacin) A substance first extracted from spinach leaves in 1941, named from the Latin word *folium* for leaf, and found to be a treatment for some types of anemia. This water-soluble compound is absorbed from the upper part of the small intestine and converted to its chemically active form by interactions with vitamin B_{12}, vitamin C and niacin.

The U.S. Public Health Service advises all women who may want to bear a child to consume at least 400 mcg of folic acid daily to reduce their risk of having a fetus affected by Neural tube defects. It is estimated that at least a 50 percent reduction in neural-tube defects, including spina bifida and anencephaly, can be achieved by this recommendation.

The American diet often fails to provide the required amount of folic acid from leafy vegetables, nuts and oranges or orange juice (see Table 15).

Sources of Folic Acid

The average American diet contains only 0.2 mg of folate. Therefore the Food and Drug Administration (FDA) has proposed fortification of various foods such as enriched breads, rolls and buns; enriched flour and self-rising flour; enriched cornmeal; enriched rice; and enriched macaroni products. Each product will be required to be fortified with folic acid equivalent to 140 mcg/100 grams of the product.

Cooking vegetables usually reduces the folate content to such an extent that in many cases the cooking water contains more of the vitamin than the cooked vegetable. In one study, samples of raw spinach averaged approximately 142.9 mcg of total folate per 100 grams of the vegetable. But after cooking, the spinach retained only 31.2 mcg of the vitamin, while the cooking water contained 92.4 mcg. However, asparagus and brussels sprouts retained approximately 84 percent and 73 percent, respectively, of their precooked folate content (see Table 16).

TABLE 15 FOLIC ACID CONTENT OF FOODS

Total Cereal	1 cup	466 mcg
Grape-Nuts cereal	1 cup	402 mcg
Lentils	1/2 cup	179 mcg
Dry beans	1/2 cup	120–160 mcg
Spinach (cooked)	1/2 cup	131 mcg
Asparagus (cooked)	1/2 cup	121 mcg
Wheaties cereal	1 cup	102 mcg
Turnips (cooked)	1/2 cup	85 mcg
Iceberg lettuce	1 cup	76 mcg

Folic Acid Deficiency

The body stores from three to six months' worth of folate. Deficiencies usually result from malnutrition or malabsorption of the vitamin in the diet. However, there are situations in which drugs or some medical disorders (see Table 17) interfere with the utilization of available vitamin. Pregnancy, some malignancies, increase folate requirements. Some liver diseases cause folate deficiency by increasing excretion of folic acid in urine and feces. Since vitamin B_{12} is required for cells to utilize folic acid, a vitamin B_{12} deficiency also causes symptoms of folate deficiency.

Approximately half of all pregnancies are unplanned. As mentioned above, neural-tube birth defects are caused by a folate deficiency. It is wise for all women of child-bearing age to have adequate folic acid in their diets. But doses of folic acid greater than 1 mg per day may mask the symptoms of pernicious anemia (vitamin B_{12} deficiency–related anemia), allowing permanent neurological damage to progress unrecognized. The dose recommended to prevent folate deficiency must be balanced against dangerous higher levels.

Dosage of Supplements

The Public Health Service (PHS) and the American Academy of Pediatrics recommend a daily dose of 0.4 mg. The pediatric group also recommends *not* taking multivitamins that contain vitamin A to achieve the required folate.

Folic Acid Toxicity

Megadoses from 5 to 15 mg may cause kidney toxicity with increased diuresis and hypertrophy, or enlargement, of the kidneys indicated by an

TABLE 16 THE EFFECTS OF COOKING ON FOLIC ACID CONTENT OF FOODS

Vegetable	Average Folic Acid Content of 4 Samples (micrograms per 100 grams of vegetable weight)		
	Raw Vegetable	After Cooking	Lost
Asparagus	174.7	146.3	16%
Broccoli	169.2	64.7	62%
Brussels sprouts	88.5	64.7	27%
Cabbage	29.6	15.9	46%
Cauliflower	56.3	42.2	25%
Spinach	142.9	31.2	78%

increase in blood urea nitrogen and creatinine levels. These abnormalities are evidence of kidney failure. Folate excesses can also cause central nervous system inflammation resulting in muscle spasms, aggressive behavior, malaise, depression, irritability and altered sleep patterns with increased dreams or insomnia.

TABLE 17 CAUSES OF FOLIC ACID DEFICIENCY

(The anemias caused by folic acid deficiency can be improved by folic-acid supplementation.)

Dietary
   overcooking of foods (folate is destroyed by heat), inadequate food intake, chronic alcoholism

Malabsorption disorders
   tropical and nontropical (celiac) sprue, scurvy (vitamin C–poor diets are usually also low in folate)

Drugs that compete for absorption
   phenytoin (Dilantin)
   primidone (Mysoline)
   barbiturates, i.e., phenobarbital
   oral contraceptives
   cycloserine (Seromycin)

Drugs that cause inadequate utilization, or a block in metabolism of the vitamin
   folic acid antagonists:
      methotrexate and related drugs (used as chemotherapeutic agents in the treatment of some cancers, certain types of arthritis and psoriasis)
      pyrimethamine (for treatment of malaria and toxoplasmosis)

   triamterene (component of the diuretic Dyazide and Maxide)
   pentamidine (protocidal drug for the treatment of pneumocystis carinii pneumonia most frequently seen in AIDS patients)
   trimethoprim (antibacterial drug used alone or with the sulfa drug sulfamextoxazole in Bactrim or Septra)
anticonvulsants
enzyme deficiencies:
   congenital
   acquired (liver diseases)
vitamin B_{12} deficiency
alcohol
ascorbic acid (vitamin C) deficiency
   amino acid excesses in the diet (glycine, methionine)
Increased requirements
   pregnancy (especially multiple pregnancies)
   malignancies (malignant tissues, especially lymphoproliferative or myeloproliferative disorders)
   infancy
   increased hematopoiesis (blood production) that occurs with hemolytic anemias, chronic blood loss, scurvy, increased metabolism (hyperthyroidism)
Increased excretion
   vitamin B_{12} deficiency that prevents the ability to incorporate folate in cells
   liver disease

food additives   Chemicals or substances added to foods and medications as coloring or flavoring agents, preservatives, sweeteners or to improve consistency. Adverse reactions are rare from the approximately 2,800 substances approved by the Food and Drug Administration (FDA). An important and potentially life-threatening reaction can occur in persons susceptible to the preservatives known as sulfiting agents. Sulfite additives can cause asthma and anaphylaxis (a form of life-threatening shock), with symptoms including a flushed feeling, drop in blood pressure and tingling sensations.

Dyes approved in the Food, Drug and Cosmetic Act (FD&C) of 1938 are derivatives of coal tar. Tartrazine, or FD&C yellow dye number 5, is frequently implicated as a cause of hyperactivity in children and asthma. However, less than 10 percent of individuals suspected of having adverse reactions to these additives reacted when challenged in a controlled study. Aspirin-sensitive asthmatic patients should be aware of the rare possibility of cross-reactivity between tartrazine and aspirin.

Parabens, a group of preservatives in creams and ointments, are strong skin sensitizers and can worsen the condition for which they are prescribed. Parabens can cause urticaria (hives) or angioedema (swelling of body tissues) when medications containing them as preservatives are injected. Oral ingestion of these substances does not seem to cause adverse reactions. Sodium benzoate, a chemically related substance, may cross-react with the parabens and can also cause asthma.

Butylated hydroxanisol (BHA) and butylated hydroxytoluene (BHT) are used in low doses as antioxidants in grain products including breakfast cereals and have not been shown to cause any allergic problems. However, since antioxidants are thought by some to prevent cancer and herpes infections and to retard aging, they are often used in megadoses in various health food preparations that may be toxic.

Nitrate and nitrite preservatives commonly used in lunch meats and hot dogs may cause migraine headaches and may be carcinogenic. Monosodium glutamate (MSG), the cause of "Chinese restaurant syndrome," may rarely cause asthma, hives or angioedema.

The azo dye amaranth (FD&C Red No. 5) was banned by the United States in 1975 because it was suspected of being a carcinogen. Aspartame (Nutrasweet) is often blamed for adverse effects, but except for a few cases of urticaria, there is no scientific proof of ill effects. Tartrazine is also frequently implicated in causing urticaria and angioedema. Well-controlled studies, such as those done at the Scripps Clinic and Research Foundation in San Diego, California, have rarely confirmed the suspicions. These dyes do play a role as sensitizers in allergic dermatitis. They are often suspected of inducing adverse effects both in the skin and when ingested. Skin reactions are relatively common; when used in foods and medications, the dyes are rarely proven to be the source of the adverse effect.

food allergy Adverse reactions to food or food additives caused by exposure to an allergen to which an individual is susceptible. However, many persons refer to any adverse food reaction as an allergy. There are basically two groups of food reactions, allergy-based or "hypersensitivity" reactions and nonallergic, or food "intolerances." When foods thought to cause allergic reaction are avoided, overall nutrition may suffer if adequate substitutions are not made in the diet. A person suffering from many food allergies is clearly at risk of nutrient deficiency, a condition that may compound distress by causing a myriad of ill effects.

Incidence

Hippocrates (460–370 B.C.) described stomach distress and hives caused by cow's milk. Galen (A.D. 131–210) recognized allergic symptoms in a child caused by goat's milk. Since early in the 20th century, medical reports carry descriptions of many similar reactions. Prevalence of true allergic reactions to food is unknown, but studies estimate the incidence of food allergy at about 1 percent of the general public. Adverse food reactions of all types, including nonallergic causes, may reach as high as 10 percent among infants if all adverse reactions are included.

Peak sensitivity to foods occurs at about age one in 3 to 4 percent of infants. Experts believe that 70 to 80 percent of babies outgrow their food allergies. In double-blind food challenges, it was demonstrated that only one-third of the patients thought to have allergies to a food actually had an adverse effect to a suspected food.

In a study of five hundred consecutive newborn infants followed over a three-year period, 142 (28 percent) were suspected of having an allergy to at least one food. However, only 27 (5 percent) reacted when challenged to that food or foods.

True allergy involves an allergen-antibody reaction. A food allergic reaction sets off a complex series of events when the food allergen comes in contact with the immune system as it is passing through or being absorbed by the gastrointestinal tract. Once absorbed into the bloodstream, the allergens attach themselves to receptors on mast cells and basophils in other target organs, the skin, respiratory tract and circulatory system, triggering

TABLE 18 FDA-APPROVED ADDITIVES THAT CAN CAUSE ADVERSE REACTIONS

Butylparaben*
Ethylparaben*
Metabisulfite
Methylparaben*
Monosodium glutamate (MSG)
Nitrates
Nitrites
Potassium sulfite
Propylparaben*
Sodium benzoate
Sulfur dioxide
Sulfur sulfite
Yellow dye #5 (tartrazine)

*Parabens are derivatives of parahydroxybenzoic acid.

the release of potent chemicals called mediators. In turn, the mediators bring on the allergic symptoms—sneezing, itching, hives, wheezing and shortness of breath or, in the most severe expression of allergy, acute shock or anaphylaxis.

Anaphylaxis, which may be fatal, seldom occurs and can usually be treated successfully if epinephrine is given immediately. Despite the fact that fatalities are rare, some experts believe that more children and adolescents die from food allergy than bee stings.

Foods That Most Commonly Cause Anaphylaxis

Only a few foods cause the vast majority of food allergic reactions. Similar properties among these food allergens are their glycoprotein composition, their water-solubility and heat and acid stability. Purified food allergens have been isolated from codfish, soybeans and peanuts. In most foods, only a small fraction of the available protein is allergenic.

Cooking may alter proteins and therefore lessen the allergenic potential of some foods, such as milk.

However, heating milk containing lactose (milk sugar) or milk altered by cooking actually increases the allergenic potential.

In children, most reactions are caused by eggs, cow's milk, and peanuts. In adults, the chief sources of allergic reactions are fish, shellfish, tree nuts and peanuts. Interestingly, various animal products do not always cross-react. Persons may be allergic to milk, but usually are not allergic to beef or inhaled cattle dander. Also, individuals with egg allergy are rarely allergic to chicken meat or inhaled feather allergens.

Many women in the United States consume large amounts of peanuts, especially in peanut butter, as a source of protein while breast-feeding. Peanut allergen in the breast milk may then sensitize the infant prone to peanut or other allergy.

Nuts, peanuts, eggs or milk were responsible for 13 fatal or near-fatal reactions in one group of allergic children. All children in the group had asthma, and most had had prior reactions to the same foods.

Outcome and Treatment of Food Allergy

Epinephrine (adrenalin) is available in spring-loaded, self-injecting syringes (Ana-Kit and Epi-Pen are two commercial brands available by prescription). Children weighing less than 30 kilograms (66 pounds) should receive a reduced dose.

Most children who died in the group mentioned above were in school or other public places at the time of the allergic reaction. Those who were immediately given an injection of epinephrine survived. Onset of a severe reaction usually occurs within minutes, but may be delayed for 30 minutes or more. In the group of 13 patients mentioned above, none of the individuals who died had received an epinephrine injection before severe respiratory distress developed. An initial reaction may be mild for an hour or more and then suddenly worsen.

In the group of fatalities, half suffered a rapid progression of respiratory difficulty before death. The other half had a two-part response: early oral itching and abdominal distress, with minimal symptoms for one to two hours before the onset of rapid deterioration and death. Therefore, it is imperative that anyone who has symptoms of a food allergy be given epinephrine as soon as possible and transported to an emergency medical facility on an urgent basis and observed for at least several hours.

Prevention of Food Allergic Reactions

Adults and children of reading age who have known food allergies should read labels carefully and become familiar with all the alternate names used for some foods. They must ask about ingredients of any foods ordered in a restaurant. Foods are often added unexpectedly; for example, peanut butter may be added to chili for flavoring. The Canadian Restaurant and Foodservice Association has a program in which designated employees of participating members are knowledgeable about all ingredients on their menu.

For persons who have had a prior food reaction and have been diagnosed with positive tests for a particular food by a qualified allergist, avoidance of that food is paramount. However, if one shows a positive allergy test but has had no past reactions to a particular food, that food does not have to be avoided.

Immunotherapy (Allergy Shots) for Food Allergy

Studies are being done to develop a safe method to desensitize food allergic persons. However, at the present time, allergy shots for food allergies should never be attempted except under research conditions. The risk of fatal anaphylaxis is great.

Testing for Food Allergy

Many individuals who have positive tests to foods can eat those same foods without having a reaction. A history of a prior food reaction usually precedes a fatal attack.

Nonallergic Food Reactions

Various other mechanisms are responsible for an individual's adverse reaction to a food: toxicity to or poisoning by contaminated foods; drug-induced effects such as those following ingestion of caffeine; and metabolic or enzyme deficiencies, such as the diarrhea induced by the inability to digest lactose (milk sugar) in a person with the lactase enzyme deficiency.

Typical descriptions of adverse reactions to a food include food hypersensitivity, food anaphylaxis, food intolerance, food toxicity (poisoning), food idiosyncrasy, anaphylactoid food reaction, pharmacologic food reaction and metabolic food reaction.

Rashes, diarrhea, colic and runny nose are often attributed to allergies, but are rarely proven to have origins in allergy.

food groups See Appendix I.

forskohlii An Ayurvedic preparation including the herb *Coleus forskohlii,* which contains the diterpene forskohlin. (A terpene is a member of the $C_{10}H_{16}$ family of hydrocarbons.) According to literature on Ayurvedic herbal products from India, this diterpene promotes nearly all pharmacological activities of the herb.

forsythia (lian qiao, weeping golden bell) A northern Chinese shrub, *Forsythia suspensa,* of the Oleaceae family, named for British horticulturist William Forsyth (1737–1800). In Chinese medicine, the fruits, leaves, leaf stalks and roots are used for preparations to treat fever, measles, skin disorders, inflammatory conditions, headache, sore throat, lymphatic tuberculosis, pinworm, jaundice and colds, among others.

foxglove (digitalis, ladies' glove, dead men's bells, purple foxglove, fairy fingers) Originally a European biennial, sometimes perennial, plant, *Digitalis purpurea,* of the snapdragon family, prized for its bell-shaped or finger-shaped (*digitus* in Latin) flowers and as a source of the drug digitalis, recognized in the United States Pharmacoepia (USP). Digitalis, made from the plant's dried and powdered leaves, contains cardiotonic glycocides, namely digitoxin and digoxin, that increase the heart muscles' ability to contract, thereby increasing the heart's output. Digitalis is used in the treatment of congestive heart failure, atrial fibrillation and flutter and paroxysmal atrial tachycardia, as well as a diuretic.

Foxglove's medicinal properties were first documented by Welsh physicians in 1250 and in William Withering's book, published in 1785.

Digitalis poisoning may develop from an accumulation of digitalis in the system. Symptoms include irregular pulse, nausea and vomiting, diarrhea, headache, partial heart block and a slowing of the heart rate. Patients on digitalis therapy should be taught to take their pulse, include high-potassium foods in their diet and be aware of the symptoms of digitalis poisoning. The treatment of poisoning may include the administration of digoxin immune Fab (fragment antigen binding), a biological substance under the trade name Digibind.

Digoxin is also obtained from *Digitalis lanata,* and is marketed as the cardiac stimulant Lanoxin.

Herbalists recommend medical direction for the use of digitalis, and add that touching the plant itself has been known to cause skin rashes, nausea and headache.

free radicals   See ANTIOXIDANTS.

fritillaria (chuan bei mu)   A western North American, European, Asian and North African bulbous herb, *Fritillaria cirrhose, verticillata* or *thunbergii,* of the Liliaceae family, whose bulbs are used in Chinese medicine to treat cough, bronchial and pulmonary conditions, colds, stomachache, breast inflammation and painful menses. *Fritillus* in Latin means checkerboard, which describes the markings on some of the plant's flowers.

fumitory (smoke of the earth)   A flowering annual found all over the world, *Fumaria officinalis,* of the Fumariaceae family, known also as *fumus terrae,* smoke of the earth. In herbal medicine, the flowering herb is dried and prepared as a remedy for liver and gallbladder conditions and scabies and other skin problems. Used also as a laxative and diuretic, fumitory in excessive doses may cause stomach pain and diarrhea.

G, vitamin An obsolete name for riboflavin or vitamin B$_2$.

galangal (catarrh root) A Southeast Asian, Chinese, Indonesian and Iranian perennial, *Alpinia galanga,* whose rootstock has been considered medicinal since the Middle Ages, when it was thought to be an aphrodisiac. Galangal prescriptions given by practitioners of herbal medicine are similar to those given for ginger.

See also GINGER.

garden nightshade A flowering plant, *Solanum nigrum,* of the Solonaceae family (see BELLADONNA) and native to regions of the United States, whose leaves are used in Native American and herbal medicine as a sedative and narcotic. Homeopathic tinctures of garden nightshade are prescribed for chorea, headache, heartburn, meningitis, night terrors, stammering, hydrocephalus, mania, peritonitis, tetanus and other ailments. The berries, poisonous until boiled, contain solanine, a toxic alkaloid, which is used to treat fever, diarrhea and heart disease and to dilate the pupils. The juice of the plant is used for kidney, liver, spleen, bladder and skin problems. Ointments and poultices are also made of garden nightshade for herpes, burns, joint pain, swellings and other irritations.

gardenia (zhi zi, cape jasmine) A popular flowering plant, *Gardenia jasminoides,* of the Rubiaceae family, originally from China and named after American physician Alexander Garden (1730–1791) who corresponded with the famous botanist Linnaeus. The fruit, seeds, flowers and roots are used in Chinese medicine as treatment for jaundice, gonorrhea, rheumatism, bleeding, abscesses and other problems.

garlic See ALLIUM.

gastrodia (tian ma) An East Asian orchid, *Gastrodia elata,* of the Orchidaceae family, whose underground stem is used in Chinese medicine to treat headache, vertigo, rheumatism, paralysis and lumbago.

gelatin A glutinous material derived by boiling collagen obtained from the skin, white connective tissue and bones of animals. Gelatin is used by the pharmaceutical industry in the manufacture of capsules for drugs and supplements.

generic products Non-brand-name drugs or supplements that contain similar active ingredients or nutrients as name-brand products and generally are less expensive. Capsules, tablets, fillers, binders or special time-release mechanisms may alter the amount of active drug absorbed and/or the time or rate at which the absorption occurs, thereby affecting the products' effectiveness. Major manufacturers claim that their brand-name products are superior to generics, but many of these same companies also make a line of generic drugs and supplements.

Theoretically, there should be no difference. But potent drugs such as heart and thyroid medications may differ significantly in their potency, and most physicians prescribe brand-name drugs. Vitamin and mineral supplements that meet United States Pharmacopoeia (USP) standards for dissolution are probably as effective as similar name brands. The USP is a legally recognized publication of standards and is updated regularly.

genetic code The biochemical basis of heredity, in which codons of DNA and RNA determine the specific amino acids sequence in proteins. Cancer may begin as an alteration in the genetic code that controls the characteristics of each cell. Antioxidants, including vitamin E, are thought by some researchers to protect a person's genetic code against these modifications. Some even feel that vitamin E can convert minor abnormalities back to normal.

See also ANTIOXIDANTS.

gentiana (gentian)   A flowering herb of temperate and arctic regions and certain tropical areas, *Gentiana macrophylla, scabra* and *triflora,* of the Gentianaceae family. Gentian is named for Gentius, king of Illyricum (the area formerly known as Yugoslavia) who allegedly discovered the medicinal plant 2,000 years ago. In Europe, gentian-root powder put in wine was considered a treatment for a number of ailments, including stomach and joint pain. In Chinese medicine, gentian is used as a remedy for rheumatoid arthritis, eye inflammations, convulsions, tuberculosis and other problems because it contains gentianine, an anti-inflammatory alkaloid. Gentian violet, from the dried rhizome and roots of *Gentiana lutea,* is the coal-tar dye $C_{25}H_{30}CIN_3$ used as a histology, cytology and bacteriology stain. It is also a topical anti-infective by the chemical name hexamethylpararosaniline chloride.

germanium (germanium dioxide or GE-132)   A mineral with dangerous adverse effects and unproven claims to boost the immune system in fighting cancer and AIDS. In 1988, the Food and Drug Administration banned importation of the substance following reports of weight loss, fatigue, anemia, kidney failure and death.

ghee   In Ayurvedic medicine, a preparation of heated, unsalted butter, used plain or varied by adding licorice, calamus root or gotu kola. Ghee is considered a flavor enhancer of foods; a tonic for increased intelligence, understanding and memory; and a digestive, laxative and detoxifier of the system. Also a remedy for peptic ulcers, colitis and wounds, ghee is said not to affect cholesterol level.

ginger (sheng jiang, sheng jiang pi, African ginger, black ginger, race ginger)   Originally a tropical Asian perennial, *Zingiber officinale,* of the family Zingiberaceae, now cultivated in many parts of the world. A popular cooking spice, ginger root, as it is commonly called, is also highly regarded as medicinal, especially as a "warming" agent that promotes digestion of fatty foods and counteracts flatulence.

In Chinese medicine, ginger tea is prescribed for colds and mucus congestion, nausea, hangover, menstrual cramps and other problems; ginger tea serves also as a bladder, kidney and uterine tonic. Ginger is also eaten as a vegetable in several Oriental cuisines.

In Ayurvedic medicine, ginger (*sunthi,* in Sanskrit) is touted as the best kitchen remedy for cough, colds, sinusitis and congestion. A paste made of ginger powder is used for relief of headache, and adding ginger to foods serves to promote digestion, elimination and body heat in cold weather.

Ginger oil, baths and compresses are used in Japan as topical applications for a wide range of ailments, including earache, flu, pain, sinusitis, kidney problems and gout, among others.

According to the *New England Journal of Medicine* in 1983, ginger capsules were discovered to be effective against vertigo and motion sickness.

ginkgo biloba (maidenhair tree)   Originally an eastern China, fruit-bearing deciduous tree, *Ginkgo biloba,* of the family Ginkgoaceae, whose fruit's kernels are eaten as a delicacy and also are said to expel intestinal worms and aid digestion. Young fruits and fruit pulp are used in Chinese medicine to treat tuberculosis and other pulmonary complaints, gonorrhea, kidney and bladder problems and vaginal discharge.

ginseng (ren shen, five finger root, sang, ninsin, panax, pannag, red berry, root of life, man root, immortality root, vidari-kanda [Sanskrit for Indian ginseng])   An Asian and North American perennial plant, both wild and cultivated, *Panax quinquefolius,* or *Panax ginseng* (*shinseng*), of the family Araliaceae, valued as an herbal medicine. Ginseng root is used in many cultures as a stimulant, general tonic and sometimes an aphrodisiac. According to allopathic (Western) medicine, evidence supporting ginseng is controversial. With its adaptogenic (antistress) properties called ginsenosides, ginseng root may be eaten raw or processed for storage as dried root (usually in the form of tea, pills or tablets) or liquid put into capsules.

Some of the acclaimed therapeutic uses of ginseng include the treatment of impotence, infertility, uterine disorders and other sexual complaints (in Chinese, Tibetan, Native American medicine), senility, hypoglycemia, arteriosclerosis, exhaustion, mental illness, stomach disorders, headache, fever and cough. Contemporary Russian scientist I. I. Brekhman's research found that ginseng may also be used as a stress reliever, because it has positive effects on the adrenal cortex of the brain, which produces hormones that fight stress. Therefore Brekhman believes ginseng may help the body resist illness.

At the Third International Ginseng Conference in Korea, ginseng was touted by Japanese scientist Dr. M. Kimura, who used it to treat patients with diabetes, and Dr. Morio Yonezawa, who reported that ginseng extract administered by injection seemed to prevent radiation-induced bone-marrow damage in patients exposed to radiation. Dr. Yoon Seok Chang, of the Seoul National University Hospital in Korea, concurred, revealing two comparative studies done on 50 patients with cervical cancer also treated with radiation. Chang reported that red panax ginseng taken orally by these patients restored their bone-marrow functions. Some scientists in the United States maintain that ginseng is a placebo, while others, like Chinese doctors and herbalists, call it "the king of medicines."

In Ezekiel 27:17, ginseng (often written as "pannag") was traded at the marketplace of Israel. Ginseng—from Asia, eastern Canada, the United States, or the ginseng plantations in Russia—is available all over the world. Homeopathic practitioners prescribe trituration and tincture of the root for appendicitis, lumbago, rheumatism, sciatica, general weakness and other ailments. Native American uses include treatment of asthma, whooping cough, nervous disorders, poor appetite, gout, cardiac weakness, indigestion, colds and neuralgia.

In Ayurvedic medicine, vidari-kanda (known as Indian ginseng) is from the plant *Ipomoea digitata,* of the Convolvulaceae family, and is used as a nutritive tonic, aphrodisiac and diuretic.

Legend has it that panax ginseng plants emit light at night, possibly attributable to the plant's alleged ability to give off organic radioactive rays like the Gartwitch rays of onions, said to promote the life processes in cells. Furthermore, ginseng plants are believed to move of their own accord during the night, possibly because their roots shift. Dr. James Duke, a researcher of the U.S. Department of Agriculture's Economic Botany Laboratory, experimented with 100 ginseng plants and discovered that about half the plants did in fact move during the night. When he replanted the ones that had been somehow disturbed, they moved again. Dr. Duke did not come to any precise conclusions about this phenomenon.

Some writers have noticed that ginseng does not seem to have an effect on individuals who are usually energetic and active. Llynn' Newman, certified nutritionist/herbalist and holistic counselor of Long Island, New York, wrote that ginseng, which supports all bodily functions, is contraindicated for those with high blood pressure and women with cysts, and it is not to be taken in conjunction with caffeine, citrus or vitamins.

gleditsia (honey locust) A Chinese deciduous tree, *Gleditsia sinensis,* of the Leguminosae family and named after the German botanist Johann Gottlieb Gleditsch (1714–1786). The roots, bark, fruits, seeds, leaves and thorns are considered medicinal by Chinese practitioners, and are made into preparations for excess mucus, intestinal worms, fever, swellings, indigestion, wounds and other ailments.

glehnia (bei sha shen) A Korean, Taiwanese, Chinese and Japanese plant, *Glehnia littoralis,* of the Umbelliferae family, whose roots are used by Chinese practitioners as a tonic for the liver and kidneys and to treat pulmonary complaints and chest pain.

glucosamine An amino-saccharide acid often combined with chondroitin and marketed as an over-the-counter treatment for the symptoms of arthritis.

See also AMINO ACIDS; CHONDROITIN.

glycemic index Physiological measure of the human body's ability to derive glucose (sugar)

TABLE 19 GLYCEMIC INDEXES OF FOODS

100%	80–90%	70–79%	60–69%
Glucose	Carrots	Bread (whole	Bananas
	Corn flakes	meal)	Beetroot
	Honey	Broad beans	Bread
	Maltose	(fresh)	(white)
	Parsnips	Millet	Mars bar
	Potatoes	Potato (new)	Muesli
	(instant	Rice (white)	Raisins
	mashed)	Swede	
	Weetabix	Rice (brown)	
		Ryvita	
		Shredded wheat	
		Water biscuits	

50–59%	40–49%	30–39%	20–29%	10–19%
All-bran	Beans	Apples	Fructose	Peanuts
Buckwheat	(canned	(Golden	Kidney	Soya
Digestive	navy)	Delicious)	beans	beans
biscuits	Orange	Blackeye	Lentils	(fresh
Oatmeal	juice	peas		and
biscuits	Oranges	Butter beans		canned)
Peas	Peas	Chickpeas		
(frozen)	(dried)	Haricot		
Potato	Porridge	beans		
chips	oats	Ice cream		
Rich tea	Potato	Milk (skim)		
biscuits	(sweet)	Milk (whole)		
Spaghetti	Spaghetti	Tomato soup		
Sucrose	(whole	Yogurt		
Sweet	meal)			
corn				
Yams				

from foods containing carbohydrate. The index is the ratio of serum glucose in the blood derived from food to that derived from a solution of pure glucose, measured over a two-hour period after ingestion.

glycyrrhiza (gan cao, kum cho, sweetwood, Chinese licorice) A Mediterranean, Asian and southern European herb, *Glycyrrhiza glabra,* of the Leguminosae family, whose roots are used in Chinese medicine to treat peptic ulcers, poor appetite, heart palpitations, weakness, dizziness, productive cough and hemorrhoids. A licorice and soybean decoction was considered an antidote for various poisons in 18th-century China. According to recent research, the roots are effective against cocaine hydrochloride and chloral hydrate, snake venom, tetanus and globefish toxins.

Cough medicines often contain licorice flavoring. In Africa, glycyrrhiza stems and roots are made into an infusion and used as a remedy for pulmonary tuberculosis, eye diseases and appendicitis. Dried, powdered glycyrrhiza root is used in Vietnam as a purgative, diaphoretic and diuretic. A glycoside called glycyrrhizine, with a licorice flavor, is found in the plant and is believed to be 50 times sweeter than sugar.

Licorice may be contraindicated for persons with hypertension because it may cause salt retention, excess potassium loss and elevated blood pressure.

goat's rue A southern European, western Asian and North American flowering perennial, *Galega officinalis,* poisonous to sheep who graze on it but considered therapeutic by herbalists. The medicinal herb is used, albeit rarely, in the treatment of diabetes, fever, worms and poisoning.

goiter Enlarged thyroid gland often caused by an iodine deficiency, usually occurring where the iodine content of a normal diet is low. Goiter was endemic to the Great Lakes region (prior to the introduction of iodized salt) and still occurs elsewhere in the world, especially in such mountain regions as the Alps, Pyrenees, Carpathians, Andes and Himalayas, where as many as 10 percent of the population have the disorder.

See also IODINE.

golden rice The genetically engineered creation of rice infused with beta-carotene, a source of vitamin A. Rice is a staple food of developing countries, where oftentimes more than 140 to 250 million children do not receive adequate vitamin A and therefore rampantly suffer from nutritional deficiencies that cause debilitation and disease, including blindness. It is believed that golden rice may reduce childhood mortality by as much as a third and eliminate half a million cases of blindness, but controversy involving risks of genetically engineered food and overdose of vitamin A has thwarted the golden-rice effort. Developed by German-born geneticist Dr. Ingo Potykus, of the Swiss Federal Institute of Technology in Zurich, Switzerland, golden rice is the result of the transference of two genes from the daffodil and one from a bacterium into the rice in order to fortify the grain with beta-carotene.

goldenrod (blue mountain tea) A North American flowering perennial herb, *Solidago canadensis* or *juncea* (two of about 100 species), of the family Compositae, whose leaves and tops are used in Native American and other herbal medicine practices for the treatment of bladder stones, hay fever and colds related to tuberculosis. Homeopathic practitioners prescribe tincture of aromatic goldenrod flowers or infusion of dried leaves and flowers for painful urination, protein in the urine, enlarged prostate, gout, deafness, croup, rheumatism, scrofula, sciatica and scanty urine. Russian herbalists used goldenrod for lack of menses, diarrhea and cystitis.

goldenseal (orange root, tumeric root, yellow puccoon, ground raspberry, jaundice root, eye balm, Indian plant) A North American fruit-bearing perennial, *Hydrastis canadensis,* of the family Ranunculaceae, whose root is valued in Native American and other herbalist medicines as a treatment for colds, stomach ulcers, tonsillitis, grippe, diphtheria, scarlet fever, smallpox, intestinal catarrh, gonorrhea, gleet, bladder ulcers and other illnesses. Homeopathic practitioners prescribe goldenseal root tincture for alcoholism, asthma, cancer, constipation, lupus, sciatica, syphilis, sore throat, uterine problems, liver disorders, including jaundice, and other ailments.

In Ayurvedic medicine, goldenseal is used for obesity, malaria, pyorrhea, hepatitis, diabetes, ulcers, infectious fever, swollen glands and various other afflictions. Like synthetic antibiotics, goldenseal's antibiotic action may be detrimental to good intestinal flora.

Goldenseal preparations are also used as a topical antibiotic and for insect bites, eczema and ringworm.

goldthread (vegetable gold, canker root, mouth root) An evergreen perennial, *Coptis groenlandica,* of the Ranunculaceae family, found in the northern United States, Canada, Siberia, India and Iceland, whose root is considered medicinal by Native American and other herbalists. Goldthread (often combined with goldenseal) is used as a tonic and relief from the desire for alcohol. Goldthread is also used to promote appetite and digestion and prevent pinworms.

gomashio A traditional Japanese macrobiotic seasoning made from sesame seeds and sea salt. Also called sesame salt, gomashio helps neutralize an excess of acid in the blood, and it is a popular ingredient in American macrobiotic cuisine.

gotu kola (brahmi [Sanskrit]) A bitter, cooling Ayurvedic herb, *Hydrocotyle asiatica,* of the Umbelliferae family, used as a nervine, rejuvenative, alterative and diuretic. Gotu kola is said to relieve stress, quiet the mind, alleviate sinus congestion, develop memory and intelligence, and promote sleep. The Sanskrit name is derived from the word *Brahma,* meaning cosmic consciousness.

grape seed (muskat) An extract made from the plant *Titis vinifera,* of the family Vitaceae, used as medicine for skin disease, eye inflammation, diarrhea, throat infection, varicose veins, cachexia, cancer, smallpox, scurvy, cholera and kidney and liver disorders. Grape seed oil has also been used to treat burns and skin ulcers and as an antacid and laxative. Grape seeds are usually obtained as a by-product in the making of wine.

GRAS list Food additives "*Generally Recognized As Safe,*" as authorized by Congress in 1958. The additives selected for this list were chosen because of their absence of known adverse or toxic effects rather than scientific proof of their safety. Motivated by the discovery that cyclamate artificial sweeteners caused cancer in laboratory animals, the Nixon administration charged the Food and Drug Administration (FDA) with the responsibility of reevaluating the GRAS list. In 1969 a panel of experts—the Select Committee on GRAS Substances of the Federation of American Societies for Experimental Biology—was assigned this task. By 1980, 305 of 415 substances studied were considered safe enough be given Class 1 status. Although additional research was recommended for 68 Class 2 substances, including vitamins A and D, they were approved for use at current levels. Caffeine, BHA, and BHT were listed as Class 3 ingredients that required additional studies within a given time frame; however, they were allowed to be used pending the outcome of those studies. Salt and four starches were placed in Class 4 with limitations on quantities or certain other restrictions. Eighteen substances were recommended for removal from the GRAS list because of insufficient evidence for safety. More than 1,700 food additives are currently on the GRAS list.

gravelroot (Joe-Pye weed, queen-of-the-meadow, purple boneset) A North American perennial, *Eupatorium purpureum*, of the Compositae family, named for Joe Pye, a Native American healer who successfully treated typhus fever with gravelroot, and for an ancient Roman king, Mithridates Eupator, who also used gravelroot as medicine. While large doses of gravelroot induce vomiting, the plant is used therapeutically to relieve calculus, or stones and gravel, in the urinary tract, rheumatism, gout, low back pain, fever and frequent nighttime urination.

green drinks and superfoods Also called formulations, green drinks and superfoods are beverages and foods to which chlorophyll has been added. Chlorophyll, the green photosynthetic pigment extracted from the chloroplasts of plants, is known to be a natural blood purifier, oxygenator and builder. Primary sources of "green" include wheat grass, barley grass, alfalfa, chlorella, aloe vera and spirulina (a blue-green algae). Green and blue-green algae, also called phytoplankton, contain large amounts of high-quality protein, fiber, chlorophyll, vitamins, minerals and enzymes, and they are a rich source of beta-carotene, vitamin B_{12}, and gamma-linolenic acid. Phytoplankton is said to help heal and detoxify the body, boost the immune system, protect against radiation and promote longevity. According to Linda G. Rector-Page, N.D., Ph.D, in *Healthy Healing: An Alternative Healing Reference*, spirulina, called "the original green superfood," contains 20 times more protein than soybeans, 40 times more protein than corn and 400 times more protein than beef, and it provides all 21 amino acids and the entire B-complex of vitamins. Spirulina grows in both ocean and alkaline waters and is easily cultivated. Chlorella contains a higher concentration of chlorophyll than any other known plant and is a complete protein food with B vitamins, vitamins C and E, and beneficial minerals. Nutritionists, herbalists and other experts tout the green formulations and may recommend them as a general tonic.

green tea A tea made from the plant *Camellia sinensis*, reported to have antioxidant properties, which neutralize harmful molecules, or free radicals, in the body, and contain a third to half the caffeine content of coffee. Some manufacturers of green tea add vitamins C and E, beta-carotene and euleuthero root to the tea. Green tea is used in the treatment of diarrhea, indigestion and motion sickness.

See also BLACK TEAS; C, VITAMIN; E, VITAMIN; ELEUTHERO; TEA.

growth factors Poorly understood compounds in food that are known to play a role in the development of some animal species, but requirements for which are unconfirmed in human nutrition. Growth factors include asparagine, bifidus factor, biopterin, chelating agents, cholesterol, coenzyme Q (ubiquinone), hematin, lecithin, lipoic or thioctic acid, nerve-growth factors, *p*-aminobenzoic acid, various peptides and proteins, pimelic acid and pteridines. It is theorized that humans synthesize these substances in sufficient amounts to satisfy normal growth.

guaiac (guayacan, lignum vitae, pockwood, guaiacum) A resin from the trees of the *Guaiacum genus*, such as *G. sanctum* or *G. officinale*, used in allopathic medicine for testing for occult blood in feces. In herbal medicine, guaiac resin (from *G. officinale*) is used as an antiseptic, diaphoretic, diuretic and stimulant, especially in the treatment of syphilis, gout, catarrh and skin diseases.

guarana (Brazilian cocoa) *Paullinia cupana*, of the family Sapindaceae and native to Brazil, Venezuela and the Amazon, a woody climbing plant with yellow flowers that turn into fruits, each carrying three nutty brown seeds, which may be dried and roasted. Guarana has long been used by Indian tribes of the Amazon, such as the Quarami and Maue, as a remedy for bowel disorders. Many South American natives harden guarana powder, then make it into a rod that may be eaten. A source of energy, guarana contains caffeine, guaranin, theobromine and theophylline. Guaranin is nearly identical to caffeine; one seed contains approximately three times the caffeine of a coffee bean. Guarana is also used to control appetite, to ease muscle cramps (including menstrual cramps) and anxiety, to elevate mood, as an aphrodisiac and as a tonic to fight the adverse effects of alcohol.

guggul (Indian bedellium) An Ayurvedic preparation made from the gum resin of the tree, *Commiphora mukul,* of the family Burseaceae, containing guggulsterones, isolated substances in the gum gugul resin, considered therapeutic as a rejuvenative, alterative, antispasmodic and expectorant. Guggul is marketed under the trade name Gugulmax.

gymnema (gurmarbooti) An Asian Indian herb, *Gymnema sylvestre,* used mainly in the treatment of Type 2 diabetes because it reduces high blood sugar levels. Gymnema is also reported to be a remedy for constipation, indigestion, water retention and liver disease.

hair analysis   Specimens of human hair may be examined chemically for the presence of vitamins, minerals and toxins in an attempt to diagnose various diseases, deficiencies or toxicities. Hair analysis is an unproven technique plagued by inconsistencies in results of hair samples from the same individual in one or more laboratories. However, there may be some validity to public health studies of hair for environmental heavy-metal exposure in various populations. Individually, great caution should be exercised in assigning any value to the results of hair analysis in determining nutritional status.

hair loss   Rarely related to vitamin or mineral deficiency. Vitamin A deficiency may cause hair loss and dandruff to occur, although vitamin A toxicity may have the same result. The anemia that results from a lack of vitamin B_6, B_{12}, folic acid or iron may cause inadequate oxygenation of blood supplying the scalp and affect the appearance of hair or its growth. Biotin deficiency, which is extremely rare, causes hair loss. Scurvy, or severe vitamin C deficiency, causes the hair to split and break below the surface of the skin, resulting in an abnormal circular hair pattern. Copper deficiency, or molybdenum toxicity that interferes with the utilization of copper, causes hair loss. Since copper is also a hair pigment, deficiency may also result in loss of hair coloring. Zinc helps maintain the oil-secreting glands attached to hair follicles, and deficiency is another correctable cause of baldness and dry scalp.

haritaki (Chebulic myrobalan)   An Ayurvedic herb, *Terminalia chebula,* of the Combretaceae family, used as a rejuvenative, astringent, nervine and laxative.

hawthorn (May bush, whitethorn, quickset, thorn-apple tree)   A British and European flowering, fruit-bearing shrub or tree, *Crataegus oxyacantha,* of the Rosaceae family, whose flowers and fruits are used by herbalists to regulate cardiac activity, myocarditis, nervous cardiac problems, insomnia and arteriosclerosis. In Ayurvedic medicine, hawthorn is considered a heating agent, stimulant, antispasmodic and diuretic. Chinese practitioners also use the hawthorn plant known botanically as *Crataegus pinnatifida,* or *shan zha.*

headaches   Acute or chronic aches or pain in the head attributable to illness, stress, strain, injury and other problems, but that also may be caused by vitamin A toxicity. Niacin can also cause headaches in therapeutic doses necessary for cholesterol reduction but probably not in doses within the Recommended Daily Allowance (RDA). Vitamin E in doses exceeding 800 I.U. may cause headaches.

See also A, VITAMIN; E, VITAMIN.

hearing loss   Diminished sense of hearing or profound loss, or absence of the sense of hearing. While aging, injury, disease processes, drug reactions and other factors may be responsible, hearing loss may result from vitamin D deficiency, which causes loss of calcium in bones. Therefore, vitamin D is essential to maintain the integrity of the small bones of the middle and inner ear. The cochlea in the inner ear is especially susceptible and may become porous and unable to transmit messages to the hearing center in the brain. Vitamin D supplementation may improve hearing in only those individuals whose loss is secondary to D deficiency. For unknown reasons, an iodine deficiency may result in a rare but correctable type of hearing loss.

heart disorders See CARDIOVASCULAR DISEASE PREVENTION AND ANTIOXIDANT VITAMINS.

hedyotis (oldenlandia) Tropical herbs of the Rubiaceae family, including *H. corymbosa* (or *Oldenlandia corymbosa*) and *H. diffusa,* used in Chinese medicine as treatments for stomach disorders and intestinal diseases, and believed by some to be a cure for cancer. Indian practitioners use hedyotis as a remedy for fever, malaria and depression.

hemochromatosis Inherited or acquired disorder in which excessive iron in the form of a complex molecule known as hemosiderin accumulates in body tissues. This potentially fatal condition causes tissue damage and disrupts function in the liver, pancreas, heart and pituitary gland. Cirrhosis of the liver, congestive heart failure, diabetes, sexual failure, loss of body hair and bronze pigmentation of the skin are symptoms.

Primary hemochromatosis is the inherited autosomal recessive form of the disorder and is more common. There are several acquired forms including one that can occur from excessive blood transfusions and excessive use of iron supplements.

See also IRON.

hemoglobin Oxygen containing pigment of erythrocytes, or red blood cells. Formed in the bone marrow as a conjugated protein consisting of an iron-containing pigment called heme and a simple protein, globulin. In the lungs, hemoglobin combines with oxygen to form oxyhemoglobin. In the tissues, oxyhemoglobin liberates oxygen in exchange for carbon dioxide. As red blood cells age, they eventually disintegrate, and liberated hemoglobin is removed from circulation by cells of the reticulo-endothelial system, especially the liver and spleen. The iron is stored and reused. The globin is converted to amino acids and also reused.

See also ANEMIA, MACROCYTIC; ANEMIA, MICROCYTIC.

hemosiderin A storage form of iron. Complex granules containing about 33 percent iron by weight, polysaccharides and proteins accumulate in tissue cells of the spleen, liver, and bone marrow (see HEMOCHROMATOSIS; IRON).

hemp seed The seed of the hemp plant, *Cannabis sativa,* of the mulberry family, that can be used whole or ground into a flour. Hemp seed is high in essential fatty acids and ranks second (soybean is first) in protein content. The psychoactive compound tetrahydrocannabinol (THC) in the leaves and flowers of the hemp plant, also known as marijuana, is not found in any appreciable quantity in the seeds, stalk or fiber.

Imperial court documents of the Han Dynasty in China indicate that since 2737 B.C. or earlier hemp was used to alleviate labor pains and as a treatment for general pain, rheumatism and fevers. As a top-notch source of protein, sterilized hemp seeds may be eaten raw or roasted (they are said to taste somewhat like sunflower seeds) or ground into flour and substituted for about one-fourth the flour called for in any recipe.

In 1794, George Washington said, "Make the most of the hemp seed, and sow it everywhere." Although the seeds, oils, paper, clothing fibers, biomass fuel and other commercial and industrial uses of hemp are relatively free of THC, hemp cultivation remains illegal: One cannot grow hemp without also growing its leaves and flowers, which contain THC, a controlled substance. Cannabis extracts and derivatives had been included in clinical and over-the-counter pain remedies until 1976, when the government pronounced marijuana illegal and decided to restrict its use to people suffering from certain diseases. Medicinal uses of marijuana leaves, particularly for the treatment of the ocular pressure caused by glaucoma; nausea and vomiting caused by chemotherapy in cancer patients; and to relieve the muscle spasms of multiple sclerosis, were banned in 1992.

Hemp agrimony (*Eupatorium cannabinum,* also called water maudlin and sweet-smelling trefoil) is a European perennial used by herbalists. The leaves are made into an infusion for treating liver ailments and rheumatism, and a decoction of the rootstock acts as an expectorant. Hemp agrimony is also thought to be effective against constipation and, as a topical remedy, against wounds, swellings and other external problems.

Hemp nettle is not of the *Cannabis* genus, but an annual weed known as *Galeopsis tetrahit,* or bastard hemp, of North America, especially Alaska and

Canada, used by herbalists for excess bronchial phlegm, anemia, spleen disorders and tuberculosis.

henbane　See HYOSCYAMUS.

herbs, general criticism of　According to the January 12, 2003, issue of *Time* magazine, "The multimillion-dollar herbal-remedy market took a hit when new studies questioned the efficacy of two of its top sellers. A six-week trial of ginkgo biloba, used to enhance memory, found that ginkgo was no better than a placebo at improving memory, learning or concentration. St.-John's-wort, which is supposed to lift your mood, didn't fare much better in a trial sponsored by the NIH [National Institutes of Health]. It concluded that a placebo was as effective as the herb for the treatment of moderately severe depression. . . . A separate study found that St.-John's-wort interferes with the effects of irinotecan, a widely prescribed chemotherapy drug."

Perhaps the most significant criticism of herbal remedies, as well as many other therapies that are considered alternative, complementary, or unconventional, is that of the American Medical Association (AMA). According to its "Report 12 of the Council on Scientific Affairs (A-97)," established at the AMA annual meeting in 1997, alternative medical systems require further scientific investigation and quality controls. Generally, the AMA states: "There is little evidence to confirm the safety or efficacy of most alternative therapies. . . . The American market for herbal remedies has doubled since 1985, to $1.13 billion in 1993 (excluding homeopathic remedies and teas). Growth is expected to continue at 10% to 15% per year through 1997. Four-fifths of all people, worldwide, still rely to a great extent on traditional medicines based on plants and their components . . ." The AMA goes on to state there is no standardization of the dose in herbal healing, and that the "safety of many of the compounds is unknown, or the potential toxicity ignored."

See also EPHEDRA; FEN-PHEN.

hesperidin　Bioflavonoid found in lemons and oranges.

See also BIOFLAVONOIDS.

hibiscus　A genus, *Hibiscus,* including about 200 species, the medicinal of which are *H. abelmoschus* (or musk-mallow), *bancroftianus, esculentus, mutabilis, palustris, rosa-sinensis, sabdariffa, sagittifolius, surattensis, syriacus* and *tiliaceus.* Muskmallow, also known as Syrian mallow, rose mallow and musk seed plant, is an annual or biennial plant of Egypt, the East and West Indies and India whose seeds are used as a nervine, stomachic, breath freshener, aphrodisiac and antispasmodic. In Chinese medicine, Chinese hibiscus (*H. rosa-sinensis*) leaves and flowers are remedies for mumps and fever, and *H. syriacus,* or rose-of-sharon, bark, roots and flowers are for dysentery, nausea and internal bleeding. Chinese practitioners also prescribe *H. mutabilis,* or cotton rose, leaves and flowers for pain, excess phlegm, copious menses, dysuria, snakesbite and inflammatory problems.

In Ayurvedic medicine, *H. rosa-sinensis,* of the Malvaceae (mallow) family, is used as an alternative, refrigerant, hemostatic and emmenagogue (to induce menses).

holistic medicine　The practice of considering all aspects of an individual—physical, emotional, cultural, spiritual, sociological and economic—in the prevention and treatment of health problems. Many branches of holism incorporate the mind-body connection, that is, the theory that patterns of thinking and behavior affect a person's physical state, traditionally known as "mind over matter." Holistic concepts have been a part of medical and health disciplines and many other human activities since ancient times. The ancient Greek physician Hippocrates said: "I would rather know what type of person has a disease than what type of disease a person has." Holistic techniques have finally begun to influence modern physicians, nurses, therapists, social workers and others, and to encourage the development of new ideas. Among the holistic leaders of today are Dr. Bernie Siegel, Dr. Deepak Chopra, Dr. Wayne Dyer, Louise Hay, Dr. Visant Lad, Thomas Moore, Dr. Dean Ornish, Dr. Andrew Weil, Melody Beattie and many others, all of whom have also become popular authors.

holly　Plants of the genus *Ilex* of the Aquifoliaceae family, including *I. pubescens* (*mao dong qing,* in

Chinese medicine), *aquifolium* (English holly), *opaca*, (American holly), *vomitoria* (Indian black drink), *verticillata* (winterberry or feverbush) and *paraguariensis* (yerba). Various species' parts are used by herbalists to treat a range of ailments, such as gout, stones, arthritis, worms, dyspepsia and other problems.

See also YERBA SANTA.

hollyhock (althea rose, malva flowers, rose mallow)   A perennial flowering Chinese herb, *Althaea rosea,* of the mallow family, found in India and southern Europe and cultivated elsewhere, whose flowers are used as a tea by herbalists to alleviate throat and mouth inflammation.

holy thistle   See BLESSED THISTLE.

homeopathy   A type of medical practice founded by Dr. Samuel Christian Friedrich Hahnemann (1755–1843), based on the theory that "like cures like," that is, a drug or other substance that can produce symptoms when given in large doses to a healthy person will in a tiny dose cure a sick person with the same symptoms. Modern homeopaths often prescribe tinctures of various herbs and combinations of herbs.

honey   From the Anglo-Saxon word *hunig,* the sweet, viscid liquid that has been used as a food, beverage (as in mead, the fermented and therefore alcoholic version of honey), flavoring, sweetener and medicine since ancient times. Bees extract the nectar of flowers and convert it into honey, which has been used as a home remedy for sore throat, diarrhea, insomnia, allergies, asthma, fever, wound infection and anxiety. One tablespoon of honey contains approximately 64 calories and 17 grams of carbohydrates. Researchers in South Africa reported that honey was effective as a treatment for salmonella, shigella, E. coli, and cholera. Ancient Egyptians, Greeks and Romans rubbed honey into wounds to help them heal, and Hippocrates recommended honey mixed with water and certain herbs as an antipyretic. Honey is also said to induce the activity of endorphins, the body's natural painkillers, and the production of serotonin in the brain, which results in relaxation

and sleep. However, the Centers for Disease Control cautions administering honey to children younger than one or two years, because bacterial spores of botulism cling to honey. Adult immune systems are strong enough to ward these spores off, but infants and toddlers do not have fully developed immune systems.

See also BEE POLLEN; BEE PROPOLIS.

hops   A perennial plant, *Humulus lupulus,* of the Moraceae family, cultivated in the United States and other parts of the world for the manufacture of beer and ale. The hops contain lupulin, a yellow, bitter, kidney-shaped grain often preferred over the hops itself. Native American practitioners prescribe lupulin tincture for delirium tremens, anxiety, worms and pain associated with gonorrhea.

In folk medicine, a root decoction of hops treats both jaundice and dandruff, and homeopathic treatments with hops include dyspepsia and gonorrhea.

Hops' conelike fruit produced by the plant's female flowers is used medicinally as a nervine. Hops tea, for example, is said to calm the nerves as well as treat diarrhea and insomnia and relieve flatulence, intestinal cramps, coughs, excess uric acid and water retention.

hordeum   See BARLEY.

horehound (marrubium)   A mostly European and North American perennial, *Marrubium vulgare,* of the Labiatae family, named from the Hebrew word *marrob,* or bitter juice. Native American, Ayurvedic and other herbal medicine practitioners use horehound as a cough remedy, expectorant, diuretic, diaphoretic, tonic and stimulant. It has also been prescribed for calming cardiac activity and to restore homeostasis (the body's natural balance) in glandular secretions.

horse chestnut (buckeye, Spanish chestnut)   An eastern European, Asian and North American deciduous tree, *Aesculus hippocastanum,* of the family Hippocastanaceae, whose leaves, bark and fruit are used medicinally by herbalists. Varicose veins, hemorrhoids, neuralgia, diarrhea, bronchitis and other ailments have been treated with horse chestnut.

horseradish A European and Asian perennial, *Armoracia lapathifolia,* or *Cochlearia armoracia,* of the Cruciferae family, cultivated in the United States and most parts of the world. The hot-tasting grated root may be mixed with vinegar and sugar or honey and used as an herbal remedy for pulmonary complaints such as asthma and coughs, gout, rheumatism and bladder infections. Horseradish, commonly eaten as a condiment, may also be made into a tincture, which homeopaths prescribe for other problems including urinary gravel and disorders, scurvy, cataract, colic, headache, toothache, protein in the urine, corneal spots and other eye afflictions and ulcers. Russian *hren* (horseradish) is a rich source of vitamin C and, in Russian folk medicine, used to treat a sluggish liver and dropsy.

horsetail (shave grass, pewterwort, bottlebrush) A perennial plant, *Equisetum arvense,* of the family Equisetaceae, whose outer layer contains silica, an astringent substance. Homeopaths and other herbalists, including Native Americans, use horsetail preparations to treat eye and skin problems, dropsy, gravel, foul perspiration, kidney ailments, urinary pain or difficulty and bleeding.

In Ayurvedic medicine, horsetail is used as a diuretic, diaphoretic and alterative.

horseweed (fleabane, butterweed, colt's tail, pride weed, Canada fleabane, bloodstaunch) A North and South American and European flowering annual, *Erigeron canadensis* or *Conyza canadensis,* of the Compositae family, used in herbal medicine as an astringent, diuretic and styptic. Ailments treated with horseweed include diarrhea, dysentery, hemorrhoids, menstrual irregularities, bladder problems, rheumatism and internal bleeding.

houseleek (thunder plant, Jupiter's beard, hens and chickens) A European flowering perennial, *Sempervivum tectorum,* of the orpine (Crassulaceae) family, whose leaves are made into infusions or decoctions for internal or external use and pre-

scribed by herbalists to treat shingles, skin problems, hemorrhoids, worms and other ailments.

human milk See MILK, HUMAN.

humulus See HOPS.

hydnocarpus (chaulmoogra tree) A tree, *Hydnocarpus anthelmintica,* of the Flacourtiaceae family, found in Burma, India and Thailand, whose seeds and seed oil are used by Chinese practitioners for the treatment of leprosy, syphilis, intestinal worms, scabies, gout and rheumatism.

hydrangea Deciduous or evergreen shrubs of the Saxifragaceae family, including *Hydrangea aspera, strigosa, heteromalla* and *macrophylla,* that are considered medicinal by Chinese practitioners. Named from the Greek words *hydros* and *aggos,* meaning water and jar, hydrangea is used in the treatment of bladder stones, wounds, malaria and certain heart diseases.

hydrogen (Active-H) A colorless, odorless, tasteless gas, a constituent of all hydrocarbons and an element that exists largely as hydrogen water (H_2O), also in use as a dietary supplement in the form of capsules and powder (trade name is Active-H). The human body needs an adequate supply of oxygen to survive. Oxygen burns hydrogen, producing energy to fuel the living system. Hydrogen and oxygen combine to produce adenosine triphosphate (ATP), the energy molecule that brings life to every bodily cell. ATP production is dependent on the production of nicotinamide adenine dinucleotide (NAD) plus hydrogen, or NADH. NAD is an enzyme that is important in metabolic reactions involving electron uptake. The billions of cells in a body must communicate with each other through electrons to maintain life. Electrons cannot move in the body without hydrogen, according to scientist Albert Szent-Gyorgyi.

The history of the development of Active-H as a supplement began more than 80 years ago, when Romanian physicist Dr. Henry Coanda found that many inhabitants of certain areas of northern Pakistan, Ecuador, Georgia, Mongolia and Peru lived active lives past 100 in remarkably good health. Coanda thought their water, derived from glaciers, contained special properties. Longevity researcher Patrick Flanagan discovered that the waters are similar to distilled water: no mineral-salt content but microscopic, colloidal (insoluble in water) minerals, particularly silica.

hydroxycobalamin   See B$_{12}$, VITAMIN.

hyoscymus (henbane, stinking nightshade)   A poisonous flowering, foul-smelling plant, *Hyoscyamus niger,* of the Solanaceae family, used as a hallucinogenic during the Middle Ages in Europe, smoked by priestesses at the Oracle of Delphi, and the contemporary source of the narcotic and antispasmodic drug hyoscyamine. While henbane is primarily a narcotic painkiller, Chinese practitioners and other herbalists use it to treat scrotal and breast swellings, gout, painful joints, headache, asthma, toothache, epilepsy and coughs.

Henbane poisoning, similar to atropine poisoning, is characterized by dry mouth; burning pain in the throat; blurred vision; thirst; hot, flushed, dry skin; rapid heart rate; palpitations; restlessness; convulsions; confusion; mania; and delirium, though death is rare. Induced vomiting, stomach lavage and intravenous administration of phyostigmine salicylate may reverse the poison's effects.

hypervitaminosis   Toxicity from any vitamin, but especially the fat-soluble vitamins A and D.

See also A, VITAMIN; D, VITAMIN; MEGAVITAMINS.

hyssop   Mainly a southern European, flowering perennial, *Hyssopus officinalis,* of the Labiatae family, named from the Hebrew word *ezeb,* referred to in Psalm 51:7 as a plant used to purify the body. In Native American medicine, the tops and leaves provide ingredients for a stimulant, aromatic, carminative, tonic and expectorant, especially helpful in treating asthma and pulmonary ailments, high blood pressure, poor circulation, jaundice, gravel, scrofula and epilepsy. In Ayurvedic medicine, hyssop is considered an anthelmintic, diaphoretic and diuretic as well.

Iceland moss (eryngo-leaved liverwort, Iceland lichen)   A lichen—a combination of a fungus and an alga living symbiotically on a surface—found in arctic and mountainous regions, including Iceland, Asia, northern North America, Great Britain and Europe. Iceland moss, *Cetraria islandica,* of the Parmeliaceae or algae family, is considered nutritive because it contains polysaccharides and iodine, but herbalists may prescribe it also as an antiemetic and demulcent. As a decoction, it is thought to be helpful for pulmonary insufficiency and other upper respiratory problems such as cough, hoarseness and bronchitis, and sometimes for tuberculosis. Iceland moss tea stimulates the flow of breast milk and regulates stomach acid. In order to be used as a food, the plant must be boiled a very long time. Prolonged usage and/or excessive amounts of Iceland moss may induce gastrointestinal and hepatic disturbances. In Ayurvedic medicine, Iceland moss is characterized as cooling, salty, sweet and astringent and used as a tonic, demulcent and alterative.

illicium (star anise, true anise, Chinese anise, Japanese anise)   A southern Chinese and northeastern Vietnamese plant, *Illicium verum* and *anisatum,* that bears star-shaped fruit used as an aromatic flavoring for liqueurs (such as anisette) and as a spice. The fruit oil of *I. verum* serves as an antidote for poisoning and a treatment for rheumatism in Chinese medicine. The *I. anisatum* plant, not used internally, is prescribed as a topical medicine for skin disorders.

immune system and vitamins   The effects nutrients have on the body's innate ability to ward off disease, such as the fact that vitamin A and beta-carotene improve immune function in measles, respiratory infections and AIDS, possibly reducing deaths. Healthy skin plays an important function in the immune system by acting as a protective barrier against invading microorganisms, and vitamin A plays an important role in maintaining the skin.

Immune function deteriorates with age. Many feel that the antioxidant vitamins C and E help preserve immune functions and prevent cancer by blocking the actions of free radicals. Free radicals appear to stimulate the production of prostaglandins, which are involved in inflammatory changes in the tissues and infection.

Vitamin C has long been promoted for its possible protection against the common cold. While this alleged benefit has not been proven, the vitamin does play a role in the production of certain antibodies and interferon. A group of Belgians over age 70 given zinc supplements had a greater immune response to tetanus vaccine and seemed to mount a better response to fighting infection. Pyridoxine, vitamin B_6 deficiency, may have a negative effect on the immune system.

See also A, VITAMIN; AIDS; ANTIOXIDANTS; ASCORBIC ACID; E, VITAMIN; FREE RADICALS.

imperata (lalang)   A weed-grass with sharp blades, *Imperata cylindrica,* of the Gramineae family, named for Italian physician and naturalist Ferrante Imperato. In Chinese medicine, the stems, roots and flowers are prescribed as treatments for ailments including kidney, lung and liver diseases, influenza, nosebleed, fever and productive cough. Extracts of lalang are said to have anticancer and antiviral properties, and herbal remedies of lalang are used in Japan, Indochina, the Philippines and Malaysia.

imperial masterwort　A wild European perennial, *Imperatoria ostruthium,* whose rootstock is used in herbal medicine for gout, cough, poor appetite, cramps, congestion, rheumatism, bronchitis and fever.

Indian turnip (bog onion, wakerobin, dragonroot)　A perennial, *Arisaema triphyllum,* native to the states east of Louisiana, Kansas and Minnesota, whose partially dried rootstock is used by herbalists after the examples set by the Pawnee and Hopi. The Pawnee made a powder of the root and applied it to the head as a remedy for headache, and the Hopi mixed it in water for temporary or permanent sterility—a surprising method of birth control. In the 19th century, Native Americans thought the Indian turnip effective against rheumatism, whooping cough and asthma.

indigo, wild (horsefly bush, rattle bush, yellow indigo)　A southern and eastern United States fruit-bearing, flowering perennial, *Baptisia tinctoria,* of the family Leguminosae, whose root bark and leaves are considered medicinal by Native American herbalists. Indigo tea was given to smallpox sufferers, and according to research done at the Flower Hospital in New York, indigo is an effective remedy for dysentery, colitis, follicular tonsillitis, quinsy, eruptive diseases and ulcerations.

Homeopathic medicine prescribes indigo in the treatment of influenza, mumps, cancer, plague, typhus, worms, variola, threatened miscarriage and hysteria, among other ailments. Indian and Pakistani practitioners use *guli* or *nil-nilika* (common and Indian indigo) to treat cardiac, liver, spleen, kidney and bladder diseases and nervous disorders including epilepsy.

See also INDIGOFERA.

indigofera　A tropical shrub, *Indigofera tinctoria,* of the Leguminosae family, known for its blue dye, used in Chinese medicine for dysentery and liver diseases. In Ayurvedic medicine, indigofera is considered an antibiotic, laxative and alterative.

infections　See IMMUNE SYSTEM AND VITAMINS.

infusion　A liquid or tea made by steeping the leaves of various herbs in boiling water.

inositol (*myo*-inositol)　Substance chemically related to glucose and essential for the growth of human cells. There are nine isomers of inositol but only *myo*-inositol is of importance to plant and animal metabolism. However, although there is no recommended daily allowance, scientists have discovered that inositol is necessary for the metabolism of calcium in cells. Therefore, it may be considered an essential nutrient in the future. The substance was first discovered in the urine of diabetics more than 100 years ago. However, it was not until 1941 that Gavin and McHenry discovered important metabolic actions in rats. Research by Eagle and colleagues demonstrated a human need by studying tissue cultures. Since bacteria in the human gastrointestinal tract and the manufacture of inositol in cells seems to be adequate, it does not satisfy the definition of a vitamin.

Uses

There are no definite indications for the use of inositol. However, there is preliminary evidence that inositol may benefit some persons with diabetic neuropathy, kidney failure and galactosemia, an inherited metabolic disorder. However, there also may be toxic effects in the latter two disorders (see below).

Inositol is present in human breast milk and may be an important nutrient for infancy. Inositol supplementation appears to be beneficial in low birthweight infants with respiratory distress syndrome.

Toxicity

Although inositol is generally considered nontoxic, in the presence of kidney failure there may be a dangerous buildup of inositol in the blood. Despite the possibility of beneficial effects of inositol as discussed above, in some cases there may be toxic effects on nerve tissues which may contribute to the development of uremic polyneuropathy. This disorder is characterized by numbness and weakness of the extremities.

insomnia　Inability to sleep.

See also TRYPTOPHAN.

International Unit (I.U.) Unit of biological material established by the International Conference for the Unification of Formulas. It is used to measure vitamins, enzymes, hormones and other substances.

intrinsic factor See B₁₂, VITAMIN.

inula Old World and Asian subtropical and temperate herbs including *Inula britannica* and *helenium,* of the Compositae family, used in Chinese and Ayurvedic medicine. The *I. britannica* plant and its roots are considered remedies for hay fever, asthma and bronchitis, and *I. helenium* roots, known as elecampane (*pushkaramula,* in Sanskrit) are used to treat cholera, dysentery, intestinal worms, malarial fever, snakebite and insect stings.

See also ELECAMPANE.

iodine A nonmetallic element of the halogen group essential in nutrition for the synthesis of thyroid hormones that control human metabolism. The halogen elements also include bromine, chlorine, fuorine and astatine, all of which form salts with sodium and other metals. Iodine is an essential mineral for all animal species. Iodine is usually in the form of inorganic iodide salts that are readily absorbed and transported to the thyroid gland for utilization and are also concentrated in salivary and gastric glands. Excretion of unused iodides are metabolized by the kidneys and lost in the urine. Organically bound iodine-amino acid complexes are less efficiently absorbed, and some are lost in the feces.

Deficiency

Goiter is the most noticeable example of iodine deficiency that causes hypothyroidism, or underactive thyroid gland. The most serious instance is cretinism, a congenital form of mental retardation. Chinese researchers found that dietary iodine given during the first and second trimesters of pregnancy reduced birth defects associated with cretinism by 400 percent. Only 2 percent of the Chinese infants given the supplement early in pregnancy had neurologic problems at birth, compared to 9 percent in those supplemented only in the last trimester.

Dietary Sources

Seafoods and water are chief sources of iodine in coastal areas. In mountainous or inland areas, sometimes called the "goiter belt," iodized salt that contains 76 mcg of iodine per gram of salt is the chief source. Milk and other dairy products absorb iodine from iodine-containing disinfectants used on cows, milking machines and storage tanks. Also, iodine is added to animal feeds.

Recommended Allowances

Levels of iodine necessary to prevent goiter are estimated by measuring urinary output. A minimum intake of 50 to 75 mcg of iodine daily is needed to maintain an adequate urinary excretion of the mineral. The U.S. Recommended Dietary Allowance (RDA) has been set at 150 mcg for adults to assure an adequate margin of safety.

An extra 25 mcg of iodine is recommended during pregnancy and 50 mcg for nursing mothers.

Toxicity

Iodine intake up to 2 mg per day has not seemed to cause ill effects in Americans. However, bread fortified with 2 to 4 mcg per gram of dry bread fed to a group of Tasmanian Islanders (where there is an endemic high level of goiters) caused a doubling of the usual incidence of thyrotoxicosis.

ipecacuanha The plant *Cephaelis ipecacuanha,* of the Rubiaceae family, grown in Brazil and used in allopathic (United States Pharmacoepia), herbal and Ayurvedic medicine as a popular emetic and source of emetine (to induce vomiting). Syrup of ipecac is used primarily to induce the vomiting of noncaustic poisons (including contaminated food and certain drug overdoses). It is also considered an expectorant in the case of intestinal amoebas and as a remedy to relieve asthma and severe congestion.

ipomoea (vidari-kanda [Sanskrit]) A tropical American plant of the Concolvulaceae family, including *Ipomoea batatas* (sweet potato), *aquatica* (kangkong) and *hederacea.* While some species of ipomoea have hallucinogenic properties, others, such as *I. batatas,* are cultivated and the tuberous roots eaten as a vegetable. The nutritious sweet potato (whose leaves are also considered a vegetable) provides feed for livestock and a stomach, spleen and kidney tonic prescribed by Chinese practitioners. Kangkong, both vegetable and medicine, is thought to be a tonic, laxative and food-poisoning antidote. The seeds of *I. hederacea* induce menses and abortion and counteract constipation, intestinal worms and scanty urine. The plant itself is used as a purgative.

In Ayurvedic medicine, vidari-kanda (*Ipomoea digitata*) provides a nutritive tonic, diuretic and aphrodisiac.

Irish moss (carrageenan)   A colloid (a substance whose particles are distributed throughout another substance), named after Carragheen (near Waterford), Ireland. The colloid is extracted from red algae and used commercially as a food stabilizer or thickener. In Ayurvedic and other herbal medicine, Irish moss—*Chondrus crispus,* of the Gigartinaceae family—is nutritive because of its iodine, amino acids, polysaccharides and other biochemical constituents, and considered an effective demulcent, emollient, tonic, antitussive and laxative. Herbalists prescribe Irish moss for patients suffering from lung irritations and diseases, dry throat and cough, ulcers and dysentery. Ayurvedic practitioners believe Irish moss to be a sweet, heating agent with nutritive, demulcent and emollient capabilities.

iron   A metallic element commonly found in soil, combined with other minerals and as salts and in mineral waters. Widely used in medicine, it is essential in humans for hemoglobin, cytochrome and other enzymes essential for life. Its chief roles are in the transport of oxygen to the tissues and in oxidation reactions in the cells.

As much as 30 percent of iron is stored in the spleen, liver and bone marrow as ferritin and hemosiderin. Iron is absorbed from the intestinal mucosa or lining and regulated by a complex balance between total iron stores, the amount and type of iron in food and by other dietary factors. Although the ability to absorb more iron increases in the presence of iron deficiency, eventually there

may be insufficient dietary supply to keep up with iron loss to prevent anemia.

Historical Background

Iron has been known since ancient times and used in tools and weapons. In the Egyptian Ebers papyrus, an ointment containing rust is mentioned as a treatment for baldness. Male impotency was treated with an iron and wine solution in early Greece. In the 17th century, chlorosis, a condition later recognized as being related to iron deficiency, was treated empirically with iron. Chlorosis, a disorder in which the skin turns greenish-yellow, frequently seen in adolescent females in the past, is rare today.

A case of iron overload was first described in 1871. Although the first nutritional study on iron deficiency was reported in 1895, it was not until 1932 that the value of iron therapy was proven.

Recommended Dietary Allowances (RDA)

The RDA for iron is based on achieving iron stores of 300 mg to meet the nutritional requirements for healthy people. That level of stored iron is sufficient for several months of an iron-deficient diet. To maintain adequate stores, the RDA for healthy menstruating adolescent and adult women is 15 mg daily. The RDA for postmenopausal women and adult men is 10 mg daily.

The daily dietary allowance of 1.0 to 1.5 mg of iron per kilogram of body weight should be sufficient for most infants. During pregnancy, an estimated total requirement of 1,040 mg of iron is needed to allow for an expanding need for mother, placenta and fetus. Although there is no need for routine supplementation during the first trimester, additional iron is necessary during the later stages of pregnancy. An average increment of 15 mg daily throughout pregnancy should satisfy the requirements of most women.

A diet needs to contain 30 to 90 grams of meat, poultry or fish, all of which provide heme iron, a complex molecule that is highly absorbed. Ascorbic acid (vitamin C) found in plant foods improves the absorption of nonheme iron and is beneficial for people not consuming adequate animal protein. However, there is probably no benefit to adding vitamin C to the easily absorbed ferrous-sulfate form of iron found in most supplements.

TABLE 20 MOST COMMON CAUSES OF IRON DEFICIENCY IN THE UNITED STATES

Stage of Life	Cause
Early childhood (6 months–4 years)	Low iron content of milk inadequate to meet needs of rapid growth
Adolescence	Rapid growth requires increasing number of red blood cells
Childbearing age	Menstrual blood loss
Pregnancy	Expanding blood volume of mother, fetus and placenta; blood loss at delivery
Women peri- or post-menopausal	Abnormal vaginal bleeding (cancer must be ruled out)
Adult men and post-menopausal women	Abnormal blood loss from gastrointestinal tract (cancer must be ruled out)

Deficiency

As iron deficiency progresses, iron stores are at first diminished without functional impairment. Eventually there is a reduction in quantity of erythrocytes, or red blood cells, and hemoglobin, and the red cells become smaller than normal. The World Health Organization has established that anemia occurs when hemoglobin concentration falls below 13 grams/decaliter in adult men and 12 grams in nonpregnant women. During pregnancy 11, 10.5 and 11 grams of hemoglobin respectively, for the first, second and third trimester, are the lower levels of normal.

Iron deficiency may result in reduced physical tolerance even before a fall in hemoglobin is seen. Changes in several constituents of the immune system may also occur, although resistance to infection is questionable. Children may experience apathy, attention deficit, irritability and difficulty learning.

Iron is also essential, with protein, vitamin E and zinc in the metabolism of vitamin A. A high calcium intake may interfere with the absorption of iron and other minerals.

Dietary Iron and Supplements

Iron supplements are preparations or natural sources of the mineral iron that are added to the diet, especially in the incidence of anemia or other indication of iron deficiency. The only times that iron supplementation are recommended for healthy people is during infancy and pregnancy. However, because of poor dietary habits, many menstruating women should probably take iron supplements also. The average American diet fails to provide adequate iron during pregnancy, and these women should receive daily supplements of 15 mg. Although menses is usually absent during lactation, nursing mothers should continue taking iron supplements for about three months postpartum because of the blood loss during delivery.

In the United States wheat flour is enriched with 20 mg of iron per pound. In Sweden and some other countries, an even greater amount of iron is added. Since ferrous sulfate imparts an undesirable taste to bread, reduced metallic iron is used. However, this form of iron is not well absorbed, and commercially available bread is now about equal to beef in iron content but only 1 to 12 percent of the iron is absorbed by normal persons. Iron-deficient individuals do absorb a somewhat greater amount.

The second National Health and Nutrition Examination Survey (NHANES II), reported in 1987, showed that not only did supplement-takers consume greater quantities of vitamin C, fruits and vegetables than non-supplement users, but users of vitamin supplements with iron did not have significantly higher levels of iron in their bodies than non-users.

Once the cause of iron deficiency has been found and corrected, the anemia is usually easily corrected by the oral supplementation of iron salts, usually ferrous sulfate. Ferrous sulfate is easily absorbed, and about 20 percent of the iron in each tablet is absorbed. This salt is the standard by which other iron salts are measured. Large quantities of vitamin C increase absorption of iron. Constipation and gastric upset are the most frequent adverse effects of iron supplements. Iron-deficient persons who require full therapeutic doses should start with one tablet daily and gradually increase to the full adult dose of three tablets daily. Most persons can tolerate the 40 to 50 mg of elemental iron required. There may be a vast difference in cost for various iron preparations, but there is little if any therapeutic benefit to the more expensive forms.

If ferrous sulfate causes sufficient gastric irritation to be intolerable, ferrous succinate, lactate, fumerate, glycine sulfate, glutamate and gluconate are absorbed almost as well as the sulfate form, but none are clearly superior. Ferric iron salts, however, are less well absorbed.

Although ascorbic acid increases absorption of iron, preparations that combine iron with vitamin C, molybdenum, copper, cobalt, folic acid and vitamin B_{12} are more expensive and may have some other disadvantages. Enteric-coated and timed-release iron preparations should be avoided, because they release the iron in the area of the small intestine with a lower rate of absorption, or may pass through the intestine too quickly to be absorbed at all.

Liquid iron preparations are available for children and the dosage requirement is generally half the adult dose for weights from 30 to 80 pounds of body weight and full adult dose over 80 pounds. Liquid iron sulfate should be sipped through a straw to prevent staining of the teeth. It is essential to take iron supplements for a minimum of six to 12 months to provide for the replenishment of the body iron stores that are diminished in the presence of anemia. In the case of chronic blood loss, continuous iron supplementation may be necessary.

Iron dextran (Imferon) injections are rarely required and should be reserved for those persons who are unable to tolerate or absorb oral tablets. Those conditions that may require the intramuscular or intravenous routes for giving iron include: malabsorption disorders such as ulcerative colitis, Crohn's disease, colostomy or ileostomy patients or those rare persons whose iron stores are so severely depleted that large amounts of iron must be administered urgently. Rarely, large doses of injected iron dextran have been reported to cause formation of a sarcoma, a form of malignant tumor. Therefore, injectable iron should be reserved for those persons whose need is absolute.

Toxicity

In normal persons, the possibility of iron toxicity from food sources is remote. In the past there were reports of poisoning from home brews made in iron vessels. However, there are approximately 2,000 cases of iron poisoning in the United States each year from supplements. Most of these occur accidently in children. Three grams of ferrous sulfate, or about nine tablets, can cause death in a two-year-old child.

Primary hemochromatosis is an inherited metabolic disorder in which excessive iron accumulates in the tissues, causing cirrhosis of the liver, congestive heart failure and bronze pigmentation of the skin. Less commonly, there are several acquired forms, one of which can occur from excessive blood transfusions (see HEMOCHROMATOSIS).

Iron supplements cause a grayish-black stool that should be distinguished from the black, tarlike stool that occurs from a bleeding ulcer.

ironweed A flowering perennial, *Veronica fasciculata*, of the Compositae family, found on prairies, riverbanks and roadsides in the eastern, southern and some western parts of the United States, whose bitter root and leaves are used in Native American medicine as treatment for various gynecological problems, chills and bilious fever, scrofula, dyspepsia and syphilis.

isoniazid Antimicrobial drug used in the treatment of tuberculosis. However, peripheral neuritis is a common adverse affect that can be prevented by taking pyridoxine (vitamin B_6).

ivy American (woodbine, Virginia creeper, wild wood vine) A flowering, fruit-bearing vine, *Vitis quinquefolia*, of the Vitaceae (grape) family, considered in Native American and homeopathic medicine to be a tonic, expectorant and astringent. The bark and twigs are prepared as a syrup, which is prescribed for scrofula, dropsy, cholera, hoarseness, hydrocele and lung diseases.

ixora Evergreen trees or shrubs, both cultivated and wild, of the Rubiaceae family, such as *Ixora chinensis*, named after a Malabar (from the Malabar Coast, a region of southwest India) god and used by Chinese practitioners to treat rheumatism, pain, abscesses and contusions.

jalap An annual vine, *Ipomoea jalapa,* of the Convolvulaceae family, native to Mexico (Xalapa), with a tuberous root that is used in herbal medicine as a carthartic.

See also IPOMOEA.

Japanese turf lily (dwarf lilyturf, creeping lily root) The plant *Ophiopogon japonicus,* of the Liliaceae family, whose bulbs are considered a nutritive "Yin tonic" by herbalists. Turf lily is prescribed for dryness in the body (membranes lacking moisture), dry cough, asthma, insomnia, anxiety and paranoia. Yin represents darkness, cold and wetness in Chinese cosmology. Also considered the "feminine passive" principle in nature, yin combines with yang ("masculine active") to produce all life.

jasmine (yellow jessamine, yasamin) A fragrant, flowering shrub, *Jasminum officinale,* of the Oleaceae family, whose oil extract is used in perfumes and whose flowers are used in herbal medicine as a calmative. In Ayurvedic medicine, jasmine flowers are also thought to promote menses and to act as an alterative, refrigerant and nervine.

Javanese turmeric See TURMERIC.

jimson weed (stinkweed, mad-apple, stinkwort, devil's trumpet, Jamestown weed, nightshade, thornapple, apple Peru) Annual shrubs and trees of the Solanaceae (nightshade) family, especially the flowering, malodorous *Datura stramonium,* found largely in North and South American fields, gardens, waterfronts and waste areas. Early American colonists discovered jimson weed growing on ship rubbish near Jamestown, Virginia, and called it "Jamestown weed." While jimson weed leaves and seeds may be considered an opium substitute for cases of epilepsy, delirium tremens, mania and general pain, herbalists have pronounced the plant dangerous. An overdose may be fatal. Tincture of jimson weed has been prescribed for hiccough, meningitis, hydrophobia, tetanus, typhus, chorea, catalepsy, apoplexy, angina pectoris, sun headache, enuresis, chronic laryngitis, spasmodic cough and asthma. Jimson weed cigarettes have been used by smokers with asthma.

External uses of the plant by Native Americans include placing crushed leaves and seeds on bruises, saddle sores and swellings and rattlesnake and tarantula bites. The plant, found in varying amounts in hay, is poisonous to horses, cattle and geese.

In October 1994, an outbreak of jimson weed use by teenagers in New Jersey, Connecticut and New York was reported in local newspapers. In New Jersey, the possession or ingestion of jimson weed is illegal, punishable by a maximum of $1,000 fine and six months in jail. One 14-year-old boy became severely ill after eating 30 to 60 jimson weed seeds, and other youngsters had to be hospitalized after eating or smoking the weed.

Not considered a narcotic, the poisonous jimson weed contains toxic chemical properties called alkaloids, which attack the body's central nervous system. Possible adverse effects include hallucinations, tachycardia, dry mouth, blurred vision, elevated body temperature, seizures and other problems that may be life-threatening.

The English settlers of Jamestown used to boil the spring sprouts of jimson weed and eat them as a vegetable. This caused hallucinations and strange, silly behavior that escalated in a matter of days to self-destructive behavior, choking and wallowing in their own waste. The victims were then confined.

jin bu huan   An herb used in traditional Chinese medicine for relief of insomnia and pain. Life-threatening heart irregularities have been reported in children ingesting from seven to 60 tablets of jin bu huan. Cases of hepatitis have also been attributed to this herb.

juglans (English walnut, Persian walnut)   An Asian and European fruit-bearing tree, *Juglans regia,* of the Juglandaceae family, named from the Latin *Jovis glans* (nut of Jupiter) and considered by the Ancient Greeks and Romans to be a symbol of fertility. Chinese practitioners and other herbalists use the walnut's kernels as a tonic and to increase the flow of urine and the kernel oil to treat intestinal worms and skin diseases. Originally, the walnut was thought to resemble the brain and thus was used in various ways to treat brain disorders.

Walnuts, commonly eaten as snack food or used as an ingredient in spreads, desserts, stuffings and many other foods, contain fats, protein and, like other nuts, the B-complex vitamins niacin, thiamine and riboflavin, and the minerals calcium, iron, copper, manganese and phosphorus.

juncus (bog rush, Japanese-mat rush)   A Japanese, Chinese, Korean and North American plant, *Juncus effusus* or *decipiens,* of the Juncaceae family, used in the making of tatami floor mats and lampwicks. In Chinese medicine, juncus pith is prescribed for the treatment of cough, pharyngitis, memory loss, insomnia and anxiety.

juniper (hapusha)   A North American, European and Asian flowering, fruit-bearing evergreen shrub, *Juniperus communis* and *oxycedrus,* of the Cupressaceae family, used in Chinese herbal medicine to treat bleeding and coughs. Other herbalists use juniper berries and twigs in preparations for the treatment of gastrointestinal cramps, gas, inflammations and infections, gout and rheumatism, tuberculosis and other ailments. In Ayurvedic medicine, juniper berries of various species of the Coniferae family, are used as a diuretic, diaphoretic, carminative and analgesic.

K, vitamin (phytonadione, vitamin K₁; menadione, vitamin K₃) A group of compounds with a common basic structure that act as a cofactor for the enzyme system essential for normal blood-clotting. Since vitamin K is produced by bacteria in the intestines, it does not strictly fit the definition of a vitamin. Only about half of the daily requirement is satisfied by intestinal flora. Dietary sources are necessary to prevent vitamin K deficiency. Vitamin K is also found in various foods of plant origin (see Table 21).

Actions

Under normal conditions, in the presence of bile, pancreatic juice and dietary fat, vitamin K is absorbed from the jejunum and ileum of the small bowel. Once absorbed, vitamin K is transported in lymphatic fluid to the liver, where it is concentrated and then widely distributed to body tissues.

In the tissues, vitamin K is associated with cell membranes, most importantly with endoplasmic reticulum and mitochondria. Normally 30 to 40 percent of absorbed vitamin K is excreted in the feces and 15 percent in the urine as metabolic products.

In the liver, vitamin K plays an important role in the actions of prothrombin (coagulation factor II), factors VII, IX, X and proteins C, S and Z. Although these proteins are still synthesized in the absence of vitamin K, they are inactive. In the presence of vitamin K, prothrombin is converted to thrombin, an enzyme. Thrombin in turn converts fibrinogen to fibrin to form a blood clot.

Other proteins that depend on vitamin K are found in bone, kidney and other tissues. Combining with calcium, these proteins help in the formation of bone crystal. Possibly they play a role in the synthesis of some phospholipids and may serve other functions.

The drug warfarin (Coumadin) is the most commonly prescribed oral anticoagulant whose action is based on its ability to counter the effects of vitamin K. Related compounds are the basis for some rat poisons that cause rats to bleed to death. Vitamin K does not reverse overdoses of the injectable anticoagulant heparin.

Vitamin Requirements

The primary criterion for determining the adequacy of vitamin K in humans is based on the maintenance of adequate prothrombin concentrations. Studies have demonstrated that individuals deprived of dietary sources of vitamin K develop clotting problems that can be corrected with resumption of an adequate diet or supplementation of vitamin K. Because there is synthesis of vitamin K by bacteria in the gut of vitamin K-deprived individuals, there is a need for dietary sources of the vitamin.

Studies have also shown that a dietary intake of about 1 mcg per kilogram (1 kilogram = 2.2 pounds) of body weight daily maintains normal blood clotting in healthy adults. Therefore the Recommended Dietary Allowance, or RDA, for a 79-kilogram (174-pound) male is 80 mcg per day and 65 mcg for a 63-kilogram (139-pound) woman.

Ill elderly patients with inadequate prothrombin respond to vitamin K supplementation, but a well-nourished, healthy geriatric population does not appear to need supplements. Trauma, physical dehabilitation, kidney failure and prolonged use of broad-spectrum antibiotics may cause vitamin K deficiency. Antibiotics often destroy the normal intestinal bacterial flora (which synthesize vitamin K) along with the pathogenic (disease-causing) germs. Malabsorption syndromes such as celiac disease disrupt the absorption of adequate vitamin

K from the gut. A relative deficiency may occur in the presence of excessive doses of other fat-soluble vitamins A, D or E.

There are insufficient data to establish the RDA during pregnancy or lactation. The diets of pregnant and lactating females appear to exceed the RDA established for adult women. Therefore no supplementation is recommended.

A healthy newborn infant has low plasma prothrombin levels, and levels in premature infants may be inadequate to prevent hemorrhage. Newborn infants are now routinely give 0.5 to 1.0 mg of vitamin K by intramuscular injection. Pre-term infants are given 1 mg or more. The dose may be repeated in one week if needed. Breast-fed infants, especially those delivered at home, may be especially prone to vitamin K deficiency. An intake of 5 mcg of vitamin K as phylloquinone or menaquinone per day is recommended for the first six months of life and 10 mcg during the second six months. The recommended amount in infant formulas is 4 mcg of vitamin K per 100 kcal.

RDA for older children is the same as adults, 1 mcg per kilogram of body weight.

Dietary Sources

Green leafy vegetables, some legumes and vegetable oils are the best dietary sources of vitamin K. However, vegetable oils lose much of their vitamin K content when exposed to light. Higher amounts of vitamin K are found in the outer leaves of vegetables while lower amounts are found in inner leaves. Climate and soil conditions may influence amounts of vitamin K in foods. Lesser amounts are found in milk and other dairy products, meats, eggs, cereals, fruits and vegetables. Breast milk is relatively poor in vitamin K content.

In the United States, the usual healthy adult diet contains an average of 300 to 500 mcg of vitamin K. Some studies suggest that these amounts are overestimated. Although a survey demonstrated that only one in 12 persons in the United States consumed green leafy vegetables on a specific day in 1977, deficiencies in Americans appear to be rare.

Preparations

There are several structurally different analogues of vitamin K. Phytonadione, or vitamin K_1, has the quickest onset of action and the most prolonged duration, and it is the most potent of all vitamin K products. It is also safer for newborns than menadione, vitamin K_3.

Toxicity and Other Adverse Effects

With the exception of patients requiring anticoagulants (in which case excessive vitamin K may neutralize the drug's effectiveness), there appears to be no deleterious effect from ingestion of large amounts of oral vitamin K.

Intravenous injections of phytonadione can cause flushing of the face, excessive perspiration, chest tightness, cyanosis, vascular collapse and shock, and severe allergic reactions, including fatal anaphylaxis. Administration of menadione to a person with glucose-6-phosphate dehydrogenase (G6PD) deficiency (a genetic disorder of metabolism) or to newborns may cause hemolytic anemia (destruction of red blood cells) and jaundice. These conditions do not occur with the use of phytonadione. Despite studies questioning the safety of vitamin K administered to newborns, scientists at the National Institute of Child Health and Human Development have concluded that there is no apparent association between vitamin K given to prevent bleeding disorders in infants and an increased risk of childhood cancers.

Herbal teas may contain coumarin derivatives, such as tonka beans, melilot, or sweet clover, and sweet woodruff, which may be dangerous in patients taking anticoagulants such as warfarin (Coumadin).

kaempferia An Old World tropical herb, *Kaempferia galanga,* of the Zingiberaceae family, whose rhizomes (underground stems) are used by Chinese practitioners to treat constipation, angina pectoris, headache, toothache and cholera. Kaempferia also serves as a flavoring agent for rice and as an ingredient in cosmetics.

kalanchoe (air plant, Mexican love plant, life plant, good luck leaf) A pantropic (though mainly African) plant, *Kalanchoe pinnata,* of the Crassulaceae family, whose leaves are used in Chinese medicine to treat coughs, headache, skin diseases and other ailments.

TABLE 21 PROVISIONAL TABLE ON THE VITAMIN K₁
CONTENT OF COMMON FOODS

Food (estimated portions)†	Vitamin K₁ (mcg/100 gm) Median (range)	Food (estimated portions)†	Vitamin K₁ (mcg/100 gm) Median (range)
Abalone (3½ oz.)	23	Cheese, cheddar (3½ oz.)	3 (2–3)
Algae		Cabbage	
Green laver	4	Raw (1½ cups shredded)	145 (46–584)*
Purple laver	1,385	Red, raw (1½ cups shredded)	44 (30–57)*
Konbu	66	Sauerkraut (1 cup)	25
Hijiki	327	Turnip	2
Amaranth, raw leaf	1,140	Cantaloupe, fresh (⅔ cups pieces)	1
Apple		Carrots	
Fleshy portion only (1 medium)	0.4 (0.1–0.7)	Raw (1⅓ medium)	5 (4–11)*
Green peel	60	Cooked (⅔ cup slices)	18
Red peel	20	Cauliflower	
Apple juice (3½ fl. oz.)	0.1 (0.01–0.2)	Raw (1 cup)	5
Applesauce (½ cup)	0.5	Cooked (1 cup)	10
Apricots, canned with skin (4 halves)	5	Celery, raw (2½ stalks)	12 (5–18)
Artichoke, globe (1 very small)	14	Cereal	
Asatsuki, leaf	190	Bran flakes (2½ cups)	2
Ashitaba, leaf	590	Corn flakes (4 cups)	0.04
Asparagus, raw (7 spears)	40	Puffed rice (7 cups)	0.08
Avocado, peeled (1 small)	40	Puffed wheat (7 cups)	2
Banana, raw (1 medium)	0.5	Shredded wheat (4 oz.)	0.7
Basella, raw leaf	160	Total brand (4 oz.)	0.7
Beans (½ cup)		Chayote	
Blackeyed, dry	5	Raw leaf	200
Kidney, dry	19	Cooked leaf (½ cup pieces)	270
Lentil, dry	22	Chicken meat, raw (3½ oz.)	0.1 (0.01–0.2)
Lima, dry	6	Chili con carne (3½ oz.)	2
Navy, dry	2	Chingentsuai, raw green	120
Pinto, dry	10	Chive, raw (33 Tbsp. chopped)	190 (130–250)
Soybean, dry	47	Chrysanthemum, garland	350
Soybean, dry, roasted	37	Clam (4 large or 10 small)	0.2
Beans, pod, raw (1 cup)	47 (40–60)*	Coffee (10 cups brewed beverage)	10 (<0.005–20)
Beef, ground, regular, raw (3 1/2 oz.)	0.5 (0.3–0.5)	Cola	
Beet, raw (½ cup)	3 (0–5)	Regular (3½ fl. oz.)	<0.005
Bell tree dahlia		Diet (3½ fl. oz.)	<0.005
Raw leaf	630	Coleslaw (¾ cup)	57
Cooked leaf	1,110	Coriander	
Blueberries, canned (⅔ cup)	6	Raw leaf (6¼ cups)	310
Bread, assorted types (4 slices)	3	Cooked leaf	1,510
Broccoli, raw (½ cup)	205 (147–230)	Corn, sweet, raw (½ cup)	0.5
Broccoli, cooked (½ cup)	270	Crackers	
Brussels sprouts, sprout (5 sprouts)	177 (175–300)	Graham (14 crackers)	0.5
Brussels sprouts, top leaf (5 sprouts)	438 (400–475)	Saltines (33 crackers)	2
Butter (6 Tbsp.)	7 (6–8)	Cranberry juice (3½ fl. oz.)	<0.005
Butterfly bream (3½ oz.)	0.2	Cranberry sauce (⅓ cup)	1

TABLE 21 PROVISIONAL TABLE ON THE VITAMIN K₁
CONTENT OF COMMON FOODS (continued)

Food (estimated portions)†	Vitamin K₁ (mcg/100 gm) Median (range)	Food (estimated portions)†	Vitamin K₁ (mcg/100 gm) Median (range)
Cucumber		Milk, cow	
Raw (1 cup slices)	19 (5–50)*	Chocolate, 2% fat (3½ fl. oz.)	0.4
Raw, peel only	360	Dry, whole (1 cup)	2
Fleshy portion only	2	Skim (3½ fl. oz.)	0.02 (0.01–0.03)
Eel (3½ oz.)	0.02	Whole, 3.5% fat (3½ fl. oz.)	0.3
Egg		Millet, dry (3½ oz.)	0.9
Yolk (5 large)	2 (0.01–4)	Mint	
White (3 large)	0.01 (0–0.02)	Raw leaf	230
Eggplant, raw (1¼ cups pieces)	0.5	Cooked leaf	860
Endive, raw (2 cups chopped)	231	Mituba, raw leaf & stalk	370
Flour (1 cup)		Miso, dry (½ cup)	11
Barley	1	Mushroom, raw (1½ cups)	0.02 (0.02–<1)
Buckwheat	7	Mustard greens, raw (1½ cups)	170
Rice	0.04	Nightshade	
Wheat	0.6 (0.1–1)*	Raw leaf	620
Fruit cocktail, canned (1/2 cup)	0.8	Cooked leaf	700
Fruit spread, assorted flavors	0.5	Oatmeal, instant, dry (1 cup)	3
Fungi		Octopus (3½ oz.)	0.07
Shitake, raw	0	Oils (7 Tbsp.)	
Shimeji	0	Almond	7
Nameko	0	Canola (Rapeseed)	141
Ginger ale		Corn	3
Regular (3½ fl. oz.)	0.01	Olive	49 (42–55)
Diet (3½ fl. oz.)	<0.005	Peanut	0.7
Grape juice (3½ fl. oz.)	0.2	Safflower	11 (9–12)
Grapes, fresh (1 cup)	3	Salad	148
Grapefruit, fresh (½ medium)	0.02	Sesame	10 (5–15)
Grapefruit juice (3½ fl. oz.)	0.2 (0.02–0.3)	Soybean	193
Honey (5 Tbs.)	0.02(0.01–0.02)	Sunflower	9
Horse, meat (3½ oz.)	2	Walnut	15
Itohiki-natto	10	Onions, (⅔ cup, chopped)	
Kaiwaredaikon, raw leaf	80	White, raw	2 (0.2–5)*
Kale, raw leaf (¾ cup)	817 (724–1139)*	Green scallion, raw	207 (170–243)
Kiwi fruit (1 medium)	25	Welsh (white)	5
Komatsuna, raw leaf	280	Welsh (green)	243
Leek, raw (1 cup chopped)	14 (10–18)	Orange, fleshy portion (1 medium)	0.1 (0.01–0.1)
Lemon, fresh (2 medium)	0.2	Orange juice, fresh (3½ fl. oz.)	0.1 (0.04–0.1)
Lemonade (3½ fl. oz.)	0.03	Osh, raw leaf	310
Lettuce (1¾ cups, shredded)		Oyster (7 medium)	0.1
Raw, heading & bib	122 (70–850)*	Pacific Saury (3½ oz.)	0.02
Red, leaf	210	Parsley	
Mackerel (3½ oz.)	5	Raw leaf (1½ cups chopped)	540 (350–730)
Malabar gourd, raw leaf	22	Cooked leaf	900
Margarine (7 Tbsp.)	51 (4–97)*	Parsnip	1
Mayonnaise (7 Tbsp.)	81	Pea	
Meatloaf (3½ oz.)	6	Raw	36 (33–39)*

Food (estimated portions)†	Vitamin K₁ (mcg/100 gm) Median (range)	Food (estimated portions)†	Vitamin K₁ (mcg/100 gm) Median (range)
Parsnip		Sardine (3½ oz.)	0.09
Pod, raw	25 (20–50)	Sesame seed, dry (11 Tbsp.)	8 (2–14)*
Green, cooked (⅔ cup)	23	Sour cream (8 Tbsp.)	1
Peaches		Soy milk (3½ oz.)	3 (2–5)*
raw (1 medium)	3 (2–3)	Spaghetti, dry (3½ oz.)	0.2
Peanut, raw (1)	0.2	Spaghetti sauce, meat-based (4 oz.)	4
Peanut butter (6 Tbsp.)	10	Spinach	
Pear, canned (½ cup)	0.5	Raw, leaf (1½ cups)	400 (240–1,220)*
Pecan, dry	10	Raw, stalk	6
Pepper, raw, green (1 cup, chopped)	17 (2–30)*	Squid (3½ oz.)	0.02
Perilla, raw, leaf	650	Squash, summer	
Pickle, dill (1 medium)	26	Fleshy portion	3 (1–4)
Pineapple, fresh (½ cup, pieces)	0.1	Peel only	80
Pineapple juice, canned (3½ fl. oz.)	0.7	Swiss chard, raw leaf	830
Pistachio nut (170 nuts)	70	Tea	
Plum, fresh, raw (2 medium)	12	Black, brewed (3½ oz.)	0.05
Pork, meat (3½ oz.)	0.07 (0.03–0.1)	Black, leaves (Dry)	262
Potato, baked flesh and skin (1 med)	4	Decaffeinated, brewed (3½ oz.)	0.03
Potato, baked skin only	0.3	Green, leaves (Dry)	1428
Potato, sweet, canned (1 cup)	4	Tofu (½ cup)	2
Potato, raw (1 potato)	0.8 (0.2–4)*	Tomato	
Potato chips (4 oz.)	10	Ripe (1 tomato)	6 (6–7)*
Potato, french fries (20 pieces)	5	Juice, canned (3½ fl. oz.)	4 (2–6)*
Prawn (3½ oz.)	0.03	Sauces (3½ fl. oz.)	7 (1–13)
Pretzel (4 oz.)	1	Top shell	3
Prune juice, canned (3½ fl. oz.)	0.6	Toumyao (Chinese)	380
Pumpkin, canned (½ cup)	16	Tuna, bluefin (3½ oz.)	0.03
Purslane, raw	381	Turkey, meat (3½ oz.)	0.02
Radish, raw (22 radishes)	0.1	Turnip	
Rice, white (½ cup)	1 (0.05–2)*	Raw	0.09 (0.09–<1)
Rice cake	0.6	Greens, raw (1½ cups, chopped)	251 (192–310)*
Roctish		Tziton, raw leaf	250
Raw leaf	290	Watercress, raw (3 cups)	250 (88–390)*
Cooked leaf	420	Wine (3½ oz.)	<0.005
Sake (3½ fl. oz.)	<0.005	Yellowtail, young (3½ oz.)	0.08
Salmon, pink (3½ oz.)	0.4	Yogurt	
Samat		Low fat (3½ oz.)	0.3 (0.2–0.3)
Raw leaf	350	Fruit flavored (3½ oz.)	0.7
Cooked leaf	960		

Source: Booth S. L., Sadowski J. A., Weihrauch J. L., Ferland G. Vitamin K₁ (Phylloquinone) Content of Foods: A provisional table. *J Food Comp Anal* 1993; 6:109–20.

†Calculated based on estimated portions to equal 100 gm from Pennington J. A., Church H. N.: *Food Values of Portions Commonly Used,* 14th & 15 Editions, J. P. Lippincott Company, 1985.

*More reliable in comparison to the other data based on the analytical quality control criteria.

(Table from Coumadin Patient Guide used with permission from DuPont-Pharm.)

kale A hardy cabbage, *Brassica oleracea acephala,* of the Cruciferae family, eaten as a vegetable or taken in tablet form as a supplement mainly for its calcium, vitamin A, ascorbic acid, thiamine, riboflavin, niacin and folacin content. The particularly high calcium content (common to dark-green leafy vegetables) has been recognized as an anti-colon-cancer agent, an antistress mineral, often called "nature's tranquilizer," and a preventive against osteoporosis in certain women.

Kamut A registered trademark of Kamut International, Ltd., used in marketing products made with an organically grown grain that is an ancient relative of durum wheat. Twice the size of common wheat, with 20 to 40 percent more protein and higher in lipids, amino acids, vitamins and minerals, Kamut provides a sweet alternative for all products that now use common wheat. New clinical studies measuring the allergenic reactivity of Kamut-brand grain products have significant implications. Many people allergic to common wheat (*Triticum vulgare*) are not allergic to a variety of wheat that is an ancient relative of durum wheat (*Triticum durum*) and is now being marketed under the Kamut trademark. This data is relevant to a growing population segment with restricted culinary choices. According to the National Institutes of Health, more than 35 million Americans suffer from food allergies, and allergic reactions to wheat are one of the most common. Eileen Yoder, Ph.D., president of the International Food Allergy Association, heads a team of physicians and scientists in the Chicago area conducting the Kamut-brand product testing. After six months of study Dr. Yoder concluded, "For most wheat-sensitive people, Kamut brand products can be an excellent substitute for common wheat." To reach this conclusion, Dr. Yoder and her team worked with two different wheat-sensitive populations—those who have immediate immune responses and those with delayed immune responses. People with immediate reactions—which may be as life-threatening as anaphylactic shock—are, fortunately, a small percentile (10 percent) of the food-sensitive population. People with less severe delayed allergic reactions comprise about 90 percent of the food allergy population.

For the delayed allergic reactions population, the Radioallergosorbent Test (IgG RAST), an in vitro assay, was employed to determine immunological reactions to Kamut-brand products and common wheat products. IgE skin testing was also administered. One hundred randomly selected food-allergy patients were tested by these methods. It was concluded that a remarkably high percentage, 70 percent, showed greater sensitivity to common wheat products than to Kamut-brand products.

Source: "Nutritional Analysis of Kamut Brand Grain," http:/www.kamut.com/index.html, downloaded 6 April 2003.

katphala See BAYBERRY.

kava kava (kawa) A Polynesian herb, *Piper methysticum,* of the Piperaceae family, whose root is considered a remedy for insomnia and anxiety by herbal medicine practitioners. It is also prescribed as a painkiller and, because it has antiseptic and diuretic properties, for urinary tract infections. Regular use of kava kava, however, may cause toxins to build up in the liver.

Pippali, an Ayurvedic medicine (*Piper longum,* of the same family as kava kava) is said to be an expectorant, stimulant and aphrodisiac. The Sanskrit word *pippali* means "long pepper."

kelp A variety of brown seaweeds of the order Laminariales, found largely in cold and temperate seas, and whose ashes are recognized as a source of iodine, potash and soda. Iodine is an essential component of thyroxine, the active substance produced in the thyroid gland. Kelp in tablet or other supplemental form is helpful in any iodine deficiency, including hypothyroidism and goiter.

Kempner's Rice Diet A treatment for psoriasis, hypertension and renal disease developed by American physician Walter Kempner. This diet, consisting of only rice, fruit juices and sugar with vitamin and iron supplements, is generally considered a nutritionally poor diet with no therapeutic value.

Keshan disease A type of cardiomyopathy, a form of heart disease primarily occurring in children on a selenium-poor diet. First recognized by Chinese scientists in 1979, in areas with soil poor in selenium, such as parts of China, New Zealand and Finland.

See also SELENIUM.

khus-khus (vetiver) A tropical and subtropical Asian and East Indies perennial grass, *Vetiveria zizanioides,* whose aromatic root is made into a tea considered to be a general tonic.

kidney disorders and vitamin requirements The process of renal dialysis removes metabolic products derived from ascorbic acid (vitamin C), folic acid and pyridoxine (vitamin B$_6$). One hundred to 300 percent of the Recommended Daily Allowance (RDA) of the nutrients should be given to renal-dialysis patients. With the possible exception of vitamin E, there are no other increased needs for vitamin supplementation with dialysis.

kidney liver leaf (choisy, noble liverwort) A flowering, evergreen plant, *Hepatica americana* and *nobilis,* of the Ranunculaceae family, used in Native American herbal medicine as a liver tonic and remedy of liver diseases. Homeopathic medicine also prescribes liver leaf for bronchitis, sore throat and dyspepsia.

knotweed (bian xu, knotgrass, pigweed, birdweed, beggarweed, crawlgrass, ninety-knot) An annual plant, *Polygonum aviculare,* cultivated throughout the world and whose flowering herb is used by herbalists as a remedy for diarrhea, dysentery, enteritis, bronchitis and other respiratory problems, jaundice, internal bleeding (including bleeding stomach ulcers), cholera infantum and other ailments.

In addition, *Polygonum hydropiper* and *punctatum,* also called smartweed, are used in decoctions for hemorrhoids and scabies, as well as for gargle and rubefacient, a local irritant that produces reddening of the skin for therapeutic purposes.

knoxia An Asian Indian herb, *Knoxia corymbosa,* of the Rubiaceae family, whose tuberous root is used in Chinese medicine for inflammation,

abdominal dropsy and excretory-system problems. The herb is named for R. Knox of Sri Lanka.

kola nut Native to West Africa, the seed of the *Cola acuminata* tree was once one of the two active ingredients in the original Coca-Cola soft drink. The other ingredient was coca, also known as cocaine, derived from dried leaves of the shrub *Erythroxylum coca*. According to American author W. Poundstone, kola nut still is one of the ingredients in Coke and Pepsi-Cola. The kola nut's active substances are caffeine, kolanin and theobromine. Kola nut is a stimulant in the digestive tract and for the combustion of body lipids and a mild aphrodisiac.

See also KOLA TREE.

kola tree (cola, kola nut, caffeine nut, guru nut) A South American, West African and West Indies tree, *Cola acuminata,* of the family Sterculiaceae, whose nuts contain caffeine and flavoring agents used in pharmaceutical preparations and in carbonated beverages. Caffeine, recognized by the United States Pharmacopoeia (USP), is an alkaloid that acts as a stimulant to the central nervous system, the stomach, fatty acids in plasma and basal metabolic rate. Caffeine, also a diuretic, decreases sleep time, may increase blood-sugar level and enhances endurance and reaction time in athletes.

Herbal medicine practitioners prescribe kola nut seeds as a cardiac tonic, pain reliever (especially of neuralgia and migraine) and antidepressant.

While caffeine is found in coffee, tea, chocolate and cola drinks, and in Anacin, Excedrin and other over-the-counter medicines, it is also available in pill or tablet form under the brand names Vivarin and No-Doz specifically for antifatigue use.

An excess of 250 mg is usually considered an overdose of caffeine that may lead to caffeine intoxication (caffeinism). Symptoms include restlessness, flushing, frequent urination, twitching, increased heart rate and/or irregularities, agitation and other problems. Delirium, convulsions, nausea, vomiting and respiratory and cardiovascular collapse may result. Treatment may include gastric lavage and the administration of phenobarbital or diazepam, and cardiopulmonary resuscitation (CPR).

Korsakoff's syndrome See ALCOHOLISM; THIAMINE.

kousso   An Ethiopian flowering tree, *Hagenia abyssinica*, whose flowers are used in herbal medicine as an anthelmintic, especially for tapeworms.

Krebs, Ernst   See AMYGDALIN.

kudzu (kuzu, ge gen)   An herb, *Radix puerariae*, containing varying quantities of the chemical daidzin in its roots, leaves and flowers. Listed in the Chinese pharmacopeia about 1,400 years ago, kudzu is reported to reduce the craving for alcohol in abusers. Studies on Syrian Golden hamsters, one of the rare instances of animals who prefer drinking alcohol to water, demonstrated a markedly decreased desire to drink alcohol in those given the extract or purified daidzin.

The root of the kudzu plant *Pueraria thunbergiana* yields a concentrated starch that is often used as a thickener in foods and for its high mineral content in tea and soup for sufferers of flu, colds and gastrointestinal ailments.

In Chinese medicine, pueraria root, or *ge gen*, is from the *Pueraria lobata* plant and used to treat chills, fever, poor circulation, high blood pressure, excessive thirst and muscle ache.

Ayurvedic practitioners use kudzu, of the *Pueraria tuberosa* plant of the Leguminosae family, as a tonic, diuretic and diaphoretic.

kumari   See ALOE.

labeling requirements   See Appendix VII.

Labrador tea (wild rosemary, continental tea, marsh tea)   A North American evergreen shrub, *Ledum latifolium,* of the Ericaceae family, whose leaves are made into a tea and considered by Native American herbalists to be therapeutic in the treatment of respiratory infections. Homeopaths prescribe a tincture of the entire plant or of the leaves and dried twigs for asthma, gout, intoxication, tuberculosis, varicella, tinnitus, ear inflammation, deafness, foot and joint pain and, in a decoction used externally, for problems including eczema, pediculosis, prickly heat and other skin eruptions and wounds. Practitioners of folk medicine also use Labrador tea for headache, stomachache, diarrhea, rickets and urinary tract weakness, among other problems.

lacto-ovo vegetarian   Person whose diet includes vegetables, milk products and eggs, but who avoids meat, seafood and poultry.
   See also VEGETARIAN DIETS.

lactovegetarian   Person who eats vegetables and milk products, but avoids eggs, meat, fish and poultry.
   See also VEGETARIAN DIETS.

lady's mantle   A North American, European, northern Asian and Greenland flowering perennial, *Alchemilla vulgaris* or *xanthochlora,* of the Rosaceae family, whose aerial portion is prepared as a tea and used by herbalists to treat menstrual problems, rheumatism, gastrointestinal disturbances, poor appetite and external problems including wounds.

Silvery lady's mantle, or *Alchemilla alpina,* is used as lady's mantle is, and for the treatment of intestinal gas.

lady's slipper (nerve root, yellow moccasin flower, Noah's ark)   European, Asian, tropical and North American orchids (Orchidaceae family), especially *Cypripedium pubescens,* whose root is valued by Native American, Ayurvedic and other herbalists and homeopaths as a nervine, tonic and antiperiodic. Lady's slipper is used as a tincture, decoction or infusion for pain relief and the treatment of anxiety, nervous headache, nervous depression and restlessness, hysteria, chorea, nervous stomach, fever, convulsions, delirium tremens, epilepsy, neuralgia, stye and other ailments.

laetrile   See AMYGDALIN.

larch   An American and European tree, *Larix europaea,* of the pine family, whose bark, resin, young shoots and needles are used by herbal practitioners to make a diuretic extract and a decoction that may be added to bath water as a stimulant. The resin, called "Venice turpentine," derives its reputation from its use in European folk medicine whereby a certain number of drops mixed with honey are used against tapeworm, suppressed menses and bloody diarrhea.

larkspur (knight's spur, lar's heel, lark's claw)   A European and North American flowering annual herb, *Delphinium consolida,* of the Ranunculaceae family, whose roots and seeds have been considered medicinal by Native American, Russian, folk-medicine herbalists and others, although extremely cautious use is advised by these practitioners because delphinium is poisonous. Limited amounts of preparations made from the larkspur herb, flower and other parts may be effective in the treatment of cramps, pleurisy, headache, convulsions, amenorrhea, Parkinson's disease, paralysis and other ailments.

laurel (bay leaves, bay laurel, sweet bay, Indian bay, Roman or Grecian laurel) An evergreen bush or tree originally cultivated near the Mediterranean Sea, *Laurus nobilis,* of the Lauraceae family, whose leaves are used in Ayurvedic medicine as a carminative, stimulant and expectorant, and by other herbalists to promote digestion.

lavender A shrub, *Lavandula vera, officinalis* and *angustifolia,* of the Labiatae family, originally from the Mediterranean area and cultivated in Europe and the United States for its aromatic flowers. In Ayurvedic medicine, lavender is used as a carminative, diuretic and antispasmodic. Other practitioners also consider lavender an antidepressant, nervine, tonic, stimulant and stomachic. Flowers and leaves are used in oil preparations for flatulence, migraine, vertigo and fainting. European herbalists find lavender an effective appetite stimulant and reliever of colic. Lavender is also a main ingredient in the Chinese medicinal oil known as "white flower oil," prescribed for headache, nervousness, upset stomach and other problems. It is also used as an external treatment of insect bites (lavender contains insect- and moth-repelling camphor), cuts and bruises. Lavender tea is considered a vermifuge, an agent that eliminates intestinal worms.

laxatives' effects on nutrients Mineral oil binds to fat-soluble vitamins A, D, E and K and linoleic acid, an essential fatty acid. This binding prevents absorption of the nutrients as they pass through the intestine and are lost in the stool. Chronic use of laxatives could result in deficiencies of these vitamins, especially night blindness from lack of vitamin A, bone disorders from inadequate vitamin D and hemorrhage from insufficient vitamin K.

Other laxatives also effect changes in the intestinal mucosa, or lining, causing poor or inadequate absorption of not only the fat-soluble vitamins but also other vitamins and minerals.

lead A metallic element, known in Latin as *plumbum,* whose compounds are poisonous. It is unknown if traces of this mineral are essential in human nutrition. If required, it is sufficiently plentiful in food, water and air to satisfy human needs.

Forty cases of lead poisoning were reported in California children in 1991 when they were given ethnic folk remedies. Most of these cases involved powders given for digestive problems in Mexican children ranging in age from eight months to five years.

lecithin A group of fatty substances (named from the Greek word *lekithos,* meaning egg yolk) called phospholipids, or phosphoglycerides, found in egg yolk, natural oils (such as soybean) and in blood, bile, nerves, brain and various animal tissue. Phospholipids are formed in all cells of the body, though the ones that enter the bloodstream are mainly produced in the liver and intestinal mucosa.

The main function of phospholipids is to maintain the structural integrity of the cells. Lecithin is also a natural bile component important in the metabolism of fat in the liver, and it helps dissolve gallstones. Of the various phospholipids, the lecithins reach the most areas of the body. As a food additive, especially in cheese, margarine and sweets, lecithin functions as an emulsifier and antioxidant.

When hydrolyzed, lecithin produces stearic acid, glycerol, phosphoric acid and choline. Lecithin is a source of the B vitamins cholin and inositol, and it is capable of breaking down fat and possibly cholesterol that clogs arterial walls.

Available in health-food stores as capsules or in granulated form, lecithin was championed by the late American nutritionist Adelle Davis as a dietary supplement for individuals who suffered heart attacks caused by high blood cholesterol. Davis believed granular lecithin, which may be added to breads, pancakes, casseroles, soups, milkshakes, meatloaf and many other recipes, is more valuable than lecithin capsules.

lemon The yellow, acid fruit of the *Citrus limon* tree, of the Rutaceae family, used as a home remedy both internally and externally. With enough of a vitamin C content to prevent or treat scurvy, lemon juice added to hot water is considered therapeutic for colds and coughs (for persistent cough, honey may be added to the mixture), headache, sore throat and rheumatism. Once commonly called a "physic," lemon juice in water was thought to promote digestion and elimination. Lemon also serves as a substitute for vinegar, spices and aromatic substances for individuals who cannot tolerate the latter, and lemon is safe for use by people with diabetes. A distinct disadvantage of drinking large amounts of lemon juice or sucking lemon juice directly from the lemon, however, is the potential erosion of tooth enamel.

Lemon juice is also used as an astringent, an enema, a hair rinse and on warts and corns. Lemon powder helps arrest bleeding.

See also LIME.

lemon balm (melissa, balm) An Old World perennial bushy herb, *Melissa officinalis,* of the Labiatae family, known for its lemony, aromatic leaves. In Ayurvedic medicine, lemon balm is thought to be a diaphoretic, carminative and nervine. Many other herbalists use lemon balm for a number of healing purposes, particularly nervous disorders, after the example set by 9th- and 10th-century Arabian physicians, who prescribed it for heart palpitations and anxiety. Because it is a mint, lemon balm infusion (tea) is prescribed for stomachache, fever, depression, tension and irregular menses. The external uses of lemon balm include the treatment of herpes simplex, rheumatism, neuralgia and wounds.

lemongrass (rohisha) A tropical grass, *Cymbopogon citratus,* of the Graminaceae family, known for its essential oil whose odor is reminiscent of lemon or verbena. Ayurvedic practitioners use the pungent, bitter herb as a diuretic, diaphoretic and refrigerant.

leonurus (motherwort, yi mu cao) An herb found in northeastern Asia, Japan and Taiwan, *Leonurus sibiricus* or *heterophyllus,* of the Labiatae family, named from the Greek words meaning lion's tail because of the plant's form. Leonurus seeds are used in traditional Chinese medicine to treat problems involving urination and menstruation and to cool the body.

lepidium (peppergrass) An herb, *Lepidium apetalum,* of the Cruciferae family, grown in temperate regions and known for its mucilage. Chinese practitioners prescribe lepidium root for colds, cough and excessive sputum production.

leverwood (hop horn beam, ironwood, deerwood) A North American tree, *Ostria virginiana,* of the Betulaceae family, whose inner wood and bark are used in Native American and homeopathic medicine for the treatment of fever, stomachache, neuralgia, headache, liver problems, lumbago and malarial anemia.

licorice (sweetwood, sweet licorice, gan cao, yasthi madhu) An Asian and southern European perennial, *Glycyrrhiza glabra,* among other species of the Leguminosae family, whose root and rootstock are well-known for their flavor when used in cough medicines, syrups, lozenges, liqueurs and candies. While licorice taken in large amounts can cause salt retention, elevated blood pressure and excessive potassium loss through the urine, it is used as a demulcent and mild expectorant, called glycyrrhiza.

Herbalists prepare the dried root of licorice as a remedy mainly for respiratory problems such as bronchitis, cough and congestion, and for stomach and intestinal complaints such as ulcers and constipation.

Licorice grows wild in India and Pakistan. In Ayurvedic practice, licorice is considered a demulcent, tonic, laxative and expectorant with cooling, sweet and bitter properties. Therapeutic use includes the treatment of hyperacidity, painful urination and general debility. Licorice, which may also be added to ghee (see GHEE), is thought to be a rejuvenative food and an agent to calm the mind, increase cerebrospinal and cranial fluid, improve vision, hair, complexion and voice, tone the mucous membranes, relieve muscle spasm and promote a sense of contentment. However, Ayurvedic practitioners do not recommend licorice for those suffering from edema, high blood pressure or osteoporosis.

life root (golden senecio, squaw weed, ragwort, false valerian, cocash weed, female regulator) North American perennial flowering herbs of the genus *Senecio,* such as *S. aureus,* of the Compositae family, whose root and herb are considered medicinal by homeopaths, Native American and other herbalists. Although senecio is mainly prescribed for a number of gynecological problems, including painful menses, adverse effects of menopause and weak ligaments of the uterus, it is also used to treat atonic, enlarged prostate, pulmonary complaints, renal colic, sciatica, pain in the spermatic cord, gravel, diarrhea, stones, gonorrhea, dysuria, kidney inflammation, angina pectoris, liver disturbances, ulcers, colitis and many other ailments.

ligusticum (lovage, chuan xiong)   Asian and European perennials of the *Ligusticum genus,* such as *L. striatum* and *L. wallichii,* whose root or rhizome is used by traditional Chinese practitioners and other herbalists to treat pain, headache, poor circulation, scanty menstrual flow, gout and rheumatism. Lovage has long been known in many countries' legends as an ingredient in love potions.

See also LOVAGE.

ligustrum (nu zhen zi, Nepal privet, glossy privet, white wax tree)   A Chinese, Japanese and Korean evergreen tree, *Ligustrum lucidum,* of the Oleaceae family, whose bark, leaves and fruits are used by Chinese and other herbalists as a diaphoretic, tonic, painkiller and treatment for coughs, swelling, vertigo, fever and headache.

lilium (lily bulb, bai he)   A Chinese flowering plant, *Lilium brownii* or *colchesteri,* of the Liliaceae family, whose bulb scales are used by traditional Chinese and Ayurvedic practitioners and other herbalists as a demulcent, nutritive tonic, nervine and treatment for urinary problems, deafness, gas and respiratory complaints.

lime   The yellowish-green fruit *Citrus acida* (also *C. aurantifolia*) from tropical citrus trees of the Rutaceae family, that is a source of vitamin C. Ayurvedic and other herbalists use lime as a refrigerant, carminative and expectorant.

Lime is also the alternate name of calcium oxide, a substance recognized in the United States Pharmacopoeia (USP) as an ingredient obtained from limestone and used in the making of mortar and cement. Lime water is an alkaline solution of calcium hydroxide in water that is used as an antacid.

linden (lime blossom, linden flower, American basswood, spoonwood, wycopy, lime tree)   Various species of trees of the *Tilia* genus, such as *T. cordata, americana* and *europaea,* whose flowers, leaves and inner bark are considered of medicinal value by Native American and other herbalists. Linden is commonly prescribed for nervous disorders including epilepsy, colds, cough, hoarseness, mucus congestion, gynecological problems, neuralgia, hives, peritonitis, rheumatism, headache, sterility and absence of menses. A combination of linden charcoal and goat's milk is administered to individuals with tuberculosis.

In addition to medicinal preparations, linden trees provide honey touted as excellent by many herbalists. Linden tar can be applied to eczema, and soft, light linden wood with its fine grain attracts carvers.

The deciduous *Tilia* species thrive in temperate climates in the north. Herbal linden flower formulas are usually made from *T. cordata,* the small-leafed European linden also known as the winter linden, and *T. platyphyllos,* the large-leafed, early blooming summer linden, with a wide fragrance range. The dried flowers are mildly sweet and sticky, and the fruit is somewhat sweet, slimy and dry. The flavor of linden tea derives from the aromatic volatile oil in linden flowers. Parts used for making herbal remedies are fresh and dried flowers, dried leaves and wood. Different parts of the *Tilia* are used in treating specific conditions and symptoms: Flowers are used in remedies for colds, cough, bronchitis, infectious diseases and headache (particularly migraine) and as a diuretic (increases urine production), antispasmodic (reduces spasm) and sedative. Leaf remedies are used to treat intestinal complaints and (topically) ulcers in the leg. Wood remedies are for liver and gallbladder disorders and cellulites, or inflammation of connective tissue. Linden is available as a flower preparation, including in teas, as a fluid extract and as a tincture. Excessive use of linden flower tea may cause cardiac complications and is not recommended for individuals with cardiac disorders. No harmful drug interactions have been reported.

lindera (wu yao)   A Chinese and Taiwanese fragrant shrub, *Lindera strychnifolia,* of the Lauraceae family, named for Swedish physician J. Linder (1676–1723), whose roots are prepared as medicine by traditional Chinese herbalists for the treatment of intestinal worms, indigestion, abdominal inflammation, hernia, asthma, cholera, menstrual pain and urinary-tract weakness.

linoleic acid   An essential fatty acid required for maintaining the integrity of cellular membranes. Human deficiency was not discovered until the early 1970s when hair loss, scaly skin and poor wound-healing was noted in a group of hospitalized patients fed intravenously with fat-free fluids. Chronic users of the laxative mineral oil and persons with chronic diarrhea, especially in cystic fibrosis, may be lacking this nutrient.

linum   See FLAX.

lion's root (cancer weed, white lettuce, prenanthes serpens)   A North American perennial herb, *Nabalus serpentaria,* of the Compositae (suborder Chicoraceae) family, whose milky juice is used by Native American and other herbalists as an astringent and antiseptic, especially in the case of diarrhea and dysentery. Homeopaths also prescribe tincture of lion's root for constipation and ophthalmia.

lipids   See FAT.

liquid liver   A liver extract, a source of iron in the form of capsules and tablets, said to support liver function and increase energy level. Extracts of beef (bovine) liver are a rich natural source of many vitamins and minerals, including iron. Liver extracts provide the most absorbable form of iron—heme iron—and other nutrients, such as vitamin B_{12} and folic acid, critical in building blood. Liver extracts can contain as much as 3 to 4 m of heme iron per gram. Although tested in people with chronic liver disease, no defined benefit from the use of liver extracts has been demonstrated, nor have side effects or adverse reactions been reported, but liver extracts are not recommended for individuals suffering from iron-storage

disorders, such as hemochromatosis. Because the liver is a major filtering organ for many potentially toxic environmental chemicals, a general concern is that consumption of liver extracts may result in increased risk of toxicity.

litchi (lychee, li zhi he)   A southern Chinese fruit of the *Litchi chinensis* tree, of the Sapindaceae (soapberry) family, with a hard reddish covering and white, sweet flesh around a large seed, also called a litchi nut. While litchi nuts are a popular addition to desserts in Chinese cuisine, Chinese practitioners use the fresh fruit as a tonic and treatment of cough and diarrhea, the seeds as painkillers and for treatment of testicular inflammation, ulcers, hernia and lumbago, and the fruit with skin and leaves as a remedy for poisonous animal bites.

lithium   A metallic element, named from the Greek word *lithos,* meaning stone. It is unknown if traces of this mineral are essential in human nutrition. If required, it is sufficiently plentiful in food, water and air to satisfy human needs. Drugs containing lithium salts are used in the treatment of bipolar disorder.

L-lysine (α, ε-diaminocaproic acid)   An essential amino acid required for the synthesis of proteins needed for optimal growth in infants and to maintain nitrogen balance in adults. Lysine has been reported to suppress herpes simplex infections but studies have failed to confirm this benefit.

lobelia (ban bian lian, Indian tobacco, pukeweed, gagroot, vomitwort, bladderpod, wild tobacco)   A tropical and temperate herb, *Lobelia chinensis* or *inflata,* of the Campanulaceae (also listed as Lobeliaceae) family, named for Flemish botanist Matthias de Lobel (1538–1616). The lobelia plant contains lobeline, a chemical derived from the dried leaves and tops of the herb that acts like nicotine, although lobelia is less potent. In Ayurvedic medicine, the pungent, heating qualities of *L. inflata* are used as an antispasmodic, emetic, expectorant and diaphoretic. Other herbalists consider lobelia one of the best emetics (hence the name "pukeweed"). Lobelia is also commonly employed in antismoking regimes. Pure lobeline relieves asthmatic symptoms and respiratory difficulties in newborns and individuals under anesthesia. There is some controversy among herbalists regarding lobelia toxicity: Some believe the herb is poisonous and in large doses may cause paralysis, vomiting and collapse, while others have not witnessed any problems resulting from lobelia. Other uses of the herb include treatment of tetany and food poisoning, and as a catalyst for other herbs in medicinal formulas.

lonicera (honeysuckle, jin yin hua) An East Asian and North American flowering plant, *Lonicera japonica*, of the Caprifoliaceae family, named for German physician and naturalist Adam Lonicer (1528–1586). In traditional Chinese medicine, the whole plant is used to treat fever and scanty flow of urine and prevent diarrhea, while the flowers are used for fever, headache, dysentery and arthritis, and the twigs for boils and pain in the bones.

lophatherum An Asian and Australian grass, *Lophatherum gracile*, of the Gramineae family, used by Chinese herbalists in the treatment of anxiety, scanty or bloody urine and fever. The root is thought to induce abortion as well as assuage problems during labor.

loquat (pi pa ye) The plant *Eriobotrya japonica*, of the Rosaceae family, whose leaves and fruit are prepared by herbalists as expectorant, anti-inflammatory and antitussive. Amygdalin, a substance in loquat leaves, is also found in apricot kernels and wild cherry bark and used in cough medicines. Herbalists also use loquat for bronchitis and lung congestion, vomiting and belching.

loranthus (mistletoe, mulberry leaf, sang ji sheng) A genus of flowering shrubs of the Loranthaceae family, such as *L. parasiticus* and *yadoriki*, that grow on host trees. Many legends are associated with mistletoe, including the Christmas tradition of kissing under a sprig of the shrub, possibly reflecting herbalists' prescriptions of mistletoe for infertility, sterility and unhappily single individuals. In traditional Chinese medicine, uses for loranthus include remedies for hypertension, threatened abortion, pain during pregnancy, bone and knee pain and excessive menstrual bleeding. Loranthus is also prescribed as a kidney and bone tonic and to induce lactation in women who have just given birth.

In Ayurvedic medicine, mistletoe (or *Viscum album*, of the Loranthaceae family) is used as a nervine, antispasmodic and emmenagogue.

Lorenzo oil Oleic and erucic acids administered as a dietary supplement to patients with adrenoleukodystrophy, or adrenomyeloneuropathy, a wasting disease caused by a severe deficiency or lack of these oils. The supplement is named for a young boy whose father researched this rare disease and discovered the missing nutrients. The 1992 film *Lorenzo's Oil* (starring Nick Nolte and Susan Sarandon) is based on the true story.

lotus (lian zi, lian xu, padma) A genus of leguminous herbs or subshrubs (also called sweet clover), such as *Nelumbo nucifera*, of the Nymphaeaceae family. Considered India's most sacred plant, the lotus blossom reflects and inspires spiritual unfoldment, hence the lotus position during yoga and meditation in which one sits cross-legged with the right foot on the left thigh and the left foot on the right thigh. Lotus seeds and root are used by Ayurvedic practitioners as tonic, remedy and food. Indications include diarrhea, leukorrhea, bleeding disorders, venereal diseases, impotence and cardiac weakness. Lotus seeds are also thought to improve concentration, help stop stuttering and open the "heart center," one of the seven *chakras* (head, third eye, throat, heart, navel, sex and root centers of the body as references to function and spirit) described in Ayurvedic (Hindu) medicine.

According to Homer's *Odyssey*, people who ate lotus fruit became the dreamy, indolent and contented population of lotusland. The fruit allegedly came from the tree *Zizyphus lotus*, of the buckthorn family.

lovage (lavose, sea parsley) A European and Asian wild, aromatic perennial, *Levisticum officinale*, of the carrot family, cultivated as a potherb, flavoring agent and home remedy. Lovage rootstock is prepared for use as a stimulant, diuretic, carminative, expectorant and stomachic, although it is believed that large doses may cause kidney damage. However, lovage is considered by herbalists to be effective against suppressed menstruation, flatulence and urinary problems.

luffa (si gua, sponge gourd, smooth loofah) An Old World tropical, annual herb, *Luffa aegyptiaca,* of the family Cucurbitaceae, whose seeds produce an edible oil and whose interior is used as a sponge commonly known as a loofah. Luffa's fruit juice is considered toxic, though it is known to be a strong purgative. In traditional Chinese medicine, luffa fruit fiber provides a remedy for pain, bleeding associated with dysentery and the uterus, testicular inflammation and piles. Ash from the fiber is prepared as treatment for jaundice, smallpox, internal bleeding and poor circulation.

lungwort (Jerusalem cowslip, Jerusalem sage, spotted comfrey, maple lungwort) A European and North American flowering perennial plant, *Pulmonaria officinalis,* of the Pulmonaceae family, whose leaves are used by Native American and other herbalists in preparations largely devoted to the treatment of pulmonary problems because of its anti-inflammatory, demulcent and mucilaginous properties. Lungwort reputedly contains vitamins C and B and iron, copper, silver, manganese, kerotin, nickel and other minerals. Lungwort tea is also prescribed as a diuretic and for external use for wounds.

lycium (matrimony vine, box thorn, Chinese wolfberry, gou qi zi) Tropical or temperate shrubs, *Lycium barbarum* and *chinense,* of the Solanaceae family, whose various uses in tradi-

tional Chinese medicine include treatment of impotence, backache, weakness, fever, diabetes, sore throat and pneumonia.

lycopene A carotenoid pigment, along with alpha- and beta-carotene, lutein and others, which occurs naturally in fruits and vegetables. Lycopene is the pigment that makes tomatoes red; redder tomatoes contain more lycopene. Numerous studies suggest that lycopene levels in the blood may be associated with reduced incidence of prostate, digestive tract, breast, lung and cervical cancer, as well as cardiovascular disease and age-related macular degeneration, the most common cause of blindness in the elderly in the Western world. Not produced naturally by the body but available through diet, lycopene is also an antioxidant that helps the body prevent and repair damaged cells. Antioxidants are compounds that fight free radicals in the body and have been shown to inhibit DNA oxidation, which some studies indicate may lead to some cancers. Tomatoes and tomato products, such as sauces, ketchup, soup and juice, constitute about 85 percent of available dietary lycopene. Other less significant sources of lycopene include guava, rosehip, watermelon and pink grapefruit. Lycopene from tomatoes is reported to be absorbed more effectively into the bloodstream if it is first heat-processed.

lygodium (climbing fern, hai jin sha) The fern of the Schizaeaceae family, named from the Greek word meaning flexible. *L. japonicum* leaves are used by Chinese herbalists to treat bloody sputum, gonorrhea, high fever and delirium. *L. flexuosum* leaves and spores are used to treat inflammation, fever and cystitis, among other complaints.

macrobiotic diet Vegetarian diet originating from the late 19th century based on a philosophy that spiritual progress is made by restricting animal-derived foods. Initially, at the "lowest" stage, the diet consists of 10 percent cereal, 30 percent vegetable, 10 percent soup, 30 percent foods of animal origin, 15 percent fruits and salads and 5 percent dessert. As spiritualism progresses, every other food except cereal is reduced until the entire diet is cereal. This diet is seriously deficient in nutrition.

See also GOMASHIO; VEGETARIAN DIETS.

macrocytic anemia See ANEMIA, MACROCYTIC.

macro minerals Minerals such as calcium and phosphorus that are required in larger quantities than trace minerals. Macro minerals include calcium, chloride, magnesium, phosphorus, potassium, sodium and sulfur.

See also MINERALS, ESSENTIAL.

macrosupplementation See MEGADOSE.

macular degeneration Deterioration of the macular area of the retina of the eye, usually related to aging or growth of blood vessels under the retina, but the cause is unknown. Macular degeneration is a common cause of impaired central vision in individuals older than 50 years of age. There is some evidence that antioxidants, especially beta-carotene, play a role in the prevention of macular degeneration. Importantly, smokers develop this serious eye disease seven years before nonsmokers. Wearing sunglasses that block out destructive ultraviolet rays is also an important preventive measure.

magnesium A metallic element whose salts are essential nutrients and required for more than 300 enzymatic reactions that are necessary for normal cell function. Magnesium functions in the conversion of carbohydrates, protein and fats to energy, and assists in the manufacture of proteins and genetic material within cells. The central nervous system is dependent on magnesium for the transmission of impulses. Muscles contract when calcium flows into muscle cells and relax when magnesium replaces calcium. Magnesium also aids in the removal of toxins such as ammonia from the body. Metabolic reactions involving thiamine (vitamin B$_1$) and biotin are dependent on magnesium.

Blood contains approximately 2 milliequivalents (milliequivalent or mEq is the number of grams of a solute contained in one milliliter of a normal solution) of magnesium per liter. Magnesium is found in both intracellular (in the cells) as well as extracellular (blood and lymph) fluids. Magnesium blood levels are regulated by the kidneys, and it is excreted in both urine and feces. Approximately 40 percent of the estimated 24 grams of magnesium present in the body is concentrated in muscle and soft tissues, 1 percent in the circulation and the balance in the skeleton.

There is some evidence that hard water containing high levels of magnesium may lead to a reduced risk of heart disease and lower blood pressure. Recent studies have failed to prove earlier reports that intravenous infusions of magnesium during the first 24 hours following a heart attack were beneficial.

Deficiency

Muscle tremors and spasms, depressed tendon reflexes, personality changes, anorexia, nausea and vomiting are signs of magnesium deficiency. Tetany, convulsions and coma may result if severe. The symptoms of hypercalcemia, or abnormally high levels of blood calcium, are similar to inadequate levels of magnesium.

Dietary magnesium deficiency is virtually unknown. However, malabsorption syndromes or other disorders in which there are significant losses of fluids and electrolytes, some kidney diseases that affect reabsorption of cations (ions carrying a positive charge because of a deficiency of electrons), states of malnutrition and alcoholism may result in magnesium deficiency. Medical therapies that can disturb electrolyte balance include nasogastric suctioning, magnesium-free intravenous feeding and some drugs, especially diuretics.

Primary idiopathic hypomagnesemia, a rare genetic disorder, is characterized by impaired ability to absorb magnesium from the intestinal tract.

Food Sources

Although all unprocessed foods contain magnesium to varying degrees, richest concentrations are found in nuts, legumes, unmilled grains, green vegetables and bananas. Removing the germ and outer layers of cereal grains results in an 80 percent loss of the mineral.

Recommended Dietary Allowances

Magnesium interacts with other nutrients in complex ways, making it difficult to establish a Recommended Daily Allowance (RDA). Nevertheless, the RDA has been established at 4.5 mg per kilogram (1 kilogram = 2.2 pounds) of body weight for adult men and women. A 20-mg daily increase is advised during pregnancy and 60 mg during lactation. Forty mg of magnesium for the first six months and 60 mg for the second six months are recommended, although there are no data on actual need for young children.

A daily intake of 6.0 mg per kilogram is sufficient for children and adolescents from one to 15 years of age.

Supplements

Magnesium supplementation may prevent the formation of oxalate kidney stones. The body seems to require a balance of calcium, magnesium and phosphorous. Therefore, some nutritionists advocate maintaining a ratio of two to one, calcium to magnesium when taking supplements. Phosphorous is plentiful in most diets and does not require supplements.

Toxicity

The large amounts of magnesium that occur in magnesium sulfate, or Epsom salts, have a laxative effect. Magnesium-containing antacids cause diarrhea in some individuals. Magnesium is toxic only to people with abnormal kidney function. Early symptoms of magnesium excess are nausea, vomiting and a fall in blood pressure. Later, slow heart rate and other heart irregularities and central nervous system depression develop. Eventually coma, respiratory distress, cardiac arrest and death may occur.

magnolia (swamp sassafras, beaver tree, Indian bark, white bay, hou po)   Evergreen or deciduous trees or shrubs, *Magnolia virginiana, M. glauca, M. acuminata* and *M. tripetata,* of the Magnoliaceae family, whose roots and trunk are used in herbal medicine. There are 35 to 40 species cultivated in the United States, especially in morasses from Massachusetts to the Gulf of Mexico, India, China and Japan.

In the past, magnolia has been listed in the United States Pharmacopoeia (USP) as a treatment for rheumatism because of its better action, greater safety and fewer side effects than quinine. Magnolia has also been used as a tonic to boost the system after chills, fever and stomachache. It is also known as a substitute for tobacco when it is desirous to break the tobacco-chewing habit.

In traditional Chinese medicine, *M. officinalis* bark is an antispasmodic and aphrodisiac, and it is given for malaria, respiratory complaints, cough, nausea, intestinal worms and other ailments.

mahabala   See MALLOW.

ma huang (ephedra, somalata)   The most popular of the ephedra shrubs, of the family Ephedraceae, a Chinese herb species prepared as medication to provide a boost for the immune system and a remedy for respiratory congestion. The drug ephedrine was first isolated from an ephedra shrub in 1887 by Nagai, although Chinese practitioners have been using ma huang and other ephedra species for more than 5,000 years. Some ephedras work as diaphoretics and antipyretics. Once ephedra's action was studied and recognized by allopathic practitioners, ephedrine became known as a sympathomimetic drug that could be synthetically produced. The action of ephedrine is similar to that of epinephrine (also called adrenaline, one of the hormones produced by the adrenal medulla), a common ingredient in medications for asthma, local hemorrhage, constricted bronchioles and cardiac arrhythmias and for use in conjunction with anesthesia.

The effects of ephedrine, although less potent, last longer, especially when given orally, whereas epinephrine is effective only by injection. Orally or by injection, ephedrine dilates the bronchial muscles, contracts nasal mucosa, elevates blood pressure (and should be used cautiously by individuals with high blood pressure) and is mainly valued for its bronchodilating properties in the treatment of asthma and for its constricting effects on the nasal mucosa in hay fever. Ephedrine sulfate (USP) is marketed under the trade name Isofedrol.

Ephedra sinica, equisetina and *distachya* branches and roots are used by Chinese and other herbalists to treat influenza, whooping cough, lung fever, allergic rashes such as hives and many other ailments. Ma huang is a popular ingredient in supplemental preparations for women, possibly because it combats night sweats usually associated with menopause and the general weakness, perhaps from loss of blood or change in hormone balance, that may be experienced during certain times of the menstrual cycle.

Ephedra is also considered medicinal according to the Vedas, the sacred scriptures of India. In Ayurvedic medicine, *E. vulgaris,* of the Gnetaceae family, works as a diaphoretic, antipyretic, antitussive, expectorant, analgesic and stimulant. Indications for the use of ephedra include arthritis, dropsy and facial edema as well as asthma, bronchitis and respiratory distress. Ayurvedic practitioners believe American ephedra (sometimes known as Mormon or Brigham tea) does not have the same diaphoretic and antitussive actions as ma huang and other Oriental species.

In 2003 the Food and Drug Administration announced plans to issue a rule prohibiting the sale of ephedra-containing dietary supplements due to apparent health risks. Ephedra has been found to contribute to cardiovascular problems such as heart attack and stroke as well as psychiatric problems.

See also Appendix IX; Appendix X.

maidenhair (common polypody, five-finger fern, rock fern) A perennial plant, *Adiantum capillus-veneris,* of the family Filices, with about 80 species, some of which are found in the deep woods of Canada and the United States. The herb of the plant is considered by herbalists to be a supplement useful in the treatment of colds, nasal congestion, hoarseness, shortness of breath, asthma, pleurisy, influenza and other respiratory problems. Ayurvedic practitioners use maidenhair fern as a demulcent, refrigerant and tonic.

malabsorption Impaired absorption of nutrients from the intestinal tract. Disorders characterized by chronic diarrhea such as celiac and Crohn's disease may cause vitamin deficiencies as well as electrolyte and fluid imbalance.

mallow (malva, high mallow) Plants of the family Malvaceae, whose herbs have been used by Native American, Ayurvedic and other herbalists as a remedy for respiratory irritation, coughs, kidney and bladder problems and other disorders. Malva leaves and flowers are claimed to soothe inflammation of the mouth and throat and help alleviate earaches.

Pliny the Elder, an ancient Roman encyclopedist known for his writings on scientific subjects, including the medicinal power of spices and herbs, wrote "that anyone taking a spoonful of mallows will be free of disease." A good amount of Pliny's information has since been discredited as incorrect. However, mallow leaves are eaten raw or boiled by the Chinese, and Native Americans made poultices for skin eruptions from mallow leaves, stems and flowers. Russian folk medicine also includes malva as a tea or nastoika (with vodka). In Ayurvedic medicine, malva is considered a demulcent, emollient and astringent. Nutritionally, malva (*M. sylventris*) contains vitamin C, minerals and sugar.

See also MARSHMALLOW.

malnutrition   Inadequate nutrition due to insufficient or unbalanced diet.

mandrake   A Mediterranean herb, *Mandragora officinarum,* of the nightshade family, said to have properties helpful in the case of chronic liver disorders and in regulating bowels. With a large forked root likened to human qualities, mandrake has been used as a cathartic, narcotic and soporific (sleep-inducer) and as a means of promoting conception. The Old Testament touts mandrake as a remedy for sterility. Mandrake is said to be highly effective and work best when combined with blackroot, senna leaves and other herbs.

American mandrake, or *Podophyllum pelatum,* of the family Berberidaceae, is also known as May or hog apple (see BARBERRY), Indian apple, raccoon berry and wild lemon. Most parts of this plant, such as leaves, berries and seeds, are poisonous in the green state; ripening takes place during the fall in North American locations. The active substance in American mandrake is podophyllum or podophyllin, capable of treating chronic liver disease, according to homeopaths and herbalists. The dried rhizome (rootlike stem) and its roots are used in the topical treatment of certain papillomas (benign skin tumors) such as verruca acuminata and other varieties of warts, polyps and condylomas. Herbalists claim American mandrake is also therapeutic in treating cancerous skin growths. Other reported clinical uses of American mandrake are for chronic constipation, gallbladder problems and abnormal conditions of the lymphatic system, spleen and blood. In Ayurvedic medicine, mandrake is used as a cathartic, alterative and toxic. Both American and European mandrake are poisonous, and homeopaths use them cautiously for fever, colic and asthma, and sometimes to promote conception. An overdose of mandrake may cause death, and if taken by a pregnant woman, it may cause birth defects.

Nonetheless, mandrake enjoys a bit of literary fame in 17th-century poet John Donne's "Song: Go and catch a falling star":

Go, and catch a falling star,
Get with child a mandrake root,
Tell me, where all past years are,
Or who cleft the Devil's foot,
Teach me to hear mermaids singing.

manganese   Metallic element essential for synthesis of mucopolysaccharides and for a number of enzymes. Manganese is concentrated in the mitochondria of pituitary, liver, pancreas, kidneys and bone. Manganese is plentiful in plant food sources; human deficiencies are virtually unknown. Toxicity has been seen only when workers were exposed to high concentrations of manganese dust or fumes. High dietary intake does not appear to be toxic.

maple (sugar maple, swamp maple, red maple)   The tree of the Aceraceae, or maple, family, touted for its rich, flavorful syrup sought by bees and people. Cultivated in many regions of the United States, the maple's inner bark and leaves are used as a decoction (see DECOCTION) to strengthen the liver and spleen, soothe the nerves and provide a tonic boost for the entire body. While maple syrup continues to be a popular form of sugar, there is a pneumonitis called maple bark disease caused by inhalation of the mold *Cryptostroma corticale,* found in the bark of maple trees. Another disease, maple-syrup urine disease, has no link to the ingestion of maple syrup, but it is named for urine and sweat that smell like maple syrup. Maple-syrup urine disease is a metabolic disorder that involves defective metabolism of the amino acids leucine, isoleucine, baline and alloisoleucine (see AMINO ACIDS). In infants, the disease induces nervous-system deterioration and death.

Tea made from maple leaves is also claimed to be a muscle toner for new mothers and to help relieve pain in the liver or spleen.

marjoram (mountain mint, wintersweet, knotted marjoram)   A native Portuguese perennial, *Origanum majorana* or *vulgare,* of the Labiatae family, used as an aromatic and fragrant cooking ingredient and thought to be effective against sour stomach, lack of appetite and general aches and pains. Marjoram, similar to oregano, is often combined with camomile and gentian when used medicinally.

In Ayurvedic medicine, marjoram is thought to be a stimulant, antispasmodic and diaphoretic. Ancient Romans prepared marjoram for calming the nerves, relieving menstrual and other pain, treating conjunctivitis and promoting urination. A European symbol of youth and beauty whose name in Greek means "joy of the mountains," the sedative marjoram was placed in closets and hope chests, made into a gargle for mouth infections or used as an inhalant or topical application for sinus congestion. Pregnant women should avoid marjoram, however, because it is a uterine irritant.

marshmallow A European perennial herb, *Althaea officinalis,* of the Malvaceae family, bearing pink flowers and mucilaginous root that is used in the making of traditional marshmallow candies. Its use in medicine is thought to help kidney and bladder function, including alleviating bladder infection, and to soothe inflammation. Ayurvedic and other herbal practitioners use marshmallow as a tonic, demulcent, diuretic and laxative.

See also MALLOW.

measles and vitamin A deficiency This dangerous viral infection has an increased severity and potential for death in children with low levels of retinol (vitamin A). It is thought that the measles virus diminishes already low levels of vitamin A and that it may be advisable to give supplemental vitamin A to patients with severe cases.

See also A, VITAMIN.

Mediterranean diet A general term for the common dietary components of several countries bordering the Mediterranean Sea set forth by the "Seven Countries Study" conducted during the 1950s by researcher Ancel Keys. According to "The Mediterranean Diet and Mortality—Olive Oil and Beyond," an article by Frank B. Hu, M.D., Ph.D., in the *New England Journal of Medicine,* "The main characteristics of the Mediterranean diet include an abundance of plant food (fruits, vegetables, wholegrain cereals, nuts, and legumes); olive oil as the principal source of fat; fish and poultry consumed in low-to-moderate amounts; relatively low consumption of red meat; and moderate consumption of wine, normally with meals." The primary rea-

sons for studying the dietary habits in Mediterranean cultures were longevity and low rates of coronary heart disease and certain types of cancer seen there, despite a high fat intake in southern Italy and Greece, especially on the island of Crete. A food pyramid designed to reflect the traditional healthy Mediterranean diet is built on a base of physical activity, noted as a beneficial lifestyle element concurrent with dietary factors in Mediterranean culture. From there up, the pyramid shows that bread, pasta, couscous, polenta, other whole grains, potatoes, fruits, beans, legumes, nuts, vegetables, olive oil, cheese and yogurt are recommended for daily consumption. Weekly recommendations include fish, poultry, eggs and sweets, and, at the top of the pyramid, a monthly intake of red meat.

A related study was conducted on the "Indo-Mediterranean diet," which indicated that an increased intake of mustard or soybean oil, nuts, vegetables, fruits and whole grains seemed to significantly lower the rate of heart attacks and sudden death from cardiac dysfunction in 1,000 patients in India with existing (or at high risk of) heart disease.

See also Appendix I; OLIVE.

megadose Doses of vitamin or mineral supplements that are 10 times or greater (for vitamin D, five times) than the Recommended Dietary Allowance (RDA) dose.

See also MEGAVITAMINS.

megaloblastic anemia See ANEMIA, MACROCYTIC.

megavitamin and megamineral therapy in childhood position statement from the Canadian Paediatric Society (Société canadienne de pédiatrie) Expresses an opinion that, ". . . as many as 10 percent of healthy children may be exposed to vitamin polypharmacy and a substantial risk of accidental overdose. Among the chronically ill, unproven megavitamin regimens may be substituted for treatments of proven efficacy and established safety.

The administration of megavitamins and megaminerals to children involves special risks for various reasons. Parents concerned for their child's health may seek simplistic remedies for difficult behavioural and developmental problems or intractable disease. Children have difficulty expressing complaints that may arise from megavitamin use. Often the symptoms of chronic megavitamin use begin with nonspecific complaints such as malaise, anorexia and fatigability; these have led parents to increase their administration of megavitamins as a tonic."

Physicians are advised to counsel parents about a balanced diet and seek consultation with registered professional dietitians and nutritionists.

[Excerpted from the report of the Nutrition Committee of the Canadian Paediatric Society entitled, "Megavitamin and megamineral therapy in childhood." *Canadian Medical Association Journal* (1990) 143:10, with permission.]

megavitamins   Use of vitamins in doses exceeding the Recommended Daily Allowances (RDA). The importance of vitamins and minerals in amounts at least equivalent to the Recommended Dietary Allowance (RDA) is unquestioned. However, alternative medical practitioners often advocate vitamins to treat a variety of disorders, including cancer, heart disease, schizophrenia and the common cold. Often vitamins and other supplements are used to replace prescription drugs. Traditionalists are not only skeptical of the benefits of such doses but also worry about toxicity and the effects of discontinuing more conventional therapy that might be life-saving or at least life-lengthening.

Studies with hyperactive, or attention-deficit, children initially seemed to indicate amazing improvements when given megavitamins. However, well-controlled studies fail to support this benefit. Improvement attributed to the vitamins by proponents of megavitamins are now thought by most pediatricians and psychiatrists to be the result of greater expectations placed on the children who were taking these substances.

It has been long been recognized that fat-soluble vitamins accumulate in the liver and can be toxic. Most excessive amounts of the water-soluble vitamins are eliminated from the body by the kidneys, and therefore large doses are not toxic. However, niacin, pyridoxine, folic acid, ascorbic acid, and pantothenic acid are water-soluble and can cause adverse effects (see Table 22).

megavitamin study of the American Psychiatric Association   A task force led by American psychiatrist and biochemist Dr. Morris Lipton to review studies conducted for the use of large doses of vitamins (known as "orthomolecular" therapy) to treat psychiatric patients, especially those with schizophrenia. They concluded that there was no evidence to support the orthomolecular theory.

See also MEGADOSE, MEGAVITAMINS.

memory loss   See ALZHEIMER'S DISEASE.

Menkes' syndrome   Inherited defect in copper absorption characterized by poor and abnormal growth, defective skin pigmentation, kinky hair, mental impairment and usually premature death.

See also COPPER.

mercury   A metallic element that, in small quantities, is not harmful. However, the flesh of fish at the top of the pelagic food chain may carry pollutants such as mercury, which can increase the risk of heart disease.

metabolism   Physical and chemical processes involved in the production, maintenance and utilization of energy in living organisms.

microcytic anemia   See ANEMIA, MICROCYTIC.

microgram (mcg)   Unit of measure equivalent to one millionth of a gram.

micro minerals   See MINERALS, TRACE.

milk, infant formula   Well-balanced cow's milk commercial products that also supply electrolytes, minerals and vitamins. These products are often more convenient than breast milk and, if consumed in adequate quantity, supply the Recommended Daily Allowances of those nutrients.

milk, human   Breast milk, available safely without cost, may strengthen resistance to infection and enhance intestinal development and bonding between mother and newborn. Although it seems

TABLE 22 THE MOST COMMON SERIOUS VITAMIN AND MINERAL ADVERSE AND TOXIC EFFECTS (USUALLY RELATED TO EXCESSIVE OR MEGADOSES)

Vitamin/Mineral*	Chief Toxic Effects**
Vitamin A (retinol) [There does not appear to be toxicity from the provitamin substance beta-carotene, which is converted to vitamin A in the body]	Birth defects if excessive maternal intake during pregnancy Liver damage Pseudotumor cerebri (increased pressure in the brain that acts like a brain tumor)
Vitamin D	Hypercalcemia and hyper-calciuria (high blood and urine calcium) that could cause calcium deposits in soft tissues and irreversibly damage kidneys and the heart Children are especially susceptible
B-Complex Components Niacin	Liver damage Worsen glucose control in diabetics
Pyridoxine (vitamin B_6)	Irreversible nerve damage
Pantothenic acid	Diarrhea
Folic acid	May mask underlying B_{12} deficiency and result in irreversible nerve damage
Ascorbic acid (vitamin C)	Kidney stones Suppression of immune response
Iron	Interferes with zinc absorption
Zinc	Suppression of immune response

*Vitamins/minerals most likely to pose a threat to health if taken to excess in normal persons.
**Individual vitamins for more complete list of adverse and toxic effects.

to contain insufficient amounts of calcium and phosphorus for optimal bone development, this does not seem to be detrimental in otherwise normal infants. Although there is a possibility of the mother passing infection or toxins to her baby, the risk of infection is greater with improperly sterilized formula. Perhaps the most common problem with breast-feeding is assuring an adequate supply.

See also MILK, INFANT FORMULA.

milk-based supplements   These liquid nutritional supplements are often made with whole milk, eggnog or instant breakfast powdered mixes. They are used by lactose-intolerant individuals and those with certain eating and gastrointestinal disorders, individuals with poor nutrient and calorie intake, individuals who must limit their fluid volume or add fiber to their system and individuals with increased nutritional needs due to multiple trauma, burns or large wounds. It is recommended that health professionals regularly evaluate the patient's daily nutritional needs.

milk thistle   See BLESSED THISTLE.

milkweed (silkweed, swallowwort, Virginia silk)   A perennial herb, Asclepias syriaca, of the family Asclepiadaceae, that produces a milky juice (some of the milkweed plants secrete latex) and umbellate flowers. Milkweed rootstock is claimed by herbalists to be a remedy for gallstones and bowel, kidney and gynecological problems. It is also said to increase the flow of urine.

TABLE 23 MINERALS ESSENTIAL TO HEALTH

Major or Macro Minerals			
Calcium	Magnesium	Potassium	Sulfur
Chloride	Phosphorus	Sodium	

Trace or Micro Minerals		
Chromium	Iodine	Selenium
Copper	Iron	Zinc

Ultratrace Minerals (probably essential to health)		
Arsenic	Lead	Nickel
Boron	Lithium	Silicon
Bromine	Manganese	Tin
Cobalt	Molybdenum	Vanadium
Fluorine		

minerals, essential Inorganic elements required for a variety of functions including giving structure to the skeleton, muscle contractions, blood formation, the synthesis of protein and the production of energy. Minerals are found in red blood cells and cell membranes. They are components of hormones and enzymes. Major or "macro" minerals include calcium, phosphorous, sodium, potassium and others. Iodine, iron and zinc are among the "trace minerals" found in very minimal quantities. Some minerals found in even more minute concentrations may be necessary for health. (See Table 23.)

minerals, trace Elements whose total body concentration does not exceed .005 percent are classified as trace minerals and include chromium, copper, iodine, iron, selenium, and zinc. (See Table 23.)

See also MINERALS, ESSENTIAL; MINERALS, ULTRA-TRACE.

minerals, ultratrace Minerals including arsenic, boron, bromine, cadmium, fluorine, lead, lithium, manganese, molybdenum, nickel, silicon, tin and vanadium that are found in the body in minute amounts even smaller than trace or macro minerals. Although they are poorly understood, since the early 1970s it has been theorized that these substances are essential for human nutrition and deficiencies of them contribute to a variety of diseases. (See Table 23.)

See also MINERALS, ESSENTIAL; MINERALS, TRACE.

mint The herbs of the genus *Mentha*, of the Labiatae family, including peppermint, spearmint and pennyroyal (*M. piperita, M. spicata, M. pulegium*) used for their menthol, an alcohol derived from mint oils, in medicinal preparations and as a flavoring agent in chewing gum, candies and toothpaste. Many herbalists believe the leaves and stems of mint plants alleviate cramps and hiccoughs in children and adults, strengthen heart muscles, avert nausea and vomiting, particularly in motion sickness, and induce cleansing and relaxation. Mint preparations are also said to be useful for headaches, intestinal gas, toothache, lung inflammation and dizziness. *Mentha arvensis,* or field mint, is used in traditional Chinese medicine as an analgesic, a diaphoretic, a digestive stimulant, a cardiovascular medicine and an antiflatulent.

Menthol, also prepared synthetically and recognized by the United States Pharmacopoeia (USP), is an antipruritic (anti-itch agent).

See also MOTHERWORT.

mistletoe See LORANTHUS.

molybdenum An essential ultratrace mineral found in all body tissues but predominantly in the liver, kidney, bones and skin. A component of the important enzymes xanthine oxidase, aldehyde oxidase, sulfite oxidase and nitrate reductase. Xanthine oxidase is associated with the formation of uric acid as a metabolic breakdown product of purine (excessive amounts of purines in the diet increase the risk for gout). Molybdenum with riboflavin (vitamin B_2) helps convert food to energy. Molybdenum is also associated with the metabolism of iron.

Deficiency

Human deficiencies of molybdenum have been difficult to demonstrate. However, there is an inherited autosomal recessive metabolic disease resulting from a deficiency of molybdopterin, a molybdenum cofactor required for synthesis of certain enzymes. The deficiency of this cofactor interferes with the production of the enzymes sulfite oxidase and xanthine dehydrogenase, causing severe neurological abnormalities, mental retardation and dislocation of ocular lenses. There is also a possibility of increased incidence of esophageal cancer in molybdenum-deficient individuals.

Dietary Sources

Hard tap water, milk, beans, breads and cereals are the principal dietary sources of molybdenum. The average American diet contains 180 mcg of the mineral daily but varies considerably, depending on where the food sources are grown. Plants grown in soils rich in the mineral may contain up to 500 times the amount found in molybdenum-poor soils. Excess copper in the diet may interfere with the absorption of molybdenum.

Recommended Dietary Allowances

A recommended daily intake of 75 to 250 mcg of molybdenum for adults and older children is easily supplied in American diets. Requirements for infants and children is based on body weight.

Ingesting more than 10 mg of molybdenum daily may increase production of the enzyme xanthine oxidase (see above), leading to overproduction of uric acid. The presence of excessive uric acid may cause gout, a condition of exquisitely painful and swollen joints, or kidney stones.

motherwort (lion's tail, lion's ear, throwwort, yi mu cao) Perennial plants, *Leonurus cardiaca* and *hetero-phyllus,* of the Labiatae family, cultivated in Europe, Asia and North America, whose tops and leaves are said to have laxative, antispasmodic and nervine properties. Motherwort can be used as an infusion (tea made with boiling water), extract or tablet to relieve heart palpitations, stomach problems, mild goiter, epilepsy, cramps, high blood pressure, suppressed menstruation, hysteria, rheumatism, sciatica, neuritis, insomnia, chest colds, convulsions, worms and liver ailments.

See also LEONURUS.

mugwort (moxa, ai ye) A North American wild herb, *Artemisia vulgaris,* of the family Compositae, whose leaves are thought to have properties useful in the treatment of colds, colic, rheumatism, menstrual problems, kidney and bladder inflammations, gout, sciatica and fever. Some herbalists also claim that mugwort counteracts the effects of opium. Native Americans found mugwort juice effective as a topical treatment for poison oak rash and wounds. Mugwort also grows in Russia and is considered a home remedy there for a number of conditions, including wounds, nervousness, female reproductive disorders, tubercular lungs and epilepsy.

In traditional Chinese medicine, mugwort leaves are used to treat headache, asthma, bleeding and menstrual problems. Several other species of Artemisia are remedies for a host of ailments including malaria, dysentery, tuberculosis, indigestion, eye diseases and fungal infections.

mullein (feltwort, Aaron's rod, candlewick, velvet dock, shepherd's club, flannel-flower, cow's lungwort, verbascum flowers) A flowering biennial plant of 300 or more species that grow in North Africa, Europe, western and central Asia and the United States. An American species is *Verbascum thapsus,* of the Scrophulariaceae family. Mullein's leaves, flowers and sometimes the roots are prepared as a medicine to relieve ailments including lung congestion, lung hemorrhage, colds, hemorrhoids, constipation, asthma, epilepsy and headache in children, nervous disorders and heart, kidney and bladder conditions. Cows may be given fresh mullein leaves as a treatment for tapeworm. Mullein contains iron, magnesium and potassium. In Ayurvedic medicine, mullein is considered an expectorant, astringent, vulnerary and sedative.

Other species of mullein, such as orange mullein (*V. phlomoides*) and black mullein (*V. nigrum*), are also used medicinally.

multivitamin and mineral supplements Proprietary products containing a variety of vitamins and minerals in varying quantities, less than, equal to or greater than Recommended Daily Allowances (RDA). In a survey of 11,775 adults and 1,877 children, approximately 3,400 different vitamin and mineral supplement products were identified. Vitamin C was found in 50 percent of these formulations, whereas calcium and iron were the most common minerals, being present in about 25 percent.

mustard Annual plants, *Brassica nigra* and *hirta* (or *alba*), of the Cruciferae family, used by herbalists as a stimulant (especially of the appetite), expectorant and carminative. However, black mustard seed is mainly used as a poultice for rheumatism, back pain and inflammations. Internal use as a carminative is limited to small doses. White mustard seeds may be antiseptic and effective against pulmonary problems. A pungent, hot spice, mustard is also considered by Ayurvedic practitioners to be a painkiller.

myristica See NUTMEG.

myrrh An aromatic gum resin derived from the tree *Commiphora abyssinica* or *myrrha,* of the Burseraceae family, that grows in East Africa and Arabia. Myrrh is used as a spice, perhaps most famous as one of the gifts of the Three Wise Men to the infant Jesus in Bethlehem. Antiseptic myrrh is used medicinally as a colon cleanser and breath freshener. Herbalists may also offer myrrh to individuals suffering from sinus problems. Ayurvedic practitioners administer myrrh preparations as an alterative, analgesic, emmenagogue and rejuvenative.

See also GUGGUL.

myrtle   See PERIWINKLE.

nails and nutritional deficiencies   Difficulties or adverse reactions shown in nails that are the result of a lack of a particular nutrient or combination of nutrients. For example, brittle, cracked, peeling, ridged, split or broken nails may indicate a deficiency of the minerals iron or copper or the vitamins B_6, B_{12}, C or folate. Spoon-shaped nails are found in persons with a long-standing iron deficiency anemia. The deformity occurs because of an inadequate supply of oxygen-rich blood to the nail beds. Other causes of nail structural disorders include hypothyroidism and psoriasis.

National Academy of Sciences (NAS)   A private, nonprofit, self-perpetuating society of distinguished scholars engaged in scientific and engineering research, dedicated to the furtherance of science and technology and to their use for the general welfare. Although not a government agency, in 1863, during the Lincoln administration, the United States Congress granted a charter to the academy with a mandate that requires it to advise the federal government on scientific and technical matters.

The NAS is made up of approximately 1,200 scientists chosen in recognition of their achievements in research. The Academy elects a maximum 60 Americans and 15 foreign associates annually. There are three other organizations—the National Research Council, the National Academy of Engineering and the Institute of Medicine—created by the NAS that cooperate with the parent academy, but elect their own membership.

National Cancer Institute   See NATIONAL INSTITUTES OF HEALTH.

National Health and Nutrition Examination Survey (NHANES III)   Data collected from the third national, population-based, cross-sectional survey, conducted by the National Center for Health Statistics of the Centers for Disease Control and Prevention, Atlanta, Georgia, from 1988–1994. The goal of the survey was providing new and current information on the prevalence of supplement use in America. With results from more than 11,000 respondents, the survey also attempted to quantify the use of folic acid and examine the relationship between supplement use and demographic factors. Based on the definition of dietary supplement as it is written in the Dietary Supplement Health and Education Act of 1994, the conclusion was published in the Archives of Family Medicine (volume 9, March 2000, pp. 258–262) and in a reprint of the article by the American Medical Association in 2000: "Consumption of vitamin and mineral supplements is a common behavior in the United States. We recommend that physicians and health professionals include questions about the use of dietary supplements when obtaining a medical history from their patients, that all dietary supplements clearly list ingredients and known contraindications to use, and that all those planning to use supplements first have their dietary practices and lifestyle evaluated by a health professional."

See also Appendix VI.

National Institutes of Health (NIH)   Federal agency that conducts or supports medical research. Part of the Public Health Service, under the direction of the Department of Health and Human Services, the NIH is located in Bethesda, Maryland. Although formally named the National Institutes of Health in 1948, its roots date back to 1887, when it was established as the "Hygienic Laboratory" at the United States Marine Hospital on Staten Island (New York).

National Research Council Council organized in 1916 by the National Academy of Sciences to act conjointly with the National Academy of Engineering in furthering knowledge and advising the federal government. The Food and Nutrition Board is a committee of the council that oversees the establishment of the Recommended Dietary Allowances.

See also NATIONAL ACADEMY OF SCIENCES; RECOMMENDED DIETARY ALLOWANCES.

natural vitamins Those vitamins obtained from nature, such as the vitamin C found in citrus fruits. With the exception of vitamin E, there is no significant difference chemically between natural or synthetic, or manmade, vitamins.

See also E, VITAMIN; SYNTHETIC VITAMINS.

naturopathy An alternative method of health care whose practitioners advocate the use of natural foods and avoidance of drugs to allow the body to heal itself.

Also known as naturopathic medicine, the word *naturopathy* was coined in America a century ago from the Greek words meaning nature and disease. The healing power of nature—*vis medicatrix naturae*—was acknowledged and employed by the ancient caregivers, including the Greek "father of medicine," Hippocrates, perhaps one of the world's earliest naturopathic and homeopathic physicians. The concept of implementing nature's healing power by using herbs, water, fasting, diet and other noninvasive, gentle treatments has now been accepted into the mainstream American culture, along with the principles that treatment for maladies should not pre-empt the body's innate ability to heal and that preventive measures promote well-being and health. Using primary and curative treatments, naturopathic physicians (NDs) conduct and make practical use of the latest biochemical research involving nutrition, botanicals, homeopathy and other natural treatments for many diseases and conditions, such as ulcerative colitis, asthma, menopause, flu, obesity and chronic fatigue. NDs also function within an integrated framework, for example, by referring patients to appropriate conventional medical specialists when necessary and using naturopathic therapies that complement conventional treatments.

Naturopathic medicine was popular and widely available throughout the United States well into the early part of the 20th century. During the 1920s there were a number of naturopathic medical schools, thousands of naturopathic physicians and thousands of patients using naturopathic therapies. But the rise of "scientific medicine," the discovery and increasing use of new pharmaceuticals, including antibiotics, and the establishment of a wide-ranging medical system primarily based (both clinically and economically) on high-tech and pharmaceutical treatments put naturopathic and other natural healing methods into a temporary decline.

By the 1970s, however, the American public felt the impact of the costs, problems and limitations of conventional medicine and began to explore other methods now referred to as integrative, alternative and complementary medicine.

According to an article, "What is the History of Naturopathic Medicine?," by Peter Barry Chowka, "Today, licensed naturopathic physicians are experiencing noteworthy clinical successes, providing leadership in innovative natural medical research, enjoying increasing political influence, and looking forward to an unlimited future potential. Both the American public and policy makers are recognizing and contributing to the resurgence of the comprehensive system of health care practiced by NDs. In 1992, the National Institutes of Health's (NIH) Office of Alternative Medicine, created by an act of Congress, invited leading naturopathic physicians (educators, researchers, and clinical practitioners) to serve on key federal advisory panels and to help define priorities and design protocols for state-of-the-art alternative medical research. In 1994, the NIH selected Bastyr University as the national center for research on alternative treatments for HIV/AIDS. At a one-million-dollar level of funding, this action represented the formal recognition by the federal government of the legitimacy and significance of naturopathic medicine. Meanwhile, the number of new NDs is steadily increasing, and licensure of naturopathic physicians is expanding into new states. By April of 1996, eleven of fifty states had naturopathic licensing laws (Alaska, Arizona, Connecticut, Hawaii, Maine, Montana, New Hampshire, Oregon, Utah, Vermont, and Washington). A number of other states are likely to enact naturopathic licensing in the near future."

In October 1996 the Natural Medicine Clinic, the first medical facility in the nation to offer natural medical treatments to the community, opened in Kent, Washington, and it is funded by the King County (Seattle) Department of Public Health. Bastyr University, one of the three American naturopathic colleges, was selected to operate the clinic.

Naturopathy, wrote Chowka, "is as old as healing itself and as new as the latest discoveries in biochemical sciences. In the United States, the naturopathic medical profession's infrastructure is based on accredited educational institutions, professional licensing by a growing number of states, national standards of practice and care, peer review, and an ongoing commitment to state-of-the-art scientific research. Modern American naturopathic physicians (NDs) receive extensive training in and use therapies that are primarily natural (hence the name naturopathic) and nontoxic, including clinical nutrition, homeopathy, botanical medicine, hydrotherapy, physical medicine, and counseling. Many NDs have additional training and certification in acupuncture and home birthing. These contemporary NDs, who have attended naturopathic medical colleges recognized by the U.S. Department of Education, practice medicine as primary health care providers and are increasingly acknowledged as leaders in bringing about progressive changes in the nation's medical system."

Naturopathy may also be useful in the treatment of animals. More information on animal homeopathy is available through the Holistic Animal Therapy Association of Australia (HATAA) at its website http://www.hataa.asn.au/.

neem   An Ayurvedic herb, *Azadiracta indica,* of the Meliaceae family, used as a bitter tonic, antipyretic and alterative. In traditional Chinese medicine, the herb is known as *Melia azedarach,* or chinaberry, pride-of-India, Persian lilac, Indian lilac, bead tree and paradise tree. While the poisonous fruits (and probably the leaves, flowers and bark as well) of the plant have killed livestock and fish, the fruits, stem and bark are used in herbal medicine to treat angina pectoris, abdominal pain, intestinal worms and as an emetic.

nelumbo   See LOTUS.

nettle   Any herb of the genus *Urtica,* of the Urticaceae (or nettle) family, particularly *U. urens,* with prickly or stinging hairs. Also known as stinging nettle, the herb contains vitamins (including C and A), potassium, protein, fiber, chlorophyll and other substances. The leaves may be used to make tea that is considered by herbalists to be a lung, stomach, urinary tract and general body tonic. Nettles are also prescribed to treat anemia, asthma, kidney and bladder inflammation, arthritis, urinary stones, rheumatism, dysentery, diarrhea, bleeding (especially caused by endometriosis) and other problems. It is said that deliberately allowing the leaf hairs to "sting" an area where there is arthritic pain will relieve the pain. Externally, the juice from heated and squeezed nettles may be applied to the scalp to stimulate hair growth, according to herbalists. A nettle powder applied to an open wound helps to stop bleeding.

Other reported uses of nettles include as a diuretic, tonic, astringent and for treating nosebleed and excessive phlegm. *U. dioica,* which grows in the United States, is often eaten as a vegetable, but one must handle nettles carefully so the bristly hairs do not sting skin or other body tissues. The roots and leaves are generally used in herbal preparations, but homeopaths prescribe tincture of the entire flowering plant for the treatment of sore throat, uremia, gout, gravel, vertigo and many other ailments.

neurologic diseases caused by vitamin deficiency Wernicke's encephalopathy of alcoholism from insufficient thiamine (vitamin B_1) and degeneration of the spinal cord from a lack of vitamin B_{12} are the only two disorders involving the central nervous system proven to result from inadequate vitamins. Polyneuropathy, delirium tremens and cerebellar degeneration, which are also associated with chronic alcoholism, are possibly related to vitamin deficiencies, but this is unsubstantiated.

See also THIAMINE.

niacin (nicotinic acid, vitamin B_3 or 3-pyridinecarboxylic acid)   A water-soluble member of the vitamin B-complex family. Although humans can synthesize small quantities of niacin, it is classified as a vitamin because the quantity made in the body is inadequate for normal function. Niacin is essential for the manufacture of the hormones cortisone, thyroxine and insulin, and the sex hormones estrogen, progesterone and testosterone. Niacin is also necessary for the normal function of the nervous system.

Dietary Sources and Supplements

Meat is high in niacin and tryptophan. Milk and eggs, although low in niacin, contain sufficient amounts of tryptophan, which is converted to niacin in the body. Cereal and many other foodstuffs contain forms of niacin bound to the food in a manner that prevents the utilization of the vitamin. To counter the poorly available niacin in those products, they are fortified with the more bioavailable synthetic niacin.

Niacin causes an intolerable flushing in many persons, and therefore the niacinamide and nicotinamide forms of the vitamin, which are free of this annoying effect, are used in many multiple-vitamin preparations.

Other Uses

Niacin has been used as a drug for many years to treat various conditions unrelated to its vitamin

properties. Doses much greater than required to satisfy its vitamin requirement are needed for these other uses.

Niacin decreases the production of low-density lipoproteins, or VLDL. This results in the production of less low-density, or LDL, cholesterol, the so-called "bad" cholesterol. Niacin also raises high-density cholesterol, or HDL, the "good, protective cholesterol." Studies have shown decreases of 15 to 30 percent in LDL and increases of 20 percent or more in HDL levels. In at least one study, heart attack survivors suffered 21 percent fewer repeat nonfatal heart attacks than a group not taking niacin. The same group had an 11 percent better long-term survival rate.

When the 1- to 3-gram doses of niacin required to significantly lower cholesterol are used, individuals should be monitored by a physician who can ascertain not only lipid (another name for the fats, cholesterol and triglycerides) but also blood-glucose and liver-function levels. High doses of the vitamin can aggravate diabetes mellitus in a patient previously controlled or can precipitate full-blown diabetes in a borderline individual. Niacin should also be avoided in patients with peptic ulcer disease and gout.

Although niacin is a very potent cholesterol-lowering drug, the huge doses required to lower cholesterol levels limit its usefulness, because only a few people can tolerate the adverse effects (see adverse and toxic effects below). There are claims that chromium combined with very small doses of niacin have a great ability to lower cholesterol, but this needs further study.

The most noticeable and common adverse effect of niacin is vasodilation, a severe flushing of the skin in which an individual feels an intense burning and itching sensation, the most common adverse effect of nicotinic acid. Often this discomfort can be prevented by taking aspirin or ibuprofen 30 minutes prior to ingesting the niacin. Starting with low doses, taking the drug with meals and avoiding alcoholic or hot beverages also lessens the "hot flashes." Less frequent but troubling side effects of niacin are diarrhea, nausea, vomiting and headaches.

Time-release niacin preparations, while reducing the flushing, may significantly increase liver

TABLE 24 RECOMMENDED DIETARY ALLOWANCES

Birth to 6 months	5 mg NE*	
6 to 12 months	6 mg NE	
1 to 3 years	9 mg NE	
4 to 6 years	12 mg NE	
7 to 10 years	13 mg NE	
	Males	**Females**
11 to 14 years	17 mg NE	15 mg NE
15 to 18 years	20 mg NE	15 mg NE
19 to 24 years	19 mg NE	15 mg NE
25 to 50 years	19 mg NE	15 mg NE
51 and older	15 mg NE	13 mg NE
Pregnant		17 mg NE
Lactating		20 mg NE

*NE = niacin equivalent (1 mg of niacin is equal to 60 mg of dietary tryptophan)

complications of niacin therapy and should generally be avoided. Although rare, fatalities have occurred from niacin-induced liver problems. The sustained-release forms are considerably more expensive than niacin tablets, which are the least expensive cholesterol-lowering drug.

Niacin, and some older drugs derived from it, have the ability to dilate some peripheral blood vessels. These drugs have been used in hopes that they would increase blood flow to areas of the body compromised by acute or chronic arterial obstruction or vasospasm. However, despite their widespread promotion and use in the past, there is no acceptable scientific evidence that they are of value in the treatment of those conditions.

Niacinamide and nicotinamide, while providing the vitamin benefits of niacin, have no lipid-lowering or vasodilating properties.

niacinamide (nicotinamide) A form of vitamin B_3 converted from niacin or the amino acid tryptophan in small, inadequate amounts to satisfy daily requirements. While supplemental niacinamide can satisfy the Recommended Dietary Allowance (RDA), it lacks the cholesterol-lowering or vasodilating properties of niacin. It also lacks the adverse itching or skin flushing of niacin.

See also NIACIN.

nicotiana (tobacco) The plant *Nicotiana tabacum*, of the Solanaceae family, named after Jean Nicot, French consul to Portugal (1530–1600), thought to be the first person to introduce tobacco to French and Portuguese courts. Cultivated by Native Americans and used in the West Indies in 1492, according to Columbus, nicotiana eventually became an addictive agent that could be smoked, snuffed or

TABLE 25 ADVERSE EFFECTS (COMPARISON OF REGULAR VERSUS LONG-ACTING NIACIN)

	Flushing	Gastric Distress	Liver Test Abnormalities	Liver Failure
Regular	severe	minimal	minimal	minimal
Sustained Release	minimal	severe	moderate	moderate

TABLE 26 TOXIC EFFECTS OF NIACIN

Toxicity can occur from 100 mg to 10,000 mg (0.1 to 10 gram) oral dose or 20 mg to 750 mg intravenously.

Acute toxic symptoms	Itching or skin flushing Headache Heartburn, nausea, vomiting
Acute and chronic symptoms	Elevated glucose (diabetes) Elevated uric acid (gout) Duodenal ulcers
Chronic symptoms	Hepatitis and liver failure Heart rhythm irregularities Rare—hyperpigmentation of the skin Hypothyroidism Optic nerve disorder Inhibition of the effects of pyridoxine (vitamin B_6) Precipitation of underlying psychosis

(See also NIACINAMIDE.)

chewed. But herbal practitioners, including the traditional Chinese, used the plant to treat sore joints, rheumatism, numbness and snakebite.

nicotinic acid Another term for the B-complex vitamin B_3 or niacin.

See also NIACIN.

nickel Trace metal with no proven human need. Nickel deficiency has been shown to decrease growth and blood production in rats, sheep, cows and goats.

night blindness A disease first recognized in Ancient Egypt in which a deficiency of vitamin A causes limited vision at night. The Papyrus Ebers recommended applying the juice squeezed from cooked liver to the eyes for a cure. The Ancient Greeks ate liver and also applied it to the eyes.

See also A, VITAMIN.

nightshade (bittersweet, scarlet berry, violet bloom, woody, fever twig, felonwort) Herbs of the Solanaceae family, including *Solanum dulcamara* and *nigrum,* whose root, bark and twigs, leaves and herb are used in herbal medicine as an emetic, diuretic and purgative, although the herbs are a mild poison and mainly used in topical applications for swellings, corns, skin diseases, herpes, gout, boils and other ailments.

See also BELLADONNA.

Null, Gary American health and fitness advocate, author, and radio and television talk-show host who promotes alternative treatments of disease and the therapeutic use of dietary supplements. Null is a highly controversial figure whose ideas are in serious question by experts.

nutmeg (jatiphala) The spice derived from the tree *Myristica fragrans,* a tropical evergreen of the Myristcaceae, or nutmeg, family. The nutmeg tree's aromatic seeds are ground into a powder, and herbalists believe small amounts may be taken to relieve cardiac and chronic nervous disorders. When added to other foods such as milk products or baked desserts, the relaxant nutmeg is said to relieve nausea and indigestion. Large doses must be avoided, however, because they can be toxic or even cause miscarriage. One of the world's major commercial producers of nutmeg (and of mace, a spice made from the dried covering of the nutmeg) is Grenada, an island in the western Caribbean Grenadines. Ayurvedic, Chinese and other herbal practitioners administer nutmeg for insomnia, sexual debility, gas, diarrhea, poor appetite, urinary incontinence and general weakness.

nutraceuticals Nutritional supplements and homeopathic, naturopathic and other nonconventional medications or remedies available over-the-counter. Although they are regulated by the Food and Drug Administration (FDA), nutraceutical manufacturers are not required to conduct clinical studies on their effectiveness. According to the website of the American Nutraceutical Association, "Nutraceuticals can be taken in many ways; following are the most common forms: Bulk herbs, available from various outlets, grown at home, or gathered in the wild, are used to make various herbal remedies. Using bulk herbs for therapeutic purposes requires a certain amount of knowledge and skill. Many plants look alike and a poisonous plant may be mistaken for a beneficial plant. Precise identification is critical in the use of wild herbs." The drying and preparation methods of bulk herbs affect their potency. Capsules and tablets (including sublingual, time-release and chewable tablets), soft-gels, powders, teas, decoctions, infusions, tinctures, syrups, compresses, liquid extracts, poultices, salves, ointments, gels, essential (aromatic) oils and lozenges can provide precise amounts of various nutraceuticals, including vitamins, minerals, herbal extracts and combinations of ingredients, and have a shelf life longer than that of dried or bulk herbs. Inert ingredients (excipients) may be used to bind the ingredients and facilitate their metabolic breakdown in the alimentary canal.

The ANA has compiled a list of brand name products that have passed clinical evaluation, with the results either published in a peer-reviewed scientific journal or reported at a recognized scientific gathering. However, some of the controlled clinical trials and studies sponsored by nutraceutical manufacturers have involved only a limited number of patients, and, in some instances, more studies may be required in order to verify results. Controlled clinical trials are studies that test the effectiveness and safety of a product when it is measured against a dummy pill (placebo) or a proven competitive product. Nutraceuticals are natural substances and therefore cannot be patented, a factor that may discourage manufacturers from sponsoring costly clinical studies.

According to "Appendix A: Resources and Guidelines on Buying and Using Nutraceuticals," in *Nutraceuticals: The Complete Encyclopedia of Supplements, Herbs, Vitamins, and Healing Foods* (Birmingham, Ala.: American Nutraceutical Association, 2003), choosing a nutraceutical is "more difficult in the United States than in countries like Germany where, by law, manufacturers of botanical medicines must guarantee that their products meet specific standards. In the United States, the U.S. Pharmacopeia, a nonprofit group, has set standards for some of the most-used herbal products (e.g., St. John's wort, saw palmetto, feverfew, among others). Manufacturers who meet the Pharmacopeia's standards can label their products with a NF, for National Formulary, or USP, for United States Pharmacopeia. They can also advertise that they meet the organization's standards. Unfortunately, Pharmacopeia standards have been set for only a handful of products."

nutrition The processes by which all living things, including human beings, animals, plants and microorganisms, obtain and use substances in their sources of food that are valuable and essential to their health. Nutrition is the end result of ingestion, absorption and metabolism—the utilization of nutrients. Studying nutrition involves identifying which nutrients create optimal well-being of the organism and which ingested substances may have harmful effects upon one's nutritional status. (See also NUTRITIONAL STATUS.) Scientists and researchers through the ages have isolated the vitamins, minerals and other substances necessary to human life and have approximated the quantities required for well-being, that is, growth, tissue repair and normal functioning, as well as therapy in the event that toxicity or deficiency of a nutrient exists. Essential inorganic nutrients that promote the growth and maintenance of living organisms are boron, calcium, chlorine, chromium, cobalt, copper, fluorine, iodine, iron, magnesium, manganese, molybdenum, nitrogen, phosphorus, potassium, selenium, silicon, sodium, sulfur, vanadium and zinc. Essential organic nutrients, the main sources of carbohydrates, proteins and fats that promote energy for living organisms requiring them are amino acids (the precursors of protein), fatty acids, glucose and other simple sugars, purine and pyrimidine and their derivatives (precursors of nucleic acids) and vitamins. Most of the essential organic nutrients for human beings must be obtained from other living organisms such as animals and plants.

All the nutrients required for human life work interdependently in order to metabolize and facilitate optimal functioning. For example, the intake of calcium also requires a certain complementary amount of magnesium so the calcium will be absorbed properly. An excess of calcium may be responsible for a magnesium deficiency; in sum, the nutrients must be balanced. The science of nutrition has not yet established irrefutable amounts of nutrients necessary to that balance, however, but has approximated amounts according to research studies and human experience. It is generally accepted that diets that do not provide adequate nutrition cause weakness possibly leading to illness and appear to impair immune defenses and psychological health.

As poor nutrition can induce disease, the state of disease can cause malnutrition. There are many factors that may adversely affect one's ability to obtain nutrients, including geographic, cultural, environmental and personal circumstances. Malnutrition is considered a world health problem.

Other adverse nutritional situations may include hospitalized patients. Practices such as prolonged infusion of intravenous fluids with glucose and/or salt solutions, failure to measure or monitor food intake, withholding meals while awaiting diagnostic tests, nutritionally inadequate meals and failure to recognize the need for increased nutritional support for some disease states or injuries or following surgery may predispose a patient to inadequate intake of nutrients.

nutritionist (dietitian) An individual with expertise in food and nutrition who instructs others in dietary matters. Registered dietitians (RD) are university-trained professionals.

nutrition therapy Adjunctive treatment advocating the use of nutritious foods, vitamins, minerals and other supplements.

It is the consensus of experts, including the U.S. surgeon general, in the *Surgeon General's Report on Nutrition and Health,* that the American diet in general, which includes saturated fats, refined starches, white flour, feedlot-fattened beef and pork, fish from polluted waters and foods treated with pesticides, preservatives, chemical additives and excessive sugar, suffers from repetition rather than variety and has a significant ill effect on our health. A poor diet can contribute to the risk of heart disease, stroke, diabetes, certain forms of cancer and other problems, such as obesity and allergies.

Among common foods and nutrients now in more popular use for their healing properties are acidophilus culture complexes; activated charcoal aloe vera, amaranth, amazake, arrowroot, astragalus, barley flour, barley grass, barley malt syrup, basmati rice, bee pollen, bee propolis, bentonite, black beans, bran, brewer's yeast, buckwheat, canola oil, carob powder, cheese, chlorella, chromium picolinate, coenzyme Q10, chondroitin sulfate A, cream of tartar, daikon radish, dashi, date sugar, dulse, egg replacer, EDTA (ethylenediamine-tetra-acetic acid), electrolyte drinks, essene bread, essential fatty acids, flax seed oil, fructose, garlic, ginger, ginkgo biloba, ginseng, glycerine (vegetable), gomashio, green magma, guar gum, gum guggul, gymnema sylvestre, kashi, kefir, kuzu, lecithin, millet, miso, mochi, molasses, mushrooms, NutraSweet, oats and oat bran, octacosanol, oils (natural vegetable), omega-3 oils, pasta, psyllium husks, pycnogenol, quercetin, quinoa, rice, rice syrup, royal jelly, sea vegetables, soy milk and cheese, spirulina, spelt and Kamut, sprouts, sucanat, tahini, teas (black and green), tempeh, tofu, tortillas, triticale, turbinado sugar, umeboshi plums, vinegars, wheat germ, and wheat germ oil and wheat grass.

Various alternative and complementary medicines—Ayurveda, homeopathy and osteopathy, among them—advocate certain types of foods and food regimens believed to promote and restore health, such as a low-salt diet.

nutritional status   Assessment of adequacy of a person's intake of calories, fluids, proteins, carbohydrates, fats, vitamins and minerals. Chronic diseases or an acute illness may cause a change in the way you eat or make it hard for you to eat, putting your nutritional health at risk. Four out of five adults with chronic diseases are affected by diet. In the elderly, confusion from memory loss may cause these individuals to forget to eat. Depression or anxiety often may cause loss of appetite. Poor dentition, alcoholism or not being able to afford a healthy diet may also be other causes of poor nutrition.

Nutritional status can be assessed using the Nutrition Checklist developed by the Nutrition Screening Initiative. Read the statements below. Circle the number in the yes column for those that apply to you or someone you know. For each yes answer, score the number in the box. Total your nutritional score.

	YES
I have an illness or condition that made me change the kind and/or amount of food I eat.	2
I eat fewer than two meals per day.	3
I eat few fruits or vegetables, or milk products.	2
I have three or more drinks of beer, liquor or wine almost every day.	2
I have tooth or mouth problems that make it hard for me to eat.	2
I don't have enough money to buy the food I need.	4
I eat alone most of the time.	1
I take three or more different prescribed or over-the-counter drugs a day.	1
Without wanting to, I have lost or gained 10 pounds in the last six months.	2
I am not physically able to shop, cook and/or feed myself.	2
TOTAL	

If your score is:	
0–2	Good! Recheck your nutritional score in six months.
3–5	You are at moderate nutritional risk. See what can be done to improve your eating habits and lifestyle. Consult a nutritionist, check out senior-citizen nutrition programs or your local health department. Recheck your score in three months.
6 or more	You are at high nutritional risk. Speak with your doctor, see a nutritionist or social service professional.

Adapted from the Nutrition Checklist of the Nutrition Screening Initiative.

See also NUTRITION AND AGING.

nutrition and aging   Certain physiological changes that occur in the elderly make them more susceptible to malnutrition. Dental losses often make chewing difficult, resulting in reduced selection of foods, digestive problems or choking. Sensory losses may result in the inability to read labels, taste or smell food that may be spoiled or cause loss of interest in eating. Reduction in the quantity of gastric acid produced may reduce the absorption of vitamin B_{12} and other nutrients.

There is growing evidence that antioxidants can reduce death from heart disease and possibly other causes in the elderly. In a nine-year study conducted at the National Institute on Aging, researchers found that older persons taking both vitamins C and E had a 42 percent lower death rate from all causes than those who did not take the supplements. Death from heart disease was reduced by 53 percent in the vitamin takers.

Aging promotes changes in body composition with a relative increase in fat and loss of muscle and bone. The metabolic rate falls with advancing age and caloric requirements fall accordingly. In addition, some drugs cause nutritional deficiencies. The malnutrition that often accompanies alcoholism is magnified in the elderly.

Nutritional supplements are frequently taken by well-nourished individuals, but those who require them, such as elderly alcoholics, rarely do.

See also NUTRITIONAL STATUS.

oak (tanner's bark, black oak, red oak, live oak, scrub oak, white oak) Trees of the *Quercus* species and the Fagaceae family, found in the United States, England and other parts of the world, whose bark and acorns have long been significant to Native American herbalists and other practitioners as remedies for diarrhea and dysentery. In his book, *Of Men and Plants: Autobiography of the World's Most Famous Plant Healer,* French herbal healer Maurice Méssegué wrote of the use of oak leaves and bark for ulcers, urinary incontinence, vaginal discharge, varicose veins, excessive menstrual flow, eczema and other ailments. A food staple of Native American tribes, acorns contain the astringent tannic acid, or tannin, a glucoside used in tanning, dyeing and the making of ink.

Homeopathic medicine employs tincture of acorns to treat alcoholism, bad breath, constipation, diarrhea, gout and other complaints. Folk medicine calls for an oak bark decoction for gastritis and tuberculosis, among other disorders. White-oak-bark infusion is also used as a treatment for goiter, sinus congestion and postnasal drip, inflammation and mucous discharges.

Also known for its strong wood for furniture, beams and other items, oak is celebrated by poet Robert Graves in *The White Goddess,* published in 1966: "Midsummer is the flowering season of the oak, which is the tree of endurance and triumph."

oatstraw (*Avena sativa*) A nerve tonic, antidepressant and anti-irritant of mucous membranes. Oatstraw is said to increase strength of mind, body and spirit; to calm and tone the nervous system; to nourish bones, teeth, hair and cartilage; to help in drug withdrawal, especially from nicotine, and to boost stamina.

oats (groats) The cereal grass *Avena sativa,* of the Gramineae family, known throughout the world as a nutritive grain usually made into oatmeal. In various herbal medicine practices, oats (also oat straw) are prescribed as a nervine, tonic, stimulant and antispasmodic. Indications for oats include convalescence from illnesses such as gastroenteritis. Oatmeal and rolled oats are considered by Ayurvedic practitioners to be a food that creates heat in the body, a premise widely accepted by nutritionists who recognize oats as a source of carbohydrates and thus energy.

ocimum See BASIL.

olive The fruit of the tropical evergreen *Olea europaea,* of the Oleaceae family, used along with leaves and bark in herbal medicine to treat fever, nervous tension and constipation, and as a base ingredient for ointments and liniments. A popular dressing for salad and a cooking component, olive oil may be applied directly to insect bites and severely itching skin. Olives contain fat, calcium and vitamin A. Olive oil is now recognized to be one of the best cooking oils, a monounsaturate containing oleic acid that resists the damaging effects of heat and light better than polyunsaturated oils. According to Joseph E. Pizzorno, Jr., N.D., and Michael T. Murray, N.D., in the *Textbook of Natural Medicine,* "Population studies routinely show a reduced risk for heart disease when the intake of oleic acid is high."

In his article, "The Mediterranean Diet and Mortality—Olive Oil and Beyond," published in the *New England Journal Of Medicine,* Frank B. Hu, M.D., Ph.D., writes: "Higher levels of consumption of olive oil are considered the hallmark of the traditional

Mediterranean diet. For centuries, olive oil has been treasured in Greece and other Mediterranean countries for its healing and nutritional properties. The use of olive oil now extends beyond the Mediterranean region. Cumulative evidence suggests that olive oil may have a role in the prevention of coronary disease and several types of cancer because of its high levels of monounsaturated fatty acids and polyphenolic compounds."

See also MEDITERRANEAN DIET.

omega-3 polyunsaturated fatty acids (fish oil)   A group of polyunsaturated fatty oils, principally eicosapentaenoic acid (EPA) and docoshexaenoic acid (DHA), obtained from fatty fishes and plants. Capsules of these fish oils are promoted and sold for the prevention of cardiovascular disease. The highest concentrations of the oils are found in salmon, mackerel, sardines, herring, anchovies, whitefish and bluefish. Other seafoods containing these oils to a slightly lesser degree are striped bass, rainbow trout, swordfish, squid and Pacific oysters.

Plant sources of a fatty acid, linolenic acid, which can be converted in the human body to EPA and DHA, are linseed oils, walnuts and walnut oil, flaxseed, rapeseed, soybeans, spinach, mustard greens and purslane.

Benefits and Claims

At least two scientifically valid studies have shown a slight reduction in blood pressure in hypertensive but not normal individuals. Serum triglyceride levels are also lowered and blood-clotting times are increased, which suggests that claims for reducing heart-attack risk may be valid. However, there is evidence that ingesting excessive fish oil, whether from natural fish sources or in capsules, may increase the risk of cerebrovascular accidents (CVA), or hemorrhagic strokes.

In a study called Fish Oil Restenosis (FORT), 8 grams of fish oil were given to patients undergoing coronary angioplasty. The supplement, which was begun 12 days before the procedure and continued for six months, failed to demonstrate benefit in preventing restenosis, or reclosure, of the arteries following the procedure. (An earlier study had reported that fish oils seemed to prevent the reclosure of coronary blood vessels following coronary angioplasty.)

Omega-3 oils have also been shown to improve the inflammatory process that characterizes rheumatoid arthritis and psoriasis. These fatty acids are thought to be essential for good health and may be important for proper vision and brain development, but the manner in which this occurs has not been confirmed. A group of kidney-transplant patients were given daily fish-oil supplements during the first postoperative year. Although there were significantly lower episodes of transplant rejection, improved kidney function and better blood pressure in the treated group, survival at one year was not significantly different from the untreated control group.

Dosage

Nutritionists believe that ingestion of a one-to-one ratio of omega-6 oils to omega-3 oils, rather than the 10-to-one omega-6 to omega-3 ratio in most American diets, is important in preventing coronary artery disease. The omega-6 oils are found in some vegetable oils including corn and safflower. It is theorized that an excess of omega-6 causes substances called prostaglandins and leukotrienes to disrupt the immune system and promote the build-up of cholesterol-containing plaque on artery walls and blood clots. These changes may lead to heart disease manifested by angina pectoris (chest pain), heart attacks and irregular heart rhythms, or arrhythmias.

The recommended intake of omega-3 fatty acids is 0.8 to 1.1 grams per day. A diet containing bony fish or shellfish two or three times a week should provide a balanced level of omega-3 oils. The ratio can also be improved by reducing the use of fatty oils other than olive and canola oil.

Toxic Effects

In addition to the increased risks of strokes from excessive omega-3 fatty oils mentioned above, fish consumed eight or more times a week may supply an excess sufficient to weaken the immune system. And paradoxically, there is evidence that these oils may actually increase serum cholesterol.

Cold-water fish may be contaminated with mercury, and therefore pregnant women should consume them in moderation.

According to American Heart Association guidelines, "Healthy people should eat omega-3 fatty acids from fish and plant sources to protect their hearts. . . . Since 2000, the AHA's dietary guidelines have recommended that healthy adults eat at least two servings of fish per week, particularly fish such as mackerel, lake trout, herring, sardines, albacore tuna, and salmon. These fish contain two omega-3 fatty acids—eicosapentaenoic and docosahexaenoic acids (EPA and DHA). A third kind, alpha-linolenic acid, is less potent. It comes from soybeans, canola, walnut, and flaxseed and oils made from those beans, nuts, and seeds." ("New guidelines focus on fish, fish oil, omega-3 fatty acid," AHA Statement, 11/18/2002, available online at http://www.americanheart.org/presenter.jhtml?identifier=3006624.)

omega-6 fatty acids (evening primrose oil) Group of fatty acids, of which gamma linoleic acid (GLA) is the most active, promoted to reduce cholesterol, thin the blood and reduce the inflammation in arthritis. There are also claims that capsules of evening primrose oil converts abnormal cancer cells to normal ones, relieves symptoms of premenstrual syndrome (PMS) and depression. Although there are no scientifically proven benefits to the supplements, they are probably nontoxic.

See also OMEGA-3 POLYUNSATURATED FATTY ACIDS.

onion A biennial or perennial plant, *Allium cepa,* of the Liliaceae family, whose bulb is a popular raw or cooked vegetable throughout the world. Ayurvedic and other practitioners consider the onion a diaphoretic, tonic and aphrodisiac. Its ammonia fumes irritate eyes and mucous membranes. Onion juice mixed with honey is said to assuage asthmatic distress, cough, nausea, vomiting, intestinal worms and spasms. Onion can also be made into a poultice for joint pain and a nasal inhalant or eye drops for relieving epileptic seizure. Onions are also credited with the ability to lower the heart rate and cholesterol.

oral contraceptives See CONTRACEPTIVES, ORAL.

orange peel The rind of the fruit *Citrus aurantium,* of the Rutaceae family, used as a flavoring agent in baking recipes and marmalades and touted by Ayurvedic practitioners as a carminative, expectorant and stimulant. Oil of the rind alleviates flatulence and is also used in the treatment of chronic bronchitis. An infusion made with the flowers is used by herbalists as a nerve stimulant.

oregano The bushy, perennial herb *Origanum vulgare,* of the Labiatae family, used widely as a

TABLE 27 OMEGA-3 CONTENT OF VARIOUS FISHES
(AMOUNT OF OMEGA-3 IN A 3½-OUNCE SERVING OF RAW FISH)

Highest (more than 1.0 gram)	Moderate (0.5 to 0.9 gram)	Lowest (less than 0.5 gram)	
Anchovies	Chum salmon	Carp	Ocean perch
Atlantic bluefish	Pacific oysters	Channel catfish	Roughy
Atlantic salmon	Pompano	Clams	Pike
Coho salmon	Rainbow trout	Cod	Pollock
Herring	Shark	Crayfish	Rockfish
Mackerel	Smelt	Eastern oysters	Scallops
Pink salmon	Spot	Flounder	Sea bass
Sablefish	Squid	Grouper	Shrimp
Sardines	Striped bass	Snapper	Whiting
Sockeye salmon	Swordfish	Tuna	
Spiny dogfish	Haddock	Mahi mahi	
Whitefish	Lobster	Mussels	

pungent spice and an herbal stimulant, carminative and diaphoretic.

Oregon grape (mountain grape)   A North American, flowering evergreen shrub, *Mahonia aquafolium,* or *Mahonia repens,* of the Berberidaceae family, whose root is used in Ayurvedic and other herbal medicine practices to treat liver disorders and liver-associated headache, indigestion, blood dyscrasias and coldness. Herbalists also report that the alkaloid berberine, found in the Oregon grape root, stimulates liver function. An infusion made of the berries is given to reduce fever.

organic (natural or health foods)   Foods grown without synthetic fertilizers, insecticides or other contaminates. However, it may be virtually impossible to guarantee that soil has not been previously exposed to those substances. Foods grown with compost, manure or other natural fertilizers, as opposed to those grown in chemically fertilized soil, are considered healthier and better-tasting. Some foods erroneously labeled as "health foods" or "natural foods" have been found to be very high in fats, salt, additives, synthetic coloring or flavoring or preservatives.

orris (Florentine iris)   A Mediterranean flowering herb, *Iris florentina,* of the Iradaceae family, whose fragrant rootstock has been used in the making of perfumes and remedies for water retention, dropsy, bronchitis, sore throat, colic and liver congestion, among other ailments. Orris root is commercially produced chiefly in Florence, Italy.

orthomolecular therapy   Theory of medical treatment utilizing doses of vitamins and minerals far exceeding the Recommended Daily Allowances. Studies have failed to demonstrate any long-term benefits to general health, cancer treatment or prevention or benefit to schizophrenia or other mental disorders. In addition, doses advocated may be toxic in some cases.

See also MEGADOSES; MEGAVITAMINS; MEGAVITAMIN STUDY OF THE AMERICAN PSYCHIATRIC ASSOCIATION.

oryza (rice)   A flowering annual plant, *Oryza sativa,* of the Gramineae family, that provides the grain known throughout the world as a food staple. Named from the Arabic word *eruz,* rice has been cultivated since ancient times and used in traditional Chinese medicine as a tonic and remedy for stomach problems. Rice water is thought to be cooling to the body.

osha   The herb *Ligusticum porteri,* of the Umbelliferae family, used by Ayurvedic practitioners as a stimulant, antibacterial and expectorant.

See also LIGUSTICUM.

osteoporosis   A condition characterized by a reduction of the mass of bone per unit of volume, which can interfere with the strength and function of the bone, especially the lower vertebrae, hip and jaw. Supplemental calcium and vitamin D may help prevent or halt the rate of bone loss, but the nutrients do not seem to be effective in restoring porous, brittle bones.

It has been estimated that at least half of American women do not absorb sufficient calcium to maintain healthy bones. There are about 500,000 fractures attributed to osteoporosis yearly, and this is expected to increase to 1 million to 1.5 million by the year 2040 because of the aging population.

While osteoporosis is related to aging, more women, particularly postmenopausal women and those who are extremely sedentary, are affected than men. Factors that appear to predispose women to osteoporosis include low body weight, consumption of alcohol, smoking, the absence of pregnancy during child-bearing years, lack of previous use of oral contraceptives and lack of regular exercise. Only direct measurements of bone density are capable of determining which women should receive preventive treatment for postmenopausal osteoporosis.

An Australian study demonstrated lower than normal bone mass in otherwise healthy young adults whose older relatives had osteoporosis. In the study, bone mineral density was determined by computed tomographic scanning (CT scan) of the spine. Bone mineral content of the os calcis (the heel bone) by single-photon absorptiometry did not predict those at high risk.

See also CALCIUM.

oxalis (yellow wood sorrel) The creeping, herbaceous weed *Oxalis corniculata,* of the Oxalidaceae family, whose triple leaves so resemble the Irish shamrock that some people claim it was wood sorrel that St. Patrick used as a symbol of the Trinity in his attempt to convert pagans to Christianity. In traditional Chinese medicine, the oxalis plant treats intestinal worms, excessive body heat, scanty urine and copious bleeding.

oyster shell calcium A source of calcium carbonate used as a supplement.

See also CALCIUM.

P, vitamin A group of substances derived from plants that were originally thought to have vitamin properties. Now referred to as "bioflavonoids," they are widely promoted as a natural source of vitamin C. However, they are probably destroyed by the acidic gastric juices before they are absorbed.

See also BIOFLAVONOIDS.

PABA (para-aminobenzoic acid) A component of folic acid, found in brewer's yeast. It has no vitamin or other nutrient properties alone. The action of sulfonamide drugs is based on their structural relationship to PABA. The antibacterial drugs compete with PABA, preventing the normal metabolism of folic acid by bacteria. PABA-containing compounds, including procaine (Novocain), may interfere with the activity of the sulfonamide drugs.

The only proven therapeutic benefits of PABA are as sunscreen and local anesthetic in products for the relief of sunburn. PABA has been used to treat arthritis. There are no proven deficiencies of PABA in humans. Products containing PABA are a frequent cause of generalized or local allergic reactions. Allergic persons may develop severe skin rashes following sun exposure. Oral doses can cause nausea and vomiting.

pai shu (bai zhu, atractylodes) The plant *Atractylodes macrocephala,* of the Compositae family, whose root, according to Chinese traditional medicine, eliminates excess electrolytes (sodium and potassium, metabolic regulators produced by the body) by inducing perspiration, thus energizing the body. Pai shu is also used as a spleen and pancreas tonic and for the treatment of diarrhea, indiges-tion, vomiting, edema, a feeling of tightness in the chest and other ailments.

panax See GINSENG.

pangamic acid (pangamate, "vitamin B₁₅") A toxic substance obtained from apricot pits, without nutritional value and no scientifically proven use; by definition, pangamic acid is not a vitamin. Furthermore, it may cause genetic mutations.

pantothenic acid (vitamin B₅, calcium pantothenate) A water-soluble vitamin converted in the body to coenzyme A. Coenzyme A acts as a catalyst (see CATALYST) interacting with vitamin B₁, vitamin B₂, niacin, vitamin B₆, and biotin in various metabolic functions, including the breakdown of carbohydrates, proteins and fats for energy. Pantothenic acid is named from the Greek word *pantos,* meaning everywhere, consistent with its widespread occurrence in animals and plants.

This vitamin is also necessary for the synthesis, or manufacture, of vitamin D, steroids and other hormones, cholesterol and other fats, bile, red blood cells, porphyrins, neurotransmitters such as acetylcholine and other vital body biochemicals. Pantothenic acid may also be necessary for the normal function of the skin.

Pantothenic acid is absorbed with other B-complex vitamins from the gastrointestinal tract. It is found throughout the body tissues, usually as coenzyme A, with the highest concentrations found in the liver, adrenal glands, heart and kidneys. There is little storage of the vitamin in the body and the vitamin is excreted unchanged by metabolic processes (70 percent in the urine and 30 percent in fecal waste).

History

Pantothenic acid was first synthesized by R. J. Williams and R. T. Major in 1940. However, it was not until 1947 that the vitamin's biological function in relationship with coenzyme A was demonstrated by F. Lipmann and others.

Deficiency

A deficiency of B_5 is virtually unknown. In an attempt to define the role of pantothenic acid, experiments have been performed with volunteers who were given a diet devoid of pantothenic acid and administered a medication that depletes tissue stores of the vitamin. These individuals exhibited many symptoms, including fatigue, heart irregularities, gastrointestinal effects, respiratory infections, skin rashes, burning sensations, lack of coordination, staggering gait, restlessness and muscle cramps.

Some researchers believe that pantothenic acid is important for normal adrenal gland function and therefore some claim the substance benefits those with Addison's disease. This research leads others to feel that B_5 is an "anti-stress" vitamin, and one study demonstrated that 10 mg daily allowed individuals to develop better tolerance to cold water stress. Since some who suffer from rheumatoid arthritis may have low levels of B_5, there is speculation that these patients may benefit from supplements.

There are as-yet-unproven claims for the role of pantothenic acid in the treatment of diabetic neuropathy, improved mental abilities, increasing gastrointestinal peristalsis, prevention of arthritis and allergies. Studies to prevent gray hair in humans based on the vitamin's ability to restore hair color in animals have been unsuccessful. Other uses, also not scientifically proven, include prevention of birth defects and some respiratory disorders; the topical use in creams, lotions or ointments to relieve itching and speed healing of minor rashes. Its value as a treatment for streptomycin and salicylate toxicities is questionable.

Recommended Dietary Allowance (RDA)

Evidence to establish an RDA is lacking, since there is no proven need for pantothenic acid alone. The vitamin biotin appears to provide for any possible effects of a B_5 deficiency. The Food and Nutrition Board of the National Academy of Sciences suggests that 2 to 3 mg is appropriate for infants and 4 to 5 mg for children seven to 10 years of age. Four to 7 mg of the vitamin daily by age 11 and for adults is probably safe and adequate.

There is no demonstrated need for increased amounts of pantothenic acid during pregnancy, lactation or old age. However, there is probably an increased need in malabsorption disorders such as tropical sprue, celiac disease or regional enteritis (Crohn's disease).

Dietary Sources

A 2,500-calorie diet from plant and animal sources provides approximately 10 mg of pantothenic acid. Richest sources of vitamin B_5 include eggs, potatoes, salt-water fish, pork, beef, milk, whole wheat, peas, beans (except green beans) and fresh vegetables. There are very high levels of the vitamin in royal jelly of bees and in the ovaries of tuna and cod. Although cooking losses are minimal, milling of grains, canning or cooking after thawing frozen foods causes up to a 50 percent loss of the vitamin. Intestinal bacteria may also synthesize some of this vitamin.

Adverse Effects and Toxicity

Although there have not been reports of toxicity, occasionally diarrhea and water retention have occurred with megadoses of 10 to 20 grams of B_5 daily.

Supplements

Synthetic D-panthothenate is available as calcium or sodium salts but panthenol, an alcohol derivative, is widely used in multivitamin formulations because it is chemically more stable. Panthenol is easily converted to the active vitamin in humans.

Supplemental doses are usually up to 100 mg daily of panthothenic acid or calcium pantothenate tablets (each 10 mg of drug being equivalent to 9.2 mg of panthothenic acid).

papaver (opium poppy) A southeastern European and west Asian flowering herb, *Papaver somniferum,* of the Papaveraceae family, linked by name to Somnus, the Ancient Roman god of sleep (also called Morpheus, and in Greek mythology, Hypnus), who created the poppy for Ceres, the goddess of the harvest, so she could alleviate her exhaustion from tending the crops. Opium comes from the sap of the poppy fruit and contains alkaloids including morphine, a powerful hypnotic and analgesic. Highly addictive morphine sulfate (USP) acts on the central nervous system, and large or excessive doses may cause life-threatening morphine poisoning. One treatment for morphine poisoning is the drug naxolone, a narcotic antagonist.

In Chinese traditional medicine, opium is a sedative, analgesic and antispasmodic, and the poppy's empty fruits (that is, after the sap has run out) are used to treat headache, toothache, diarrhea, asthma and spasms.

papaya (pawpaw, custard apple, melon tree)
The tropical American tree *Carica papaya,* of the Caricaceae family, whose fruit, leaves and seeds are used by herbalists to treat intestinal worms and digestive ailments. Papaya contains papain, an enzyme that digests proteins and is similar to pepsin produced in the stomach.

Paraguay copper tea   A stimulating beverage, also called yerba mate, made by steeping the leaves and stems of the *Ilex paraguariensis,* of the Aquifoliaceae family, in boiling water.

parsley   A Mediterranean, biennial herb, *Petroselinum sativum* or *crispum,* of the Umbelliferae family, whose leaves, roots and seeds are used by herbalists as a diuretic, laxative and expectorant. The essential oil of parsley, apiol, can substitute for quinia, given for intermittent fever, and ergot, as a parturient (administered after giving birth to stimulate contractions of the uterus). A popular kitchen herb that was once associated with Hercules, the Greek god of strength, because it seemed to give racehorses more stamina, parsley with its chlorophyll works as a breath freshener and neutralizer of gastric juices. Parsley also contains vitamins A and C, niacin, riboflavin, thiamine, potassium and calcium. Psoralen in parsley may have some ability to fight cutaneous T-cell lymphoma (a type of skin cancer). Parsley is also thought to block histamine formation and therefore ward off allergy attacks, particularly of hives and hay fever. Apiol and another chemical, myris-

ticin, in parsley produce laxative and diuretic effects.

While it may deplete the body's potassium supply, parsley's major fame lies in its role in the Passover Seder as the bitter herb eaten as a symbol of new beginnings. Native American and other herbalists prescribe parsley for kidney and bladder inflammation or stones, epilepsy, jaundice, venereal diseases and other ailments. Homeopathic uses include the treatment of intermittent fever and night blindness.

passion flower (maypops, purple passion flower)
A flowering, climbing vine, *Passiflora incarnata,* of the Passifloraceae family, whose plant and flower are used by herbalists to treat nervous conditions such as headache, shingles, insomnia and hysteria. Passion flower is also considered an antispasmodic and diaphoretic.

patchouli (pogostemon)   The fragrant southeast Asian plant *Pogostemon cablin,* of the Labiatae family, whose leaf oil is used in perfumery and in Chinese medicine to treat headache, gas, vomiting and diarrhea.

pau d'arco (lapacho, tabebuia)   A Brazilian tree, lapacho (also grown in Argentina) or *Tabebuia haptaphylla,* of the Bignoniaceae family, whose inner bark is considered by herbalists to have antibacterial, antifungal, hypotensive, tonic, antidiabetic and antitumor properties. Prescribed for inhibiting the growth of cancers and tumors and for skin diseases, the immune system–supporting pau d'arco must be aged in order to be as potent as possible. Immature or outer bark is not believed to have the same effectiveness as the properly aged inner bark.

The Calaway tribe descended from the Incas had long used pau d'arco before it came to the attention of medical professionals in Brazil and Argentina. Allegedly, pau d'arco was responsible for curing cases of leukemia and other viral diseases in those countries. Other testimony has been given to the effectiveness of lapacho, but the substance has not yet been recognized or documented in allopathic literature.

pellagra   Syndrome caused by a deficiency of the vitamin niacin or a metabolic error in which the body is unable to convert tryptophan to niacin. The disorder is characterized by rashes, inflammation of the mucous membranes, diarrhea and mental symptoms including confusion, depression, anxiety, delusions and hallucinations. Supplemental niacin cures this disorder (see NIACIN).

pennyroyal   See MINT.

peony (paeonia, white peony, bai shoa yao)   Eurasian and North American shrubs or herbs, including *Paeonia lactiflora* and *suffruticosa*, of the Ranunculeae family, known for their flowers and named after Paeon, the Greek physician who first used peony for medicinal purposes. Among the peony's history of uses are the peony-seed necklaces made by children of the Elizabethan era to ward off witches. According to Chinese practitioners, *P. lactiflora* roots are said to increase menstrual and urinary flow, work as an intestinal antiseptic and expectorant, and treat tuberculosis, stomach problems and other ailments. *P. suffruticosa* root bark is used as a remedy for convulsions, bloody vomitus related to fever, scarlet fever and other problems. An extract of the rootstock of *P. officinalis*, the common peony, is used by other herbalists as a sedative, diuretic and antispasmodic. A decoction made of the root is administered in minute doses for gout, asthma and other problems, although a tea is not to be made from the peony plant or flowers because they are poisonous and ingestion may be fatal.

peppermint   See MINT.

periwinkle   European, particularly British, and American creeping shrubs or perennial herbs, including *Vinca major* and *minor*, of the Apocynaceae family, utilized by herbalists for diarrhea, excessive menstruation, nosebleed, bleeding in the mouth, toothache, seizures and other nervous conditions.

pernicious anemia   Potentially fatal anemia caused by vitamin B_{12} deficiency.
     See also B_{12}, VITAMIN.

peyote (mescal button, devil's root, dumpling cactus, sacred mushroom)   A southern Texan, Mexican and Central American spineless, succulent cactus, *Lophophora williamsii*, from which mescaline is derived. Mescaline is a poisonous alkaloid that causes hallucinations and an intoxication known as mescalism. In certain Native American tribes, peyote's flowering heads, called buttons, are used in religious ceremonies to produce altered states of consciousness. Peyote is classified as a narcotic whose use is restricted to scientific research.

Phen-fen   See FEN-PHEN.

phenylalanine (α-amino-β-phenylpropionic acid)   An essential amino acid, most of which is converted by enzymatic reaction to tyrosine. When combined with aspartic acid it forms the artificial sweetener Aspartame.

Unproven Uses
Some claim that phenylalanine supplements can suppress the appetite, increase libido (sexual desire), improve memory, mental alertness, relieve depression and enhance the pain-killing ability of endorphins. Endorphins are narcotic-like hormones produced by the body in response to injury or disease.

Dietary Sources
Found in all protein-rich foods, phenylalanine content is also especially high in soy, cottage cheese, dry skim milk, almonds, peanuts, lima beans, pumpkin and sesame seeds.

Adverse Reactions and Toxicity
In the absence of the enzyme phenylalanine 4-monooxygenase, phenylalanine accumulates, causing the serious disorder phenylketonuria. Supplements should not be taken during pregnancy nor by those with skin cancer. This amino acid also may cause blood pressure elevation.
     See also AMINO ACIDS; PHENYLKETONURIA; TYROSINE.

phenylketonuria   An inherited disease, expressed by an autosomal recessive trait, known as PKU, in which a defective enzyme, phenylalanine

4-monooygenase, causes the failure of the amino acid phenylalanine to oxidize to tyrosine. This reaction causes brain damage with severe mental retardation, convulsions, tremors and tumors. Other symptoms include hypopigmentation of the skin and hair, eczema, spasticity, contorted position of the hands and mousy odor in sweat and urine. If the disease is not detected at birth by a diagnostic test, brain damage may occur within the first three years of life.

If the disease is recognized at birth by a simple urine test, all symptoms of PKU are preventable by strict dietary restriction of phenylalanine. Therapy adherence in young children with PKU allows normal bone development. However, older patients with poor dietary compliance are at risk for low bone-mineral concentration.

See also PHENYLALANINE.

phosphorus   Essential element in the diet found in all tissues and involved in almost all metabolic processes. Phosphorus is the second most abundant mineral in the body and the average adult contains 1 to 1½ pounds of the substance. It is a major component of bones and teeth, occurring in a ratio of 1 part phosphorus to 2 parts calcium. Approximately 85 percent or 700 grams (of the mineral) is found in the adult skeleton. This mineral helps maintain the acid-base balance of blood, or pH.

Phosphorus is found in nearly all foods, and dietary deficiency is virtually unknown. One exception is a low-birth-weight infant fed exclusively breast milk for which supplementation is required to prevent rickets. Chronic users of antacids containing aluminum hydroxide may become deficient because aluminum interferes with phosphorus absorption. This deficiency causes bone loss, weakness, anorexia (loss of appetite) and pain.

Recommended Dietary Allowances

For children one to 10 years and adults after age 24, 800 mg per day is recommended. For ages 11 to 24 years and during pregnancy and lactation, 1,200 mg is recommended. Phosphorus is adequate for full-term infants fed breast milk. Formula-fed infants should be given 300 mg through six months of age and 500 mg from six to 12 months.

Toxicity

In normal diets with adequate calcium and vitamin D, phosphorus is unlikely to have adverse effects. However, excess phosphorus may lower blood-calcium levels to unsafe levels.

pica   Compulsive eating of substances that lack nutrients including dirt, ice, gravel, flaking paint or plaster, clay, hair, wood, laundry starch. Pica is common in persons deficient in iron or zinc, but may also occur during pregnancy, when craving for certain foods frequently occurs.

piper (long pepper, bi ba, pippali)   The pungent herbs *Piper longum, nigrum* and *sarmentosum,* of the Piperaceae family, used in Ayurvedic medicine as a stimulant, anthelmintic, expectorant and aphrodisiac, and in other herbal practices for various illnesses. *P. nigrum,* or black pepper (*maricha,* in Sanskrit), which is native to Sri Lanka and southern India and cultivated elsewhere in the tropics, is commonly used as a cooking and table spice. The fruits are used in Chinese medicine to treat colic, headache, gas, scanty urine and menstrual pain. Other species are used whole or in part to aid digestion, treat stomach disorders and sunstroke.

See also RED PEPPER.

pipsissewa (ground holly, prince's pine, wintergreen, zimolubka)   An evergreen of temperate zones whose herb bears fragrant, purple flowers, including *Chimaphila umbellata,* of the Ericaceae family. Roots and leaves of the plant are made into a tincture and prescribed by homeopaths and folk-medicine practitioners for cataracts, diabetes, fever, enlarged glands, gonorrhea, kidney, bladder and liver disorders, syphilis, malignant ulcers, scrofula and other ailments. Ayurvedic practitioners use the plant as a diuretic, astringent and alterative. Pipsissewa is not to be confused with *Gaultheria procumbens,* also called wintergreen.

PKU   See PHENYLKETONURIA.

plantain (ribwort, Englishman's foot, greater plantain)   An herb of the Plantaginaceae family, particularly *Plantago* varieties of green-flowering plants such as *P. lanceolata* and *major*. Not to be confused with the plantain tree that produces a starchy fruit of the banana family, the plantain herb is prescribed by herbalists to treat bladder and kidney infections, hepatitis and bacillary dysentery. Externally, plantain is used on insect bites and stings and to promote the healing of wounds.

platycodon (jie geng, balloon flower, Chinese bell flower)   A Chinese and Japanese flowering shrub, *Platycodon grandiflorus*, of the Campanulaceae family, whose roots are used in traditional Chinese medicine for excess gas, congestion, tonsillitis, stomach ulcers, intestinal worms, influenza, sore throat, dysentery and other ailments.

pleurisy root (butterfly weed, flux root, orange swallow-wort, tuber root, wind root, white root, Canada root)   A North American perennial plant, *Asclepias tuberosa*, of the Asclepiadaceae family, used by herbalists as a carminative, diuretic, diaphoretic and expectorant. Ayurvedic herbalists also use pleurisy root as a febrifuge. Native Americans either chewed the dried root or made tea from the root to treat respiratory infections and dysentery.

plumeria (frangipani)   Fruit-bearing, flowering trees of the tropics, particularly *Plumeria rubra*, of the Apocynaceae family, named after Marquis Muzio Frangipani, who in the 16th century invented perfume for scenting gloves with this plant, and French botanist C. Plumier (1646–1706). While the plant's viscous white latex is toxic, the flowers are used by Chinese and other herbalists to treat diarrhea, dysentery and cough. Buddhist, Hindu and Muslim legend has it that even if the plumeria is uprooted, it continues to bear flowers and leaves and therefore is a symbol of immortality. In addition, planting a plumeria tree at a gravesite is a Malay custom.

PMS   See PREMENSTRUAL SYNDROME.

pogostemon   See PATCHOULI.

poke (pokeroot, pokeweed)   An American perennial herb, *Phytolacca americana*, of the family Phytolaccaceae, used by herbalists for blood and lymphatic purification, swollen glands, arthritis and rheumatism. Ayurvedic herbalists also use pokeroot as an emetic, alterative and cathartic.

polygonum   See KNOTWEED.

polypharmacy, women and   The concurrent use of medications and dietary supplements and the possibility of increased risk, particularly for women, of adverse drug reactions involving such use, according to the Society for Women's Health Research. Women are reported to be more inclined to combine both prescription and/or over-the-counter drugs with supplements, such as St. John's wort, and, because of sex-based metabolic differences between men and women, to experience side effects from the substance interactions. An estimated 7,000 deaths per year in the United States are attributed to the adverse side effects caused by multiple-medication and supplement use.

Source: *Advance for Nurses*, Greater New York/New Jersey, 3, no. 2 [January 20, 2003]: 8A.

pomegranate   A southern Asian and tropical shrub, *Punica granatum*, of the Lythraceae family, that bears a thick-skinned fruit about the size of an orange. The fruit has many seeds and an acidic red pulp, and is used in Ayurvedic medicine as an astringent, tonic, alterative and anthelmintic. Tapeworm has been treated with pomegranate seeds since the Ancient Greeks, and the rind with its high tannin content makes both an internal and external astringent for skin conditions, a vaginal douche, a remedy for diarrhea and a gargle.

poppy   See PAPAVER.

potassium   Principal cation (ion carrying a positive charge) of muscle and most other cells. Adult bodies contain about 250 grams of potassium. It is essential in maintaining the fluid balance in our cells and is required for all cell reactions. Most of the potassium is concentrated in cells at a concentration more than 30 times greater than in the plasma and interstitial fluid. Cells contain 145 milliequivalents (mEq) of potassium per liter of fluid, plasma, 3.8 to 5.0 mEq per liter (1 mEq of potassium equals 39 mg). Although the concentration of potassium in the blood is small, it is of great significance. Potassium is needed in the conversion of glucose into glycogen for storage, for the transmission of nerve impulses, for skeletal muscle contraction and the function of hormones. Potassium may also play an important role in maintaining normal blood pressure. Populations that consume large amounts of dietary potassium have a lower incidence of hypertension. Animal studies have shown that potassium may have the ability to prevent strokes and protect the kidneys from the effects of hypertension even if the blood pressure itself is not lowered by potassium.

Potassium is absorbed from the gastrointestinal tract, and blood levels are kept in balance by kidney regulation. Although most potassium is lost in the urine, some is also lost in the stool and minimal amounts in the sweat.

Deficiency

Potassium deficiency can be caused by severe malnutrition, alcoholism, prolonged vomiting or chronic diarrhea. Diabetic acidosis, the most severe form of diabetes mellitus, and some forms of chronic kidney disease can also lead to severe deficiency. Low blood levels of potassium can also cause nausea and vomiting, which might in turn worsen the deficit. Anorexia (loss of appetite), listlessness, apprehension, drowsiness and irrational behavior are signs of serious potassium depletion. Fatigue, muscle weakness, spasms and cramps, tachycardia, or rapid heat rate, and if severe, heart arrythmias, or irregular heart beat and eventually heart failure, potentially fatal, occur as potassium deficit progresses. Sudden death that can occur during prolonged fasting, such as occurs in persons with anorexia nervosa or starvation, may be a result from potassium deficiency.

Severe burns or trauma to large areas of the body and prolonged high fever deplete potassium. The beneficial action of diuretics, drugs used to treat high blood pressure and congestive heart failure, increases urine output and sodium excretion. Unfortunately, there is also a considerable loss of potassium. This loss is minimized by some diuretics such as amiloride, triamterene or spironolactone, called "potassium-sparing" diuretics.

Other drugs that can cause significant loss of potassium include laxatives, especially those containing phenolphthalein such as Ex-Lax and Feen-A-Mint, bisacodyl (Dulcolax) and senna (Senokot), corticosteroids, the anti-Parkinson drug L-DOPA, salicylates, the antibiotic gentamicin and the antifungal drug amphotericin B.

Potassium deficiency may lessen a person's desire for water, worsening cases of dehydration.

Dietary Sources

Many dairy products, except for cheese; meats; poultry; fish; legumes; fruits; vegetables; and whole grains are rich in potassium. Although bananas, oranges and tomatoes are reputed to contain large quantities of potassium, ingesting them is not an efficient method of maintaining adequate potassium levels in the body.

Unfortunately, the processing of food has resulted in an increase in sodium and decrease of potassium in the diet of many persons. Potassium is also lost in cooking.

Supplemental Potassium

The average American diet contains 2 to 6 grams of potassium daily. A Recommended Dietary Allowance (RDA) has not been established and normal individuals do not require supplemental potassium. However, most persons taking diuretics that are not potassium-sparing should take supplements if they have normal kidney function. Because of a potential for toxicity, potassium supplements should not be taken except under the direction of a physician. Supplements of potassium chloride require a prescription and come in tablet, capsule or liquid form. Potassium supplements must also be taken very cautiously with antihypertensives called "ace inhibitors," including captopril, enalapril and others. These drugs have potassium-sparing properties and may cause the potassium to rise to unsafe levels in patients who have compromised kidney function.

Toxicity

Daily intake of 18 grams of potassium or more can cause signs of toxicity. Blood levels can become elevated from excessive use of potassium-containing salt substitutes, kidney failure, acidosis, serious infections, gastrointestinal hemorrhages and severe muscle trauma. Signs of hyperkalemia (excessive levels of potassium) include muscle weakness, heart irregularities, heart failure and death by cardiac arrest. Toxicity can occur from smaller amounts of potassium, and may be fatal in persons with kidney failure.

pregnancy vitamin and mineral requirements
One of the most important times that normal women require vitamin and mineral supplements is during pregnancy. Over the past 150 years, the female reproductive span has increased to nearly 40 years, from menarche at about age 12.5 years to menopause after age 50. Unfortunately, the U.S. Department of Health and Human Services reports that between 25 and 30 percent of all pregnant patients do not enter into prenatal care before the second trimester of pregnancy. About 40 percent of pregnancies are followed in the public sector and average fewer than eight visits versus the recommended standard of 14 prenatal visits. There is a possibility that supplements taken by all women of child-bearing potential might reduce the risks for various pregnancy complications or birth defects. For instance, it is known that dietary iodine prevents cretinism (congenital hypothyroidism), and folic acid reduces the number of neural tube defects such as spina bifida. Some experts express concern that there will be a false sense of nutritional security in women relying too heavily on supplements rather than good dietary habits. There is also worry about excessive intake of some vitamins or minerals resulting in harm to either the women or her fetus (see Toxicity, below).

At the first prenatal visit, the pregnant woman should have a total nutritional assessment, including a physical examination of the body and skin for evidence of nutritional deficiencies. A dietary food intake assessment should be made based on a dietary history of a three- to seven-day food intake. Measurements of height, weight and, if indicated, skin-fold thickness should be done. Blood and urine tests to assess suspected deficiencies should be ordered. If even a minor deficiency is suspected, nutritional counseling from a professional trained in the special needs during pregnancy should be arranged immediately.

Additional dietary or supplemental calcium has been reported to reduce blood pressure and the development of pregnancy-induced toxemia.

Added zinc has been associated with less incidence of abruptio placentae, fewer preterm deliveries and a lower rate of perinatal mortality.

Iron requirements of pregnancy are high. Loss of iron in the urine, stool and sweat amounts to an estimated 170 mg for the gestational period. The fetus requires about 270 mg and 90 mg are contained in the placenta and cord. Iron is needed for the increase in red blood cells that occurs during the last half of pregnancy. However, much of this is recovered when the red blood cell volume returns to normal after delivery.

Lactation contributes about 0.5 to 1 mg of iron per day. Therefore, the total iron loss for an uncomplicated pregnancy ranges from 420 to 1,030 mg or 1 to 2.5 mg per day over the 15 months of pregnancy and lactation. Iron lost by bleeding at delivery is approximately equal to that saved by not having menses during pregnancy.

Zinc requirement increases during pregnancy, and there are some reports that low zinc levels have been associated with congenital malformations, preterm birth and maternal complications in otherwise healthy women.

Pregnancy increases the demand for vitamin D, especially during the last trimester. Therefore, the Recommended Dietary Allowance is increased to 400 I.U. daily.

Folic acid is among the most important vitamins to be supplemented during the child-bearing years. Neural tube defects, including anencephaly, spina bifida and encephalocele, are among the most common serious birth defects. They occur in approximately one of 1,000 births in the United States. The U.S. Public Health Service has recommended that all women of child-bearing age should consume at least 0.4 mg of folic acid daily. The evidence is so strong that these defects can be prevented by taking folic acid supplements before conception and through the first trimester that the Food and Drug Administration has proposed requiring folic acid fortification of bread, rolls and buns, enriched flour and enriched self-rising flour, enriched cornmeal, enriched rice and enriched macaroni products. Since approximately half of all pregnancies are unplanned, this plan would lessen the dependence on behavioral changes to assure adequate folate levels in women.

During the last half of pregnancy, the fetus removes approximately 0.2 mcg of vitamin B_{12} daily. Therefore additional B_{12} is needed.

The fetus drains vitamin C from the mother as blood levels may be 50 percent higher in the fetus. An additional 10 mg of vitamin C daily to the recommended dietary allowance should suffice for this loss.

Toxicity

Vitamin/mineral supplements containing less than twice the RDA are presumed to be safe for both mother, fetus and breast-fed newborn. However, vitamin A in doses only slightly higher have been shown to be teratogenic, or cause birth defects. Taken during early pregnancy, higher doses of vitamin A may cause permanent learning disabilities, spontaneous abortions and birth defects.

Although there is a serious need for adequate folic acid to prevent the birth defects mentioned above, daily intake in excess of 1,000 mg per day could mask pernicious anemia (associated with vitamin B_{12} deficiency), possibly resulting in irreversible nerve damage.

See also B_{12}, VITAMIN; FOLIC ACID.

premenstrual syndrome (PMS) An ill-defined variety of physical and emotional symptoms that occur on a regular basis starting a week or so prior to the onset of the menstrual period, or the luteal phase. For years women were told that the various symptoms were "all in their heads" and that they were "hysterical." But women consistently complained of more than 150 different symptoms. The most frequent complaints of PMS are bloating, headaches, mood changes, breast tenderness, weight gain and abdominal cramps. Despite the doubts of many, the myriad symptoms are probably legitimately explained by fluctuations in levels of the hormones estrogen and progesterone interacting with electrolytes and biochemicals called neurotransmitters that regulate the nervous system, and dietary factors such as poor nutrition, caffeine, smoking and alcohol. Reinforcing this theory, researchers in New Zealand reported that 15 of 21 women given fluoxetine (Prozac) experienced significant relief from their PMS symptoms. Prozac, an antidepressant, enhances levels of the neurotransmitter serotonin in the brain. When this

drug was switched to a placebo for three months, only three of the group continued to show an improved response. However, similar symptoms that appear on and off throughout the month are probably not related to the menstrual cycle and should not be considered PMS.

There may be marginal vitamin deficiencies associated with the symptoms. A balanced diet may offer some improvement, and some advocate the use of various supplements. Magnesium, vitamin B_6, vitamin A and zinc have been reported to relieve PMS. Vitamin and mineral users must be cautioned that exceeding Recommended Dietary Allowances for some vitamins may be toxic. There have been studies in which placebo or sugar pills reduced symptoms as well as a diversity of supplements, reinforcing the possibility that psychological factors may indeed predominate in this syndrome.

Nutritionists recommend a well-balanced diet, with a vitamin-mineral supplement containing vitamin B_6; regular aerobic exercise; adequate sleep; and avoidance of caffeine, smoking and excessive alcohol. The symptoms can be so distressing in some women that hormonal suppression of ovulation may be necessary. However, Prozac and other antidepressants that affect the delicate chemical balance of the brain may provide a real breakthrough in the relief of this troublesome disorder.

preservatives Substances added to foods or supplements to prevent them from spoiling. There are about 100 preservatives in common use. Antioxidant vitamins such as ascorbic acid, or vitamin C, are used to preserve frozen fruits, dry milk, beer and ale, flavoring oils, apple juice, soft drinks, candy, artificial sweeteners, canned mushrooms, processed meat products, jellies and preserves.

prickly ash (yellow wood, toothache tree) A North American shrub or tree, *Zanthoxylum americanum,* of the Rutaceae family, whose bark and fruit are used in herbal medicine. Native Americans believed the bark alleviated toothache. Ayurvedic practitioners use the pungent and bitter prickly ash as a stimulant, carminative and anthelmintic.

primrose (butter rose, English cowslip) A European perennial plant, *Primula vulgaris* and *officinalis,* of the Primulaceae family, whose flowers, herb and rootstock are used in herbal treatment of migraine, insomnia and other nervous problems, weakness, mucus congestion, respiratory infections, rheumatism, gout and blood dyscrasias, or diseases.

princes' pine   See PIPSISSEWA.

probiotics   Bacteria that thrive in the intestines and are considered "friendly," or beneficial, because they promote the absorption and assimilation of nutrients throughout the body. Examples of probiotics are *Lactobacillus acidophilus* and *Bifidobacteria.* Supplements of these may be required if the body is deficient in probiotics, such as those found in fresh vegetables.

processing of foods   The preparation of the ingredients of food products, such as the milling of grains, that greatly reduces vitamin and mineral content. Processing wheat to make white flour results in the loss of up to 40 percent of vitamin C, 65 to 85 percent of B-complex vitamins, almost 60 percent of magnesium and 70 percent of zinc. In addition, fiber, protein and other vitamins for a total of 26 nutrients are reduced or removed. Only traces of iron, calcium, niacin, thiamine and riboflavin are added to make "enriched" bread.

The addition of sodium bicarbonate to green beans and peas to preserve their green color or to dried beans to soften them alters the pH to greater than 8, inactivating thiamine. High temperatures in cooking and canning also destroy thiamine, but freezing does not affect levels. Thiamine is also destroyed by X-rays, ultraviolet irradiation and the addition of sulfite preservatives used for dehydrated fruits.

Heat reduces availability of pyridoxine. The presence of ascorbic acid increases the loss of pyridoxine and vitamin B_{12} in processes requiring heat.

See also COOKING METHODS.

prostate cancer   Malignancy of the walnut-sized gland present at the base of the male bladder. Although 13 percent of all men will eventually be diagnosed with this cancer, as many as 50 percent have microscopic evidence of the malignancy at autopsy. High-fat diets, especially those rich in the types of fat found in meat, have been blamed for increasing the risk for prostate as well as many other cancers. There is an almost 50 percent lower rate of prostate cancer in Florida when compared with Maine. It has been theorized that the difference is caused by an as-yet-unexplained protective effect of vitamin D that is present in warmer climates with more sun exposure. (Sunlight produces vitamin D in human skin.)

protein   A nitrogenous compound found in plants and animals that, when hydrolyzed, converts to amino acids required for the development and repair of body tissues and the source of heat and energy. The word protein is derived from the Greek word *protos,* meaning first—a particularly apt definition in view of the necessity of protein to human and animal life.

Different food protein sources influence the utilization and possibly the requirements for other nutrients. Therefore, it is very difficult to determine rational and safe dietary requirements for individuals or different populations.

Deficiency

Protein deficiency is usually linked to a lack of adequate calories and results in malnutrition. This condition, called kwashiorkor, is usually seen in infants and children as a result of poor diet, infections, intestinal parasites and other factors. Protein deficiencies are rare in the United States.

Toxicity

There is no strong evidence that ingestion of excessive protein up to twice the Recommended Dietary Allowance (RDA) is harmful in persons with normal kidney function. However, there may be significant risk to persons with kidney disease in even normal quantities of proteins.

See also AMINO ACIDS.

provitamin   Any compound that can be converted, or metabolized, to a vitamin in the body. An example is the carotenoid beta-carotene, a fat-soluble pigment in orange, dark-yellow and dark-green vegetables and fruits. When ingested, it can be converted to vitamin A. Other provitamins are vitamin D_2, ergosterol and D_3, 7-dehydrocholesterol, which are converted to vitamin D.

See also A, VITAMIN; D, VITAMIN.

prunella (heal-all, self-heal) A Eurasian perennial, flowering herb, *Prunella vulgaris,* of the Labiatae family, whose stem, leaves and flowers are used in Chinese medicine to treat lymphatic tuberculosis and fever, and whose fruits are made into remedies for eye inflammation, headache, vertigo, nervousness and other ailments.

pseudotumor cerebri An uncommon cause of increased intracranial pressure that may result in severe headaches and visual disturbances. Among the many causes of this rare condition are very high and prolonged doses of vitamin A.

See also A, VITAMIN.

pseudovitamins A group of compounds that do not satisfy requirements for classification as vitamins but are nevertheless promoted as vitamins by some. These substances include orotic acid (vitamin B_{13}), inositol, choline, methione, para-aminobenzoic acid (PABA), carnitine (vitamin B_4), amygdalin or laetrile (vitamin B_{17}), bioflavonoids (vitamin P), pangamic acid or pangamate (vitamin B_{15}) and gerovital (vitamin H_3).

psoriasis Common, chronic, inflammatory skin disorder characterized by reddened, dry, scaling patches of various sizes, covered by grayish-white or silvery-white scales. There may be small areas of bleeding under the lesions, which are most commonly found on the extensor surfaces of the extremities, such as the elbows and knees, scalp, genitalia and lumbosacral region. The nails may become pitted and a particularly severe form of arthritis may accompany the rash.

Various dietary measures and vitamin supplements have been promoted for psoriasis, but it is very difficult to assess the results because the disorder waxes and wanes. Some report that a very low-fat and modified-protein diet is successful in a limited number of patients. Dr. Kempner's Rice Diet was popular in the 1940s, but adherence is difficult. Two articles published in 1986 reported disappearance of psoriatic lesions on the rice diet. The rice diet has severe limitations nutritionally and must be supplemented with at least the Recommended Daily Allowance (RDA) for vitamins and minerals. The diet also is deficient in protein and must be closely monitored by a physician or nutritionist.

Vitamin A has been promoted for the treatment of psoriasis, but it is safer to use the provitamin form, beta-carotene, which is nontoxic. Vitamin D taken by mouth or applied topically seems to have some benefit, as reported in the British medical literature. However, large oral doses of vitamin D are toxic.

A diet deficient in the essential fatty acid linoleic acid may contribute to the occurrence or severity of psoriasis. This nutrient is found in safflower and other vegetable oils, nuts and seeds. An inadequate supply of zinc, required for absorption of linoleic acid, may play a role by limiting the availability of the essential fatty acid.

Leukotrienes are biochemicals in the body that contribute to the inflammatory process of psoriasis. The omega-3 fatty acids found in fish oils seem to limit production of leukotrienes, and there have been reports of improvement in the skin disorder with the use of fish-oil supplements.

Capsaicin, a substance derived from chili peppers, has been used as a cream to relieve the pain and itching of psoriasis. For severe cases of psoriasis, a chemotherapeutic drug called methotrexate may be helpful. Methotrexate is chemically related to the vitamin folic acid. However, while its chemical structure is similar enough to fool cells to take up this substance, it lacks the vitamin's ability to promote cell growth and therefore may have a limiting effect on the skin disorder and some cancerous tumors.

A well-balanced diet, regular exercise, stress reduction and a multivitamin-mineral supplement may be beneficial for those who have psoriasis.

psyllium (isaphgul) A laxative, demulcent and astringent derived from *Plantago psyllium,* of the Plantaginaceae family.

See also FIBER.

pyridoxine (pyridoxal, pyridoxamine or vitamin B_6) A group of chemically related structures that are converted in the liver to the active form of the vitamin. The Council on Pharmacy and Chemistry has assigned the name *pyridoxine* to the vitamin. B_6 acts as a coenzyme (see COENZYME) by participating in more than 60 enzymatic reactions involving amino acids and essential fatty acids. Amino acids are the building blocks of proteins, and therefore B_6 is essential for the growth and maintenance of almost all of our body functions.

The vitamin stimulates the conversion of amino acids to carbohydrate or fat to be utilized for energy or stored for later use. It is also essential for the enzymatic reaction that releases sugar from storage in the liver. B_6 is essential in the conversion of tryptophan to niacin (see TRYPTOHAN). B_6 is also involved in the synthesis of hormones, the red-blood-cell protein hemoglobin and formation and maintenance of the nervous system. It helps in the manufacture of some neurotransmitters that regulate nerve impulses and prostaglandins that help regulate blood pressure, muscle contractions and the heart and other processes.

History

Vitamin B_6 was first discovered in 1926 in rats fed a diet deficient in vitamin B_2, which caused a rash. However, it was not until 1936, when György recognized that it was another substance that caused the rash, that it was named vitamin B_6. The chemical structure was determined in 1939.

Deficiency

Rarely seen alone, B_6 deficiency usually occurs in individuals also lacking other B-complex vitamins. Skin rashes, seizures, carpel tunnel syndrome and, rarely, anemia are the most characteristic features of pyridoxine deficiency.

Some infants who are born with a defect in B_6 metabolism develop mental retardation and seizures, or convulsions. B_6 levels may be low during pregnancy, and in the past the vitamin has been used to treat the nausea and vomiting of pregnancy. It has also been used to treat the depression that accompanies the use of oral contraceptives by some women.

Recommended Dietary Allowances

The RDA for adult men is 2.0 mg and 1.6 mg for women. These values are based on the anticipated average quantities of protein consumed of 100 grams. However, if a person eats huge amounts of protein, these allowances may need to be increased.

Dietary Sources

The highest concentrations of vitamin B_6 are found in chicken, fish, kidney, liver, pork and eggs. Unmilled rice, soy beans, oats, whole-wheat products, peanuts and walnuts are also good sources of the vitamin. Up to 70 percent is lost during freezing and processing luncheon meats, and up to 90 percent in milling cereal.

Drug Interactions

Up to 40 drugs are known to affect the availability or metabolism of vitamin B_6. Foremost among these are prolonged use of the antituberculosis drug isoniazid; penicillamine, a chelating agent used in the treatment of copper, mercury and lead poisoning and rheumatoid arthritis; cycloserine, an immunosuppressant drug; and hydralazine, an antihypertensive. The administration of vitamin B_6 may alleviate some adverse effects of those drugs. B_6 speeds up the metabolism of levodopa and thus lessens the effectiveness of the drug, used in the treatment of Parkinson's disease.

Toxicity

Chronic toxicity from vitamin B_6 to the central nervous system may result in ataxia, or an unsteady gait, and muscle weakness. Some have had withdrawal symptoms of dependency after chronic use of as little as 200 mg.

Doses of 200 mg intravenously or 200 to 600 mg orally may result in adverse drug interactions with the anti-Parkinson drug levodopa, the heart drug quinidine and penillamine, a chelating agent used to treat Wilson's disease, a potentially fatal inherited disorder in which copper accumulates in the liver, and severe rheumatoid arthritis.

See also COPPER.

pueraria   See KUDZU.

pumpkin   The roundish, usually bright-orange fruit of the *Cucurbita pepo* vine, of the Cucurbitaceae or gourd family, whose pulp is eaten as a vegetable or made into pies and other foods, and whose seeds are considered of medicinal value by herbalists. Ayurvedic practitioners, as do most herbalists, prescribe them as a diuretic and anthelmintic. The seed oil is also used for chapped skin, wounds and burns.

pyrola   See WINTERGREEN.

quassia (bitter ash, bitter wood) A tropical American and West Indian tree, *Picraena excelsa*, of the ailanthus family, named after Quassi, an 18th-century Surinam slave who discovered the quassia heartwood's use as a remedy for roundworms in children and its value as an insecticide. Herbalists also use quassia-wood infusion for fever, indigestion and rheumatism. If the infusion is used as an enema, it is effective against pinworms.

queen of the meadow See GRAVELROOT.

quercetin A bioflavonoid derived from blue-green algae, used therapeutically as an anti-inflammatory agent, particularly for the treatment of allergies and asthma, because it suppresses the release and production of histamines and leukotrienes that cause allergic symptoms.

quercus (daimyo oak) A Korean, Japanese and Chinese tree, *Quercus dentata*, of the Fagaceae family, named from the Latin word for tree. Its acorns are used by Chinese practitioners as a remedy for diarrhea and excessive menstrual flow; leaves are used to stop bleeding, quench thirst and treat hemorrhoids and dysentery; its bark is thought to expel intestinal worms.

quick weight-loss programs Drastic and prolonged reduction of caloric intake to stimulate weight loss. Diets below 800 calories per day have many shortcomings, and they may cause potassium deficiency, which may lead to heart irregularities. Diets of less than 1,200 calories may be deficient in thiamine, pyridoxine, vitamin B_{12}, iron, magnesium and zinc. Very-low-calorie diets use protein as a source of energy. In fact, diets of less than 1,000 calories, with protein content greater than carbohydrate, are actually deficient in protein. These diets may also contain excessive fat and cholesterol.

The safest and most sensible weight-reducing diet is based on a balanced intake of the four food groups. Four servings of whole grains and four of fruits and vegetables, two milk and two meat or legume will provide about 1,600 calories. The high-fiber content of this diet probably reduces drastic fluctuations in blood-sugar levels and thus usually reduces hunger.

Weight loss should be slow and gradual, averaging 1 to 2 pounds per week. Weight loss that exceeds 2 pounds results in loss of water and lean body tissue rather than fat. A multiple vitamin-mineral supplement and exercise, of at least 30 minutes of aerobic activity (treadmill is best) every other day, should be an integral part of all diet programs. If weight loss does not occur, then exercise time should be increased instead of further reducing calories. To avoid toxicity, supplements should not exceed two or three times the Recommended Dietary Allowances.

Group diet programs such as Weight Watchers offer emotional support and behavioral modification. However, once the desired goal has been reached, it is important to stay on a maintenance program. The majority of patients in these programs regain lost weight after dropping out of the program. An individual's weight gain may even exceed what was lost, within a short time of going off a diet.

quinoa A gluten-free supergrain of ancient Incan derivation rich in protein from amino acids and complex carbohydrates that can be used as a dietary staple akin to rice.

quisqualis (rangoon creeper) A Burmese, Malaysian, Philippine and New Guinean climbing shrub, *Quisqualis indica,* of the Combretaceae family, whose name in Latin means "What is this?" Chinese practitioners use the fruits and seeds as a roundworm remedy, and the seeds in oil for skin diseases and eruptions.

radish (raphanus, lai fu zi)   An annual or biennial Eurasian plant, *Raphanus sativa,* of the family Cruciferae, with a pungent, fleshy root that is eaten as a vegetable and used in herbal medicine to aid digestion and treat cough, rheumatism and gallbladder disturbances. The leaves are used for headache, and the whole plant treats diarrhea, dysentery and intestinal worms. Radishes contain small amounts of calcium and vitamin C.

rasayana   The Sanskrit word roughly meaning "give life," referring to certain herbal nutritional supplements used to rejuvenate, strengthen, balance, restore and purify the body. In Ayurvedic medicine, herbs and minerals are used separately or in combination as rasayanas. Amla (Indian gooseberry, the highest natural source of vitamin C), guggul, ashwaghanda, ginseng, licorice, aloe vera, saffron, gotu kola, elecampane and honey are examples of rasayanas, which are more closely associated with Indian food than medicine. One brand of rasayana preparation is Biochavan, either as a jam or tablets made by Ageless Body, Timeless Mind products (Quantum Publications).

raspberry   A European and North American prickly perennial or biennial plant, *Rubus idaeus* and *strigosus,* of the Rosaceae family, whose fruit (not true berries but aggregates with several drupelets) and leaves are used in Native American, Ayurvedic and other herbalist practices as an astringent, stimulant, laxative, tonic and emmenagogue. Raspberry leaf tea is said to prevent miscarriage. Raspberry is also a remedy for diarrhea, dysentery and irritation of the urinary tract, and is widely utilized as a flavoring agent for syrups and other preparations. Nutritionally, raspberry contains vitamins A and C, calcium and traces of other minerals.

RDA   Abbreviation for Recommended Dietary Allowance.
See also RECOMMENDED DIETARY ALLOWANCE.

recommended dietary allowance (RDA)   The levels of intake of essential nutrients that, on the basis of scientific knowledge, are judged by the Food and Nutrition Board to be adequate to meet the known nutrient needs of practically all healthy persons (see Appendix IV).

The Food and Nutrition Board is a subcommittee of the National Research Committee and has developed RDAs since 1941. The board has offered 10 revisions of its recommendations since their first publication in 1943.

The RDAs are not minimal requirements but are published to set standards for good nutrition. The RDA serves as the basis for the United States Recommended Daily Allowances (USRDA) established by the Food and Drug Administration (FDA) for labeling purposes.

See also NATIONAL RESEARCH COMMITTEE.

red pepper (cayenne, chile pepper, capsicum, Spanish pepper, Zanzibar pepper, la jiao)   A tropical perennial plant, *Capsicum frutescens* or *anuum,* of the family Solanaceae, whose fruit is used in herbal-medicine practices as an appetizer, digestive, stimulant, irritant and tonic. It is prescribed to build up the body's resistance for a cold that is just beginning, and it can be made into an infusion to treat stomach or intestinal cramps.

Large amounts of cayenne can cause damage to the gastrointestinal tract and kidneys. As a spice used on foods, cayenne is thought to stimulate the appetite.

rehmannia   A northern Chinese perennial herb. *Rehmannia glutinosa,* of the family Scrophulariaceae, named after Russian physician Joseph Rehmann (1779–1831). Rehmannia root is an herbal Chinese remedy for bleeding, fever, anemia, sore throat, mouth ulcers, bloody vomitus, vertigo, irregular menses and premature ejaculation.

reishi mushroom   A traditional Chinese medicine, *Ganoderma lucidum* (also known as *ling zhi* or reishi) is a rare, hard, bitter-tasting, difficult-to-cultivate mushroom not eaten as food outside of Asia. A medicine with a long history of use, reishi promotes longevity, vitality, good blood circulation, normal blood pressure and healthy blood vessels, hair and skin; helps fight insomnia; relieves allergies and arthritis and helps enhance sports performance. Classified as one of the "superior herbs"—those considered capable of promoting overall well-being and enhancing bodily vitality—in ancient Chinese medical texts, reishi increases disease resistance, normalizes bodily functions and acts as either a tonic or a sedative. According to "Reishi Mushroom," http://www.chinese-herbs.org/reishi/, reishi contains "polysaccharides and triterpenoids that are known to enhance the functioning of the immune system. Studies have also shown that these ingredients suppress the growth of implanted tumor cells. Especially continuous intake of reishi achieves the best results." Also an adaptogen, with properties similar to ginseng, reishi is prepared as a supplement and used in nutrition therapy. In *Eating Well for Optimum Health, The Essential Guide to Food, Diet, and Nutrition* (New York: Knopf, 2000), Dr. Andrew Weil writes: "the polysaccharides in mushrooms . . . are very large, long-chain sugar molecules that are structural components of many cells . . . They resemble the constituents of bacterial cell walls and for that reason may be immunologically active." Weil adds that beneficial polysaccharides are not in the American "button" mushroom but in wild and Asian varieties.

retinaldehyde, retinoic acid, retinol   Substances found in animal fats that are active forms of vitamin A.

See also A, VITAMIN.

rheumatoid arthritis (RA)   Chronic, crippling form of arthritis, characterized by inflammation of the lining, or synovial tissue, of the joints. All joints may be affected, but the small joints of the fingers and feet are the most commonly involved. Inflammatory changes can involve the heart, lungs and other vital organs. The cause of RA is undetermined, but probably involves an impairment of the immune system. RA differs from osteo- or degenerative arthritis in that the latter is a degeneration of cartilage.

Many supplements have been promoted as treatments or cures for RA; however, symptoms of this disease come and go, and it is difficult to prove benefits for supplements as well as for traditional treatments. Selenium has antioxidant properties and is involved in the production of prostaglandins, hormonelike compounds that regulate the inflammatory process. Blood levels of selenium, as well as pantothenic acid, have been found to be lower than normal in some patients with RA. While preliminary studies have suggested some improvement in joint pain in those given supplements, benefits have been inconsistent. Pantothenic acid alone has never been proven to be of value in treating any disease. Vitamin E alone or in combination with selenium has also been reputed to have benefits for RA.

Although copper bracelets have been promoted for the relief of arthritis, high copper levels have been seen in some persons with RA and other inflammatory disorders. Paradoxically, drug compounds containing copper may be effective in treating some of these disorders. Omega-3 fatty acids, or fish oils, have been found to improve some patients with RA. Penicillamine, a drug used to treat rheumatoid arthritis, increases the elimination of pyridoxine (vitamin B_6) in the urine.

rhubarb (rheum, da huang)   Asian plant, *Rheum tanguticum, palmatum* and *officinale,* of the Polygonaceae family, named from the Greek word, *rha,* meaning rhubarb. In herbal medicine, the roots are used to treat constipation, jaundice, fever, infectious hepatitis, diarrhea, amenorrhea related to blood clotting, internal bleeding, dysentery, worms and menstrual pain.

rhus (sumac) East Asian temperate-zone trees or shrubs of the *Rhus* genus, including *R. verniciflua* (varnish tree or Japanese lacquer tree) and *R. succedanea* (wax tree). In Chinese traditional medicine, rhus is used to treat bleeding, diarrhea, dysentery, intestinal worms and tuberculosis. Lacquer is a product of the wax tree.

riboflavin (vitamin B$_2$) Formerly called vitamin G, water-soluble component of the vitamin B complex. Riboflavin is converted by the body to two coenzymes, flavin mononucleotide (FMN) and flavin dinucleotide (FAD), which are necessary for normal tissue respiration (transport of oxygen to the cells) and the metabolism of lipids such as fatty acids. This vitamin is also required for the activation of pyridoxine (vitamin B$_6$) and the conversion of tryptophan to niacin. Riboflavin may also play an important role in maintaining the stability of erythrocytes (red blood cells).

In healthy individuals, the B vitamins including riboflavin are readily absorbed from the gastrointestinal tract, mainly in the duodenum. However, this is not the case for those suffering from malabsorption disorders or alcoholism. Vitamin B$_2$ is metabolized or broken down by the liver, and its metabolites are eliminated by the kidneys. The vitamin or its breakdown products are found in all body tissues, especially the liver, spleen, kidneys and heart, and in breast milk. Excess B$_2$, beyond the body's requirements, is excreted mostly unchanged in the urine and feces. Riboflavin is found in retinal pigment and appears to be essential in the eye's ability to adjust to light.

Deficiency

Ariboflavinosis, or vitamin B$_2$ deficiency, is a rare form of malnutrition or malabsorption that causes angular stomatitis and cheilosis (soreness in the mouth and tongue and cracks in the corners of the mouth), corneal vascularization and dermatosis (rashes in the genital area and dryness of the skin on the face). Severe deficiency may interfere with the production or cause premature death of red blood cells, resulting in anemia and neuropathy.

Animal studies suggest that a lack of riboflavin may inhibit the production of antibodies to protect against infections and increase susceptibility to esophageal cancer. Persons highly sensitive to light and those with cataracts may have B$_2$ deficiency, and increasing intake may improve or prevent these troublesome problems.

Supplementation

Riboflavin may be of value in physical stress situations and tissue repair, including burns, following gastrectomy, hepatic-biliary tract disease (alcoholism and cirrhosis or obstructive jaundice), phototherapy by blue light in the treatment for hyperbilirubinemia in newborns that causes photo-decomposition of the vitamin, hyperthyroidism, prolonged infection, chronic fever, diseases, including celiac, tropical sprue and Crohn's, in which there is severe diarrhea, malignancy and prolonged emotional stress.

Studies in China conducted by the collaborative efforts of the National Eye Institute and the Chinese Academy of Medical Sciences have demonstrated the protective effects of riboflavin and niacin in preventing a type of common cataract. Riboflavin is part of the enzyme system that maintains a supply of the antioxidant glutathione in the eye.

Other Possible Uses

Claims of riboflavin's benefit in the following disorders or situations are unsubstantiated: acne, burning foot syndrome, migraine headaches or muscle cramps. Higher than RDA doses of vitamin B$_2$ and other vitamins and minerals have been reported to strengthen the immune system. A combination of vitamins B$_2$ and B$_6$ may improve carpal tunnel syndrome. Depression and anxiety have been attributed to inadequate B$_2$.

Precautions

There have been no confirmed abnormalities or other problems during pregnancy or breast-feeding with normal daily requirements.

Adverse Effects/Toxicity

There is no known toxicity or other side effects of large doses of riboflavin, although the urine may turn dark yellow or orange with very high doses. However, in some animals high doses of riboflavin have increased the growth of some tumors.

The United States Pharmacopeia (USP) maintains that cooking generally does not alter the availability of riboflavin. Some authors dispute this, claiming that cooking meat causes a 25 percent loss, and milk loses 10 to 12 percent of vitamin B_2 following pasteurization and irradiation for vitamin D.

Storing milk in clear glass bottles increases loss of riboflavin up to 75 percent in three and a half hours. Blanching of vegetables before they are canned or frozen can destroy up to 40 percent of this vitamin. Milling of grains destroys a large percentage of the B vitamins, but many of the processed products are enriched by replacing riboflavin and other vitamins and minerals.

Supplements

There are no studies available in geriatric patients to determine their increased need for riboflavin. See Table 28 for dosage to treat riboflavin deficiency.

See also EYE DISEASES.

TABLE 28 RECOMMENDED DIETARY REQUIREMENTS (RDA) FOR RIBOFLAVIN[1,2]

Infants and children	
birth to 6 months	0.4 mg
6 to 12 months	0.5 mg
1 to 3 years	0.8 mg
4 to 6 years	1.1 mg
7 to 10 years	1.2 mg
Adolescent and adult females	
11 to 50 years	1.3 mg
51 years and older	1.2 mg
Pregnant females	1.8 mg
Lactating females	
first 6 months	1.6 mg
second 6 months	1.7 mg
Adolescent and adult males	
11 to 14 years	1.5 mg
15 to 18 years	1.8 mg
19 to 50 years	1.7 mg
51 years and older	1.4 mg

[1] Adequate diet generally provides sufficient riboflavin without need for supplementation

[2] Use of the following drugs may increase the requirement for riboflavin: phenothiazines, tricyclic antidepressants and probenecid.

TABLE 29 BEST FOOD SOURCES OF RIBOFLAVIN

Milk and dairy products	Fish
Meats	Green leafy vegetables
Whole grain and enriched cereals and bread	

---

rice See GOLDEN RICE; ORYZA.

rickets Disruption in the growth plate of bone caused by vitamin D deficiency, called osteomalacia in adults. Children with rickets have poor appetite and grow slowly. They have weak muscles, deformed bones that buckle or appear "bow-legged" or "knock-kneed," a bulging forehead and may have pelvic and spinal deformities. Misshapen breastbones can cause "sunken" chests that can lead to breathing difficulties. In addition there may be bone pain, fatigability, growth retardation and convulsions and tetany in its most severe form. These children have delayed dentition and are especially susceptible to tooth decay.

Vitamin D is synthesized by the skin upon exposure to sunlight. It is essential for the utilization of calcium and phosphorous to make normal bone. Rickets has been recognized for thousands of years and was first described scientifically in the mid-1600s. In the early 1800s, air pollution from the industrial revolution reduced sun exposure, and rickets become a serious health problem in northern Europe and England. However, it was not until the 1930s that vitamin D was demonstrated to be the cure.

See also D, VITAMIN.

rose hips The ripe accessory fruit or seed pods of the *Rosa* species of the Rosaceae family, recognized as a rich source of vitamin C. In addition to widespread popularity as a vitamin supplement, usually in tablet or capsule form, rose hips are used in Ayurvedic medicine as a stimulant, carminative and astringent. Flowers and hips of roses are of medicinal value, especially *Rosa californica, centifolia, damascena, eglanteria, gallica, laevigata* and *roxburghii*.

rosemary Originally a Mediterranean evergreen shrub, *Rosmarinus officinalis*, of the family Labiatae, cultivated throughout the world as an aromatic seasoning. The leaves and flowering tops are useful in herbal remedies for indigestion, headache, arthritis, nervous stomach, insomnia, colds, suppressed menses, hypotension, poor circulation and, externally, for wounds, eczema, sores and baldness. Excessive amounts of rosemary may be toxic.

rue (herb-of-grace, German rue) A southern European, North American and northern African flowering, perennial plant, *Ruta graveolens,* of the Rutaceae family, whose herb is valued by herbalists for the treatment of palpitations related to menopause, painful gas and colic, gout and rheumatic pain. Because it is also prescribed to promote the onset of menstruation, rue should not be used by pregnant women. Ayurvedic practitioners use rue as a nervine and anthelmintic as well.

rutin A bioflavonoid obtained from buckwheat and other plants.

See also BIOFLAVONOIDS.

safe and adequate intakes   Levels that are considered nontoxic for nutrients and for which there is inadequate knowledge to establish RDAs. Prior to the 10th edition of the book *Recommended Dietary Allowances* (1989), the Food and Nutrition Board of the National Research Council listed vitamin K, biotin and pantothenic acid; trace elements copper, chromium, fluoride, manganese, molybdenum and selenium; and electrolytes sodium, potassium and chloride in that category. By the 10th edition of the publication, RDAs have been established for vitamin K and selenium, and minimal requirements have been given for electrolytes.

safflower (dyers' saffron, false saffron)   A European, especially Mediterranean, and North American annual plant, *Carthamus tinctorius,* of the Compositae family, whose flowers can be made into a tea that induces perspiration, considered effective against colds and certain cases of hysteria. In Ayurvedic medicine, pungent safflower is prescribed as an alterative, emmenagogue and carminative. An edible oil is made from the seeds of the safflower; it is high in linoleic acid and low in saturated fatty acids. The flower heads yield a red or orange dye.

saffron (autumn crocus, Spanish saffron)   A perennial flowering plant cultivated largely in France, Spain, Sicily and Iran, *Crocus sativus,* of the Iridaceae family, was used as a perfume and dye by the Ancient Greeks and Romans. From the 14th to 18th centuries, spice dealers were called "saffron grocers," because saffron was an important commodity. The plant's dried flower stigmas serve as antispasmodic, aphrodisiac, expectorant, sedative and emmenagogue in herbal medicine. Ayurvedic practitioners also use saffron as a carminative. A food flavoring and coloring agent (Spanish rice is typically yellow because of the saffron), saffron is used as a remedy for cough, stomach gas, gastrointestinal disturbances, whooping cough and insomnia, although its high price prohibits its accessibility, and it takes some 40,000 flowers to produce one pound of saffron. Furthermore, it contains a toxic substance that affects the central nervous system and may cause kidney problems.

sage (salvia, dan shen, sauge [French])   A wild and cultivated perennial shrub, *Salvia officinalis,* of the Labiatae family, named from the Latin *salveo,* meaning "I heal" and *salvus,* to save. Sage leaves in herbal medicine are believed to be capable of arresting perspiration (such as night sweats related to tuberculosis), stopping the flow of breast milk, soothing nervousness, counteracting diarrhea and inflammations of the stomach and intestines, relieving mucus congestion and assuaging menstrual difficulties. Overdose or prolonged use of sage may be toxic. Thought to temper grief when laid on graves, sage also served as a fortune-telling device for single girls in medieval England. Sage's grayish-green, aromatic leaves are also a meat flavoring. According to an old English proverb, "He that would live for aye must eat sage in May." And 17th-century English author John Evelyn wrote that proper intake of sage could make a man immortal, following the prehistoric and ancient use of sage as a means of promoting longevity.

The leaves, flowers and dried roots of the Asian species *Salvia militorrhiza* and *japonica* are recognized by traditional Chinese practitioners as treatment for menstrual and uterine problems; liver and gastrointestinal ulcers; stomach pain; internal abscesses; insomnia; inflamed kidney, bone or breast; parasitic worms; enlarged organs; and malarial fever.

While Chinese herbalists believe sage increases mental alertness and physical strength, the English surgeon and herbalist John Gerard wrote in 1597: "Sage is singularly good for the head and brain, it quickeneth the senses and memory, strengtheneth the sinews, restoreth health to those that have the palsy, and taketh away shakey trembling of the members."

St. Benedict thistle   See BLESSED THISTLE.

St. John's wort (amber, goatweed, Klamath weed, Tipton weed)   An eastern North American and Pacific coastal shrubby perennial, *Hypericum perforatum,* of the Hypericaceae family, used by Ayurvedic and other herbalists as an antispasmodic, astringent, nervine and expectorant. During the medieval, customary St. John's Eve (June 23) fires—to "purify the air" of evil spirits and thereby protect people, animals and crops—St. John's wort, along with ivy, mugwort, figwort, vervain, lavender and others, was smoked and hung in homes and other buildings to ward off evil powers. Some people even wore the smoked herbs around their necks.

With an odor like turpentine, St. John's wort is believed to have medicinal use for nervousness, bedwetting, insomnia, depression and other ailments. Oil extract from the herb treats stomachache, intestinal distress and lung congestion, while St. John's wort tea is prescribed for menstrual cramps. The herb may be toxic to animals and may cause photosensitivity of the skin.

salt, table, versus sea salt   Sea salt is proclaimed in health food stores to be beneficial; however there is no significant benefit, although sea salt may contain small quantities of other minerals such as magnesium and calcium. Sodium chloride is the basic ingredient in both, and the negligible quantities of other minerals are not worth the additional cost. Ordinary table salt is fortified with the mineral iodine. Iodized salt has resulted in the reduction in cases of goiter (enlarged thyroid glands) from areas of the United States formerly called the "goiter belt," caused by iodine deficiency.

See also IODINE.

sandalwood (white saunders)   A tree native to India, *Santalum album,* of the Santalaceae family, whose wood is used in herbal medicine preparations for the treatment of bronchitis, indigestion, fever and nervousness. In ancient Burma, India and China, Hindus and Buddhists burned sandalwood in funeral pyres and as incense, and used it also as a perfume and an embalming substance. After sandalwood trees were cut down and the branches removed, they were left to the termites, who devoured the superfluous outer layer of wood. The valuable, aromatic heartwood was then available for commercial use.

sanicle (pool root, wood sanicle, black snakeroot)   An American perennial plant, *Sanicula marilandica,* of the carrot family, long thought to have healing powers as an anodyne or astringent. The rootstock is prepared as a remedy for sore throat, mouth sores, ulcers, hemorrhage, intermittent fever, chorea and excessive menstrual bleeding. Leaves of *S. europaea* yield an astringent, styptic and expectorant, used especially for chest congestion and, externally, as a treatment for wounds and skin eruptions.

Homeopaths also prescribe sanicle for such problems as night terrors, foot sweat, crusted nose, neuralgia, diabetes, sore coccyx, ulcerated cornea, potbellied children, itching, emaciation and premature ossification.

sarsaparilla (smilax, greenbrier, spignet, quay, quill, zarzaparilla)   A Central American, Mexican, northern South American and West Indian perennial, *Smilax officinalis,* of the Liliaceae family, whose rootstock is used by herbalists as a carminative, diaphoretic, diuretic and tonic, particularly in treating gout, rheumatism, colds and gas. In Chinese medicine, the *S. glabra* species yields a cooling tonic and purgative, as well as an insecticide and an external preparation for boils and abscesses.

Following Swedish anthropologist Alfred Metraus's discovery that Amazon Indians took sarsaparilla as a cure for general weakness, the plant—named from two Spanish words, *zarza*, bush, and *parilla*, little vine—became a sensation in the United States in the mid-1800s. Sarsaparilla was known as a spring tonic that purified the body, especially after various winter infections and ailments. Today, sarsaparilla is a sweet, carbonated beverage flavored with sassafras oil and distilled European birch oil.

sassafras (saxifrax, saloop, ague tree, cinnamon wood) A North American deciduous tree, *Sassafras albidum* or *Laurus sassafras*, of the Lauraceae family. A tea made from sassafras bark is used in herbal medicine as a blood-purifier and promoter of perspiration and urination. Native Americans drank sassafras tea to reduce fevers and relieve pain.

saw palmetto (fan palm, sabal) A North American, fruit-bearing shrub, *Serenoa serrulata*, of the Palmae family, with berries of medicinal value. Herbalists use either an infusion or a tincture made with the berries as remedies for respiratory irritation such as bronchitis, kidney and prostatic problems and diabetes. Ayurvedic practitioners also prescribe saw palmetto as an aphrodisiac.

savory (bean herb) A Mediterranean annual, aromatic plant, *Satureja* or *Satureia hortensis*, of the Labiatae family, whose herb serves as a seasoning, and an astringent, expectorant, carminative, stimulant and stomachic. Savory tea is the most popular form of the herb as a medicinal supplement.

schisandra (schizandra, magnolia vine, wuweizi, limonnik, omicha, gomishi) In traditional Chinese medicine, the herb *Schisandra chinensis* (also identified as *Fructus Schisandrae*), of the family Schisandraceae or Magnoliaceae, is prepared as an important tonic. It is said to prolong youth, increase stamina, prevent fatigue, supplement deficiency, boost male potency and treat asthmatic cough, night sweats, insomnia, amnesia, heart palpitations, dehydration symptoms, cholera, influenza, snakebites, bone fractures, frequent urination and other ailments.

Schisandra products are made from the red berrylike fruit of a hardy vine of the magnolia family and are often combined with other herbs, such as ginseng and biota seeds, as remedies for coronary heart disease, bronchitis and other respiratory congestion, constipation and spermatorrhea. Schisandra is native to China, Japan, Korea and Russia. Two dozen additional species of schisandra also exist, all indigenous to Asia, except for the relatively rare schisandra vine, which is native to woody areas of North Carolina and neighboring states. Schisandra is touted in early medical texts of China as one of the "superior herbs," capable of promoting overall well-being and enhancing bodily vitality, perhaps even athletic performance. Some hunting tribes of northern China often ate dried schisandra berries to increase their energy. The Chinese have long considered schisandra ideal for lack of energy and for nervous exhaustion from stress. Schisandra has also traditionally been taken to beautify the skin, strengthen the sex organs, and promote mental function. As a topical medicine, schisandra is applied to sores or skin abrasions. In traditional Russian folk medicine, schisandra is considered a treatment for diabetes.

Dennis J. McKenna, Ph.D., and his coauthors explain in *Botanical Medicines: The Desk Reference for Major Herbal Supplements*, second edition, that "[s]o far, the most extensive data on schisandra supporting clinical application concerns hepatoprotective activities, especially in infectious or toxin-induced hepatitis, and as an aid for liver tissue regeneration after liver surgery/hepatectomy, and hepatitis. . . . Anecdotal reports from China include the use of schisandra in the treatment of mild spastic paralysis resulting from stroke, as well as in cerebellar ataxia and Parkinson's disease."

schizophrenia, vitamin therapy in There have been reports for many years that large amounts of niacin were beneficial in the treatment of mental illness, especially schizophrenia. There have been attacks and counterattacks by proponents of megadoses (doses exceeding by 10 times or more the Recommended Dietary Allowances) of vitamins, especially niacin, and by traditional psychiatrists, most of whom are adamant about its detriments. Each side in this controversy claims the other is being either narrow-minded or "unscientific."

There is no question that niacin has marked pharmacologic (druglike) effects that differ from its vitamin activity. However, most of the benefits demonstrated by proponents of the supplements were observed on patients who also required the use of tranquilizers.

See also MEGAVITAMINS; ORTHOMOLECULAR THERAPY.

scurvy Nutritional disease caused by an ascorbic acid, or vitamin C, deficiency and it can be cured by vitamin C supplementation. Symptoms have been described since ancient times by the Egyptians, Greeks and Romans. In children, scurvy causes poor bone and tooth structure. However, the human toll of suffering and death was probably greatest among the sea explorers of the 16th to 18th centuries, A.D. Within months of departing for journeys across the seas, sailors experienced symptoms including bleeding and rotting gums and the bad breath that accompanies it, loosening of teeth, painful swelling of joints, dark blotches on the skin from bleeding under the skin, muscle weakness and loss of energy. From 1740 to 1744, six British ships set out to circle the globe. On these expeditions 1,051 men died, most from scurvy, and only Admiral Anson's flagship returned. Although James Lind, a Scottish surgeon, is credited with discovering in 1747 that citrus fruits can prevent or cure scurvy, it was probably recognized by others much before this time. However, Lind's nutritional experiments led to the dramatic cure of the disorder. Lind gave six different diet supplements to six pairs of sailors suffering from scurvy. Those sailors given oranges, lemons, limes and apple cider improved. Lind incorrectly reasoned that the citrus fruits counteracted the poisonous and noxious "putrid humors" resulting from blocked perspiration from the damp, salty sea air. Unfortunately, it was not until 40 years later that the British made lemon or lime juice a routine part of sailors' diets.

Captain James Cook should be credited with first proving that long sea voyages could be completed without the dread of scurvy. During his voyages from 1768 to 1775, he insisted that his crew eat local greens and other available foods when on land and maintain good hygienic practices.

Despite the findings that led to the prevention of scurvy at sea, scurvy continued to plague the 19th-century populations on land. Scurvy was ever-present in soldiers of the United States Civil War and other conflicts, found in miners during the California gold rush and was widespread during the potato famine in Europe.

It was not until almost 1930 that vitamin C was isolated as the factor that cured scurvy, by Albert Szent-György and Glen King.

See also ASCORBIC ACID.

seawrack (bladderwrack) A type of seaweed, *Fucus vesiculosus,* used by herbalists as an antirheumatic, a weight-reduction aid and a thyroid regulator. It is also used in the preparation of kelp and as a manure.

selenium Nonmetallic element principally obtained as a by-product in the refining of copper, named from the Greek word *selene,* meaning moon. Selenium is an essential mineral required as a constituent of the enzyme glutathione peroxidase and may be vital to the functions of the antioxidant vitamin E. Current research is identifying other evidence of important functions.

Deficiency
It was not until 1979 that Chinese scientists associated selenium deficiency with a fatal cardiomyopathy called Keshan disease (named for Keshan, one of the provinces of China where the disease was studied in relation to selenium deficiency) that occurs most frequently in children and in women of child-bearing age. Dietary deficiencies occur in areas with soil poor in selenium, such as parts of China, New Zealand and Finland. A study in which several thousand Chinese children were given selenium supplements seemed to support this conclusion. However, some scientists feel that selenium-deficient persons are more susceptible to a virus, not selenium deficiency itself, that actually causes Keshan disease.

Patients intravenously fed total parenteral nutrition (TPN), which is deficient in selenium, have occasionally experienced muscular discomfort or weakness that responded to supplements. Rarely, those on TPN developed a cardiomyopathy suggesting a human requirement for this mineral.

Dietary Sources

Meats, especially kidney and liver, and seafoods are the most consistent sources of selenium. Grains and other seeds are dependent on the soil for selenium content. During water and fruits and vegetables contain minimal amounts of the mineral. Although organically bound forms of selenium seem to be more bioavailable, this form did not significantly change glutathione peroxidase activity tests when compared to the activation by inorganic sources. American adult diets provide on average 83 to 129 mcg of selenium per day.

Requirements

By studying the amount of selenium needed to prevent Keshan disease in Chinese people and New Zealanders, it has been estimated that North American adult males require 70 mcg based on 79 kilograms (174 pounds) of body weight and females weighing 63 kilograms (139 pounds), 55 mcg.

By accounting for weight changes, dietary absorption factors and milk production, it has been estimated that an average increase of 10 mcg during pregnancy and 20 mcg of dietary selenium during lactation would be needed to assure adequate levels of the mineral in the mother and breast milk.

Ten mcg of selenium allows for 5 mcg as calculated from adult values with an additional 5 mcg to allow for growth in the first six months of life. This need for selenium increases to 15 mcg from six to 12 months of age. These amounts provide a level of safety from deficiency when compared to the lower and average levels available to breast-fed infants in New Zealand and Finland who do not seem to suffer ill effects from those levels. Recommended selenium levels for older children is based on adult values because insufficient information is available to determine needs.

Toxicity

In a selenium-rich soil of one Chinese region, approximately 5 mg per day of dietary selenium causes hair loss and changes in fingernails. Thirteen Americans developed nausea, abdominal pain, diarrhea, nail and hair abnormalities, peripheral neuropathy (pain, numbness or weakness in one or more peripheral nerves), fatigue and irritability when they were accidentally poisoned by taking nonstandardized tablets containing more than 27 mg of selenium per tablet. Some plants accumulate levels toxic to grazing animals from the soil rich in this substance.

self-heal   See PRUNELLA.

senna (sana)   Dried leaves, leaflets or pods of various senna plants, such as *Cassia acutifolia* and *angustifolia,* of the Leguminosae family, widely used in allopathic and herbal medicine as a cathartic. Some varieties are grown as ornamentals.

sesame seeds   Seeds of the tropical and subtropical annual herb *Sesamum indicum,* of the Pedaliaceae family, used as a source of an edible oil, a flavoring agent and a nutritive tonic, demulcent and rejuvenative.

shark cartilage   Gristle, or dense connective tissue, obtained from sharks, powdered and marketed as a natural anti-cancer substance that allegedly reduces tumors. Shark cartilage is one of the various alternative treatments for cancer patients whose conditions have not responded to other treatments and who are considered to be in the final stage of the disease. Only scant data exist on the effectiveness of shark cartilage. It was popularized by Dr. I. William Lane, a biochemist and head of Cartilage Consultants, in Short Hills, New Jersey, and author of the book *Sharks Don't Get Cancer.* Other scientists and cancer researchers claim sharks do get cancer and that Lane's book exaggerates the substance's effects.

However, the unadulterated shark cartilage products (that is, *not* cartilage derivatives filled with sugar) available in stores have gained popularity and have been approved for study by the federal Food and Drug Administration (FDA).

shatavari (Indian asparagus)   The Ayurvedic herb *Asparagus racemosus,* of the Liliaceae family, used as a nutritive tonic, demulcent, emmenagogue and rejuvenative. Chinese traditional practitioners use the roots of *A. cochinchinensis,* or shiny asparagus, as a treatment of phlegm in the respiratory passages, scanty urine, chronic cough, bloody sputum and fever.

shepherd's purse (cocowort, St. James' weed, mother's heart, case wort, toywort, pickpocket) A common annual, malodorous plant, *Capsella bursa-pastoris,* of the Cruciferae family, that tastes like cabbage, although it has not been used as food since American pioneer roasted the seeds and ate the herb. Herbalists and folk-medicine practitioners believe shepherd's purse effective against stomach and intestinal disturbances, venereal disease, pulmonary disease, internal bleeding, diarrhea, intermittent fever and bedwetting.

shiitake (black mushroom, xiang gu) The Oriental mushroom *Lentinus edodes,* of the family Agaricaceae, eaten as a vegetable and considered by Chinese and other herbalists to enhance the immune system, promote circulation, lubricate the intestinal tract and thereby relieve constipation.

Widely cultivated for its edible and flavorful caps, shiitake also contains properties shown to dissolve fat, help lower blood cholesterol levels and aid in recovery from stomach and cervical cancer.

See also REISHI MUSHROOM.

Siberian ginseng The herb *Eleutherococcus senticosus,* of the Araliaceae family, prescribed by herbalists for increasing energy and endurance (see GINSENG).

silicon Nonmetallic element essential for normal development of long bones and skulls in chickens. Although no human deficiency has been identified, some scientists feel that silicon and other trace minerals (see TRACE ELEMENTS) may play a role in human enzyme systems, specifically in the development and maintenance of bone and in the formation of connective tissue.

Elevated levels of silicon have been found in persons with atherosclerosis but evidence of a role in its development has not been found. Whole grain products, vegetables, dried beans and peas provide adequate silicon and supplements are not recommended.

skin The integument, or outer covering of the body, that is a major body organ and essential to life, composed of the epidermis, or outer layer, and the thicker dermis, which rests against the subcutaneous tissues. The skin's main functions are to protect the body against injury and parasites, regulate body temperature, help in eliminating bodily waste (perspiration), prevent dehydration, serve as facilitator of the cutaneous senses (such as heat, cold, pain, etc.) and provide a reservoir for water and nutrients, such as vitamin D (which emerges when the skin is exposed to the sun).

A wide variety of skin disorders occur from deficiencies of several nutrients, such as vitamin A, essential for growth and maintenance of the skin. Vitamin A deficiency can cause a condition known as follicular keratosis, hyperkeratosis or xeroderma, in which there is excessive production of keratin, a hard protein. The excess keratin causes keratin deposits to form around hair follicles, resulting in a rough texture to the skin suggestive of "goose-flesh" or "toad-skin." Niacin deficiency causes cracked, scaly, deeply pigmented skin. These changes are especially seen in areas of the skin exposed to sunlight. Riboflavin deficiency (vitamin B_2) and protein-energy malnutrition (PEM, which includes kwashiorkor, marasmus or a combination of the two) may also cause rough, scaly, spotty, "sandpaper" and sore skin.

Facial skin that is scaly, off-color, cracked or dry to the point of flaking may be attributable to PEM, lack of vitamin A or iron deficiency. A skin rash may occur in persons taking high doses of pyridoxine (vitamin B_6) when they are exposed to the sun. The skin also gives rise to nails that should be firm and pink and hair that should be shiny and firmly attached to the scalp. Dull, loose, brittle hair may be caused by PEM, and irregularly shaped, brittle or ridged nails may indicate poor iron status. Paleness may be caused by anemia (severe anemia can cause ashy skin) or general malnutrition. Bronzing of the skin may indicate the early stages of pellagra, a niacin-deficiency disease. Some anemias and gastrointestinal disorders induce a sallowness in the skin. Jaundiced, or yellow, skin may be caused by excessive intake of carotene or by liver disease.

See also NIACIN.

skullcap (scutellaria, hoodwort, mad dog weed, side flower, blue pimpernel, helmet flower, huang qin) An East Asian bitter herb, *Scutellaria baicalensis,* of the Labiatae family, whose root is utilized by Chinese, Ayurvedic and other herbalists as treatment for high blood pressure, bloody vomitus, constipation or diarrhea, dry cough, high fever, jaundice and breast inflammation. Skullcap is also considered useful in preventing miscarriage.

slippery elm (moose elm, red elm, Indian elm) A Central and North American and Asian deciduous tree, *Ulmus fulva,* of the Ulmaceae family, whose inner bark is used as a demulcent, emollient and nutritive by herbalists, particularly Native American practitioners. The fresh or dried bark is usually powdered and prepared as an emulsive drink for any inflammatory, gynecological, digestive, catarrhal and cancerous diseases. Slippery elm is also made into lozenges for sore throat and laryngitis. Tincture of the bark prescribed by homeopaths treats constipation, hemorrhoids, pain, syphilis, herpes and other ailments.

smoking See CIGARETTE SMOKING'S EFFECTS ON VITAMINS AND MINERALS.

sodium Alkaline metallic element that is the chief cation (an ion—an atom or group of atoms—with a positive charge) of the extracellular body fluids and the primary regulator of body-fluid volume. Sodium regulates the osmolarity, or concentration of body fluids, as well as their acid-base balance. Sodium is involved in an active transport across cell membranes and must be pumped out in exchange for potassium (called the "sodium pump") in order to maintain a proper balance of fluids and other substances within body cells. Sodium homeostasis, or balance, is controlled primarily by the hormone aldosterone's action on the tubules in the kidneys. Aldosterone levels increase when sodium levels are low and urinary levels are practically zero. The hormone is decreased when sodium levels are excessive, increasing the excretion of sodium in the urine. Despite the kidneys' ability to conserve sodium, some of this electrolyte is lost in sweat and fecal waste.

TABLE 30 SODIUM BALANCE IN THE BODY

Consumption of a fatty meal → sodium concentration in the blood increases → stimulates thirst → consumption of water is increased → blood sodium is diluted back to normal → kidneys excrete excess water and sodium in the urine

Sodium is very active and chemically combines with many substances and is widely found in nature. Salts of sodium are commonly used in medicine.

Deficiency

If blood concentration of sodium becomes too low and water is replaced without sodium, water moves from the blood into the cells and symptoms of water intoxication may develop. These symptoms include headaches and muscle weakness. Despite losses of sodium in sweat, depletion is rare, except in disorders such as chronic diarrhea, severe trauma or some kidney diseases. Deficiency is rare in persons on salt-restricted diets.

Requirements

The minimum average adult requirement is 5 milliequivalents, or 115 mg of sodium or 300 mg of sodium chloride (table salt) per day. To accommodate various levels of physical activity, a safe minimum intake is probably about 500 mg per day. Most American diets exceed this amount easily, even in the absence of "added" salt. Since there is no benefit to the consumption of high levels of sodium, the Food and Nutrition Board recommends a limit of 6 grams of sodium chloride per day.

Toxicity

Excessive salt intake increases the extracellular space pulling water from cells to maintain sodium concentration. This process can lead to edema, congestive heart failure and hypertension. Increasing water intake in many cases will allow the kidneys to remove the excess sodium.

See also WATER INTOXICATION.

sodium ascorbate A soluble salt of ascorbic acid, or vitamin C, used for injectable forms of the vitamin.

See also ASCORBIC ACID.

soft drinks   Popular beverages that contain large amounts of phosphorous in the form of phosphoric acid. High phosphorous intake impairs the absorption of calcium, increases the loss of calcium in the urine and reduces the calcium in bones. These changes may result in osteoporosis.

See also CALCIUM; PHOSPHOROUS.

solanum   See NIGHTSHADE.

Solomon's seal (sealwort, drop berry, yu zhu)   Various *Polygonatum* species of the perennial herbs of the Liliaceae family, especially *P. odoratum, multiforum, biflorum* and *commutatum,* found in the north temperate zone. The name refers to various folklore, such as a description of the cut rootstock: "Scars" on that inner surface resemble Hebrew characters. The 16th-century herbalist Gerard said the herb "sealed up" wounds and fractures. Inked and pressed onto paper, the flower yields a Star of David (a six-pointed star) that is also called the Seal of Solomon.

The rhizome has medicinal value as an astringent, demulcent and tonic in herbal medicine. Treatments include gastrointestinal inflammations, hemorrhoids, erysipelas, neuralgia, ruptures and gynecological problems and pain.

sophera   Trees of the *Sophera* genus, of the Leguminosae family, such as *S. japonica* (Japanese pagoda tree, Chinese scholar tree) and *S. subprostrata,* whose flower buds, fruits, seeds and root are prepared by Chinese traditional practitioners as remedies for ailments including many types of bleeding, high blood pressure, intestinal worms, sore throat and tumors.

sorrel (sourgrass, meadow sorrow, red top sorrel)   A European and North American plant, *Rumex acetosa,* of the Polygonaceae family, characterized by sour or acid sap or juice, whose leaves are used in Native American, homeopathic and other herbal medicine practices as a diuretic, antiscorbutic, refrigerant and vermifuge. Sorrel may be eaten in salad or as a pot herb. Fever, thirst, cardiac weakness, jaundice, kidney and bladder stones, scurvy, excessive menstruation, convulsions and other ailments are treated with sorrel preparations.

spearmint   See MINT.

spelt   A 9,000-year-old wheat grain, *Triticum aestivum spelta,* that originated in the Fertile Crescent and became popular in the Western world. In Germany, spelt is referred to as *Dinkel* and is used in foods and beverages from bread to beer. In Italy, *farro* is an ingredient in soups, pizza dough, breads and cake. Because of its high water solubility, spelt's nutrients are easily absorbed by the body and include certain carbohydrates that aid blood clotting and stimulate the immune system. Spelt is also a rich source of fiber, B-complex vitamins and protein (reported to be from 10 to 25 percent greater than most commercial wheat).

spikenard (old man's root, wild licorice, petty morrel, life-of-man)   A Himalayan aromatic plant, *Nardostachys jatamansi,* of the valerian family, and an American herb, *Aralia racemosa,* of the ginseng family. The American perennial herb root and rhizome were used by North American Indians as a food, and herbalists use them as an alterative, diaphoretic and expectorant. Spikenard is also believed to strengthen and purify the blood, alleviate pain of childbirth and alter the course of uric acid disorders. Homeopaths prescribe spikenard for asthma, cough, diarrhea, hay fever and other ailments.

sprue   See MALABSORPTION.

squaw vine (partridgeberry)   The herb *Mitchella repens,* of the Rubiaceae family, used by herbalists as a treatment for menstrual problems and to strengthen the uterus for childbirth.

stevia leaf powder (sweet leaf of Paraguay, azucacaa, erva doce, capim doce)   The herbaceous perennial *Stevia rebaudiana,* usually used as a natural herbal sweetener. It is indigenous to Brazil, Venezuela, Colombia and Paraguay, where the native Guarani have long used stevia (*caa-ehe*) to sweeten bad-tasting liquid medicine. Stevia and its extracts may be used as supplements in weight-loss programs because of their ability to decrease one's cravings for sweets and fatty foods. Stevia has also been used as a remedy for diabetes, hypoglycemia, candidiasis, high blood pressure and skin abrasions and to inhibit growth and reproduction of bacteria-like plaque. Reported to be 30 times sweeter than sucrose, dry stevia leaf has economic potential as a natural alternative to artificial sweeteners, such as aspartame or sodium saccharin.

sticklewort   See AGRIMONY.

stress   The body's response to emotional disturbances, or physical injuries caused by severe burns, illness, starvation, surgery, or exercise. Stress often initiates changes in metabolism, including the metabolic rate itself, hormone levels, energy reserves, immune response, blood-glucose levels, negative nitrogen balance, fluid and sodium retention and increased elimination of potassium. Stressful situations have also been linked to low levels of vitamins A, B-complex and vitamin C and the minerals selenium, zinc and magnesium. Deficiencies of vitamins B_1, B_6 and B_{12} can cause symptoms including depression, confusion and mental disturbances, but they have no bearing on the psychological stresses of everyday life. In New York State the attorney general took action to force a major vitamin producer to stop advertising the vitamins for relief of emotional stress. However, the metabolic alterations caused by stress serve, importantly, to signal the body against further depletion, damage or diminished organ function. The better a person's nutritional status, the better chance he or she has to recover as quickly as possible from the many forms of stress. Some nutritionists and health professionals refer to this as a "bank account" for good health, with vitamins and minerals in adequate supply to be drawn upon when necessary.

Nutrition counseling to assure a well-balanced diet is important for many people but especially essential for those under stress. Unfortunately, some situations inhibit adequate nutrition, e.g., malabsorption disorders such as ulcerative colitis or Crohn's disease, in which diarrhea prevents the absorption of vitamins and minerals, and nutrient imbalances may prevail. When food and nutrient intake becomes altered by illness—loss of appetite, dry mouth, difficulty swallowing, nausea or the like—an individual is at risk of malnutrition. The illness may extend into problems with digestion and absorption of nutrients; surgery involving the stomach or intestines, radiation enteritis or diseases characterized by diarrhea can intensify nutrient loss. Metabolic changes, such as a loss of energy, and changes in the excretion of nutrients, such as loss of fat-soluble vitamins and calcium in the feces of persons with certain cancers that affect enzyme secretion, may contribute to malnutrition and malabsorption. Malnutrition in the elderly may involve a combination of mental or physical illness and deteriorating motor skills and senses, especially an impaired sense of taste and smell that often leads a person to eat less or eat only foods with strong flavor. In general, illness may lead to malnutrition, and malnutrition may lead to illness.

sugar (saccharum, sugarcane)   An Old World tropical perennial grass, *Saccharum officinarum*, of the family Graminae, named from the Greek word *saccharum*. Sugarcane was brought by Columbus to America, where the crop thrived and became a major industry, especially in the West Indies and other Caribbean islands. Sugar is known throughout the world as a sweetener and energizing nutrient. Chinese herbalists use sugarcane juice to treat excess phlegm in the respiratory tract, to stimulate the stomach and, externally, for wounds, ulcers and other skin conditions.

sulfur   Nonmetallic element found in all body tissues especially those high in protein content. Sulfur is a constituent of the amino acids cystine, cysteine and methionine, building blocks of protein. It is also found in the B-complex vitamins thiamine, pantothenic acid and biotin. Sulfur is an important component of hair, muscle, skin, the connective tissue that holds cells together, bones and teeth. This mineral is involved in the clotting of blood and the activation of some enzymes and is a component of insulin.

A sulfur deficiency is unknown. Dietary protein supplies adequate sulfur. There are no recognized toxic effects of dietary sulfur.

suma (Brazilian ginseng, para toda)   The plant *Pfaffia paniculata*, of the Amaranthaceae family, whose root is considered by herbalists to be a nutrient, demulcent, and energy tonic adaptogen similar in effect to other ginsengs. Suma preparations are prescribed by homeopaths and other herbal practitioners for chronic fatigue and low energy level. It has also been given to cancer patients, but there is insufficient research to assume the herb an effective anticancer agent.

sumac   See RHUS.

sunflower   A tall, common plant, *Helianthus annuus,* of the family Compositae, said to have been cultivated in pre-Columbian America, with large, yellow flowers and black or brownish disk, and bearing nutritious seeds. Sunflower—the state flower of Kansas and a symbol of Peru—contains phosphorus, calcium, iron, fluorine, iodine, potassium, magnesium, sodium, protein, thiamine, niacin and vitamin D. Herbalists use sunflower preparations as a diuretic and expectorant, as a decoction for the treatment of jaundice, heart conditions, diarrhea, malaria and in various topical preparations such as ointments and liniment for pain associated with rheumatism.

sunlight and vitamin D   See D, VITAMIN.

supplements, vitamin and mineral   In a 1986 survey, the United States Health and Nutrition Examination Survey (NHANES II) reported that about 35 percent of adult Americans took vitamin-mineral supplements regularly. In 1987, the National Health Interview Survey showed that 51.1 percent of adult Americans from 18 to 99 years had taken a vitamin-mineral supplement in the previous year. However, only 23.1 percent took them daily. Whites, women and the elderly were more likely than blacks, men and younger persons

to do so. Most took multivitamin products, with vitamin C, calcium, vitamin E and vitamin A supplements the next most commonly consumed. Users took a mean of 2.15 supplements in 1980, but only 1.77 in 1986. Interestingly, and unfortunately, the most likely people to take the supplements were also the most likely to be well-nourished, those with higher income and education levels. It was also determined that the vast majority of persons taking supplements take them in quantities considered to be safe.

The American Dietetic Association estimates that 60 million Americans spent $4 billion on supplements in 1993. These figures were basically unchanged since earlier studies in the 1970s, when the first National Health and Nutrition Examination Survey (1971 to 1975) was conducted. A follow-up survey approximately 10 years later indicated no statistically significant increase in longevity among vitamin users in the United States.

See Appendix V.

sweet flag   See CALAMUS.

synthetic vitamins   Supplemental products manufactured rather than obtained from natural sources. Studies conducted by the United States Department of Agriculture (USDA) demonstrated that equal blood levels of vitamin C were obtained when comparing the vitamin obtained from oranges, orange juice, cooked broccoli or vitamin C tablets.

The only naturally occurring vitamin that may be somewhat more potent than a similar dose of the synthetic vitamin is E. Probably of greater importance is the dissolution time of the product, which determines its ability to be absorbed into the blood stream.

See also ABSORPTION; E, VITAMIN.

tamarind A tropical, flowering evergreen, *Tamarindus indica,* of the Leguminosae family, whose fruit is eaten and made into beverages, and whose fruit and leaves are used by herbalists as a laxative, anthelmintic and refrigerant.

tansy (bitter buttons, parsley fern, hindheal) A European and North American perennial, aromatic herb, *Tanacetum vulgare,* of the Compositae family, considered by Ayurvedic and other herbal medicine practitioners to be an anthelmintic, emmenagogue and tonic. Tansy leaf tea, also prescribed for nervousness and anxiety, may be toxic if taken in large doses.

tarragon (estragon) A perennial North American, southern Asian, European and Siberian shrub, *Artemisia dracunculus,* of the Compositae family, named from the Latin *dracunculus,* or little dragon. A seasoning with a slight licorice flavor, especially popular in French cuisine, tarragon has healing properties, according to herbal practitioners, effective against pain (it acts like a local anesthetic, for such things as toothaches), intestinal gas, irregular menses, arthritis, rheumatism and gout and worms. Tarragon tea is said to stimulate the appetite and help alleviate insomnia.

Other *Artemisia* species, including mugwort, are used in Chinese traditional medicine.

See also MUGWORT.

taurine A nonessential, sulfur-containing amino acid that functions with glycine and gamma-aminobutyric acid as a neuroinhibitory transmitter. A potent antiseizure nutrient, taurine is incorporated into one of the most abundant bile acids and is therefore significant in bile-acid metabolism and digestion. Taurine also aids in rehabilitation from drugs or alcohol, treatment of epilepsy, hyperactiv-ity, high cholesterol, circulatory and cardiac disorders, hypothyroidism, edema and high blood pressure. Sources of taurine include breast milk, shark and abalone.

tea A beverage made by steeping the leaves or other parts of various herbs or plants in boiling water. Many teas contain caffeine, tannin and a volatile oil that gives the tea its flavor and aroma. Caffeine is a stimulant also used in the manufacture of painkillers. Green tea, prepared by heating the leaves in an open tray, has nearly twice the amount of the element fluoride as black tea, which is made from fermented, then dried, leaves. Herbal teas, made from herbs, barks, grasses, flowers and other plant parts, are widely used throughout the world as remedies for any number of ailments or symptoms. Some herbal teas may be harmful.

See also BLACK TEA; CAMOMILE; GREEN TEA; INFUSION; PARAGUAY COPPER TEA.

tempeh A complete-protein food made by the controlled fermentation of cooked soybeans with a *Rhizopus* mold fungus and eaten in parts of Asia. The *Rhizopus* mold binds the soybeans into a compact white cake. Tempeh has a firm texture and a nutty mushroom flavor. It is sold fresh, refrigerated or frozen. A staple source of protein long established in Indonesia, tempeh can be used as an ingredient in soups, spreads, salads and sandwiches. In addition to providing all essential amino acids and isoflavones, tempeh has been touted for its bone-building effects and for helping to reduce the risk of coronary heart disease and some cancers.

thiamine (vitamin B₁) Water-soluble member of the B-complex vitamins, whose deficiency is the cause of beriberi. Thiamine is an important coenzyme required for the intermediary metabolism of carbohydrates and some amino acids. It is especially vital for a normally functioning central nervous system. Thiamine also is vitally involved in the conversion of fatty acids into steroids and is essential for normal growth and skin integrity. Thiamine may also exhibit anti-oxidant properties (see ANTIOXIDANTS). Vitamin B_1 deficiency causes beriberi.

Historical Background

Beriberi was first described in 2697 B.C. by the ancient Chinese in the Neiching, a medical book. A Japanese surgeon, Tomoe Takaki, attributed the disorder to an improper diet in 1884. In 1912, chemist Casimir Funk isolated an extract from rice bran which he called "vitamine," but despite claims that it would cure beriberi, it did not. However, Dutch chemists Pierre Janssen and Willem Donath, again working with rice bran extracts, did isolate the factor effective against the disease. In 1934, American scientist Robert Runnels Williams isolated and determined the structure of thiamine, and in 1936 it was synthesized. The active coenzyme form of thiamine was determined in 1937.

Deficiency

The characteristic manifestations of beriberi change with age and systems of the body involved. The disease is most common in infants between the ages of two and three months. Afflicted babies exhibit a distinctive cry that varies from a loud piercing cry to hoarseness or aphonia (a total loss of voice). They become cyanotic, short of breath, vomit, have tachycardia (a rapid heart rate), develop an enlarged heart and may convulse. Death may result in a matter of hours, unless thiamine is administered.

Older children and adults may have the dry, paralytic or nervous form of beriberi; the wet or cardiac type; the cerebral type; or subclinical, with minimal or no apparent symptoms.

In dry beriberi there is a symmetrical, or bilateral, peripheral neuropathy (a wasting of the nerves) in which the distal, or lower, segments of limbs are affected more severely than the proximal, or upper, ones, with calf tenderness and difficulty raising from a squatting position. These symptoms also are found in wet beriberi, as well as congestive heart failure, with an enlarged, poorly

functioning heart muscle that causes fluid retention in the lungs and extremities.

Thiamine and vitamin B_{12} are the only vitamins whose deficiencies have proven causes of neurologic disease. It takes only three weeks of total dietary lack of thiamine to see the first signs of deficiency. Malnourished patients, especially those with severe alcoholism, are likely to develop the Wernicke-Korsakoff syndrome, or "cerebral beriberi." Wernicke's syndrome is characterized by ocular abnormalities such as paralysis of the muscles controlling the movements of the eyes; dysfunction of the cerebellar or vestibular regions of the brain causing ataxia, or a staggering gait; and generalized confusion, with the patient appearing listless and spatially disoriented. Lethargy is common but stupor and coma are rare.

> COLLOQUIAL DESCRIPTION OF SEVERE
> THIAMINE DEFICIENCY:
> "HOT AS A HARE; BLIND AS A BAT;
> DRY AS A BONE;
> RED AS A BEET; MAD AS A HATTER"

If the patient survives Wernicke's syndrome, symptoms of Korsakoff's psychosis may develop. The state of amnesia that denotes this condition may be recognized by confabulation, in which the patient relates imaginary stories to fill in gaps in memory.

Although anyone deficient in thiamine may develop this serious disorder, alcoholics have both a diminished dietary vitamin supply and decreased ability to absorb thiamine in the gastrointestinal tract. Furthermore, alcoholic liver disease impairs the conversion of thiamine to its active form, thiamine pyrophosphate, and the ability of the liver to store thiamine. It is critical to administer thiamine before glucose is given in any alcoholic or malnourished patient, since carbohydrate loading may trigger the Wernicke-Korsakoff syndrome.

Even persons with a subclinical or minimal thiamine deficiency may exhibit behavioral changes such as irritability, frequent headaches and fatigue. Oral thiamine has been reported to have mosquito repellent properties.

Recommended Dietary Allowances

One mg of thiamine daily is recommended for adults. Maximum absorption is 8 to 15 mg daily, and absorption is enhanced by taking supplements in divided doses with food. An additional 400 mcg, or 1.4 mg, is recommended during pregnancy to allow for increased maternal caloric intake and fetal growth. During lactation, 1.5 mg is recommended to allow for increased energy consumption and the 200 mcg of thiamine secreted daily in breast milk. There is only limited information on thiamine requirements for infants and children (see Table 31).

Dietary Sources

Thiamine is widely found in plant and animal food sources but there are significant amounts in only a few. Meat, especially liver and pork; dried beans; peas; soybeans; peanuts; whole grains; egg yolk; poultry; and fish are the richest dietary sources of thiamine.

Food processing destroys much of the thiamine in foods. Alcoholics not only have a vitamin-deficient diet but alcohol actually interferes with the absorption of thiamine.

There are factors in the diet that may interfere with the bioavailability (ability of the body to utilize dietary substances or drugs) of thiamine. These are called antithiamine factors (ATF). Tea, coffee (both caffeinated and decaffeinated) and the chewing of betel nuts or tea leaves deplete thiamine. Citrus fruits high in ascorbic acid, or vitamin C, have a protective effect on thiamine. Thiamine is also poorly absorbed by persons with folic acid or protein deficiencies.

TABLE 31   RECOMMENDED DIETARY ALLOWANCES FOR THIAMINE (VITAMIN B_1)*

	Age	Dosage
Infants	birth to 6 months	0.3 mg
	6 to 12 months	0.4 mg
Toddlers	1 to 3 years	0.7 mg
Children	4 to 6 years	0.9 mg
	7 to 10 years	1.0 mg
Males	11 to 14 years	1.3 mg
	15 to 50 years	1.5 mg
	over 50 years	1.2 mg
Females	11 to 50 years	1.1 mg
	over 50 years	1.0 mg

(*Food and Nutrition Board, National Academy of Sciences–National Research Council, 1989)

Adverse Effects and Toxicity

Oral doses of thiamine up to 500 mg daily are easily eliminated by the kidneys, and there are no reports of oral toxicity in adults. However, one study has reported toxic effects of large doses in infants. There have also been reports of allergic reactions from intravenous administration of thiamine, ranging in severity from itching and hives to deaths from anaphylactic shock (the most severe form of an allergic reaction).

See also ANTITHIAMINE FACTORS; BERIBERI; PROCESSING OF FOODS.

thuja (arborvitae, tree of life, yellow or white cedar)   A North American evergreen pine tree, *Thuja occidentalis,* of the family Cupressaceae, whose branchlets, leaves and bark are used in herbal medicine as a diaphoretic and emmenagogue. Thuja is also said to be effective against muscular and joint pain, headache and pain in the heart. Thuja is a dangerous herb, however, because it contains a toxic oil, and its use is restricted to medical supervision.

thyme   Eurasian herbs of the Labiatae family, such as *Thymus vulgaris,* with pungent, aromatic leaves that are used as a seasoning and as herbal-medicine preparations for cough, colds, intestinal gas, indigestion, diarrhea and, as a tea, for nightmares.

thymus extract   A product of the thymus gland of the immune system used as a nutritional supplement for individuals with chronic upper respiratory tract infections, AIDS, hepatitis B, allergies and insufficient thymus gland function.

Most often derived from young calves (bovine), the extract Thymomodulin (its trade name) is prepared so that it concentrates small proteinlike molecules, or polypeptides, and may help prevent recurrent upper respiratory tract infections. Preliminary studies suggest that Thymomodulin may also be helpful in improving one of the T-cell defects in patients with human immunodeficiency virus infection (HIV), in treating acute and chronic hepatitis-B infections, in restoring the number of peripheral white blood cells in cancer patients undergoing chemotherapy or radiation and in relieving allergies, including asthma, hay fever and food allergies, in children. The effectiveness of Thymomodulin may be the result of improved thymus gland functioning or of the presence of hormones or other biologically active substances in the extract. In addition to releasing several hormones, such as thymosin, thymopoeitin, and serum thymic factor, that regulate various immune functions, the thymus gland is responsible for cell-mediated immunity (immune mechanisms not controlled or mediated by antibodies), which helps the body resist infections by yeast, bacteria, fungi, parasites and certain viruses, such as Epstein-Barr and herpes simplex. The thymus also produces T lymphocytes, white blood cells that participate in cell-mediated immune activity, which overall help protect against the development of cancer, allergies and autoimmune disorders, such as rheumatoid arthritis.

tin   A metallic element whose organic compounds exhibit varying levels of toxicity. It is unknown if traces of this mineral are essential in human nutrition. If it is required, it is sufficiently plentiful in food, water and air to satisfy human needs.

tincture   A basic medicinal alcohol solution to which can be added powdered or liquid herbs. Homeopaths prescribe a certain number of drops of tinctures of various herbs for the treatment of ailments.

tocoferols   See E, VITAMIN.

tooth development   See DENTES.

total parenteral nutrition (TPN)   Nutritional support given intravenously to individuals unable to eat, be fed or absorb nutrients through the gastrointestinal route. Amino acids must be supplied in adequate amounts for protein synthesis as well as glucose and fats. Vitamin supplements are essential in these patients, although excessive amounts of vitamins A and D should be avoided. In addition to a daily multivitamin formula, additional supplemental folic acid must be given initially and weekly and vitamins K and B_{12} every three weeks. A biotin deficiency may occur in infants on TPN characterized by acidosis, rash and hair loss.

The electrolytes sodium, chloride, potassium, magnesium, calcium and phosphorus are essential components for TPN. If TPN exceeds one to two weeks, zinc, copper and chromium should be supplemented.

toxicity   Ability to cause poisonous effects, such as damage to tissues or disturbance of body function, that may cause illness or death. All nutrients at some level become toxic. Some adverse effects result from a pharmacologic, or drug type, of activity. High amounts of water or salt can be fatal. The fat-soluble vitamins A and D may cause significant and well-recognized toxicity if taken to excess. However, water-soluble vitamins such as niacin and pyridoxine (vitamin B_6) can also cause adverse effects in large amounts.

TPN   See TOTAL PARENTERAL NUTRITION.

trace minerals   See MINERALS, TRACE.

triticale   A blend of *Triticum*, a genus of wheat, and *Secale*, a genus of rye, creating a wheat-rye hybrid with a high yield and rich protein content produced mostly in the United States, Russia and Australia. The first cross was reported in 1875, and the first fertile cross in 1888. The name *triticale* first appeared in scientific literature in 1935 and is attributed to E. Tschermak von Seyseneg. Although not suitable for bread-making, triticale flour may be combined with wheat flour.

tryptophan (L-tryptophan, α-amino-β-3-indole propionic acid, proteinochromagen [obsolete term])   One of nine amino acids essential in the human diet. In the presence of thiamine (vitamin B_1), riboflavin (vitamin B_2), and pyridoxine (vitamin B_6), tryptophan is converted to niacin in the body (approximately 1 mg of niacin is formed from 60 mg of dietary tryptophan). Tryptophan is also required for growth in infants and for nitrogen balance in adults. It is also necessary for the formation of the neurotransmitter serotonin.

Uses

In the absence of adequate niacin, tryptophan may lessen the symptoms of pellagra. Tryptophan has questionable therapeutic value as a supplement for the relief of insomnia and depression and in reducing sensitivity to pain (including migraine) and premenstrual tension (PMS). There are also unproven claims of its ability to reduce dependency on alcohol.

Deficiency

Tryptophan deficiency is rare. However, an inherited disturbance in tryptophan metabolism interferes with the conversion of this amino acid to niacin in the body. This disturbance may result in the symptoms of pellegra despite the presence of adequate niacin. Abnormal metabolic breakdown of tryptophan may result in carcinoid syndrome (a group of symptoms characterized by cyanotic flushing of the skin, diarrhea, wheezing, sudden drops in blood pressure and edema caused by the secretion of chemically active substances from a tumor in the stomach or intestines). The drug isoniazid, used in the treatment of tuberculosis, causes a deficiency in the coenzyme pyridoxal phosphate required for the conversion of tryptophan to niacin.

Dietary Sources

A 3-ounce serving of fish or meat will satisfy the 200-mg minimum daily adult requirement. Dairy products, turkey, bananas, dates, peanuts and other protein-rich foods are good sources of tryptophan.

Supplements

L-tryptophan supplements have been withdrawn in the United States and Canada because of toxicity resulting from contaminated batches (see below).

Toxicity

Eosinophilia-myalgia syndrome (EMS) is a serious and life-threatening adverse effect caused by impure L-tryptophan supplements. In 1989 physicians in New Mexico reported three cases of severe muscle pain and very high blood eosinophil (white blood cells that are elevated in allergic and some other disorders) counts linked to L-tryptophan. After many other cases were reported, on November 17, 1989 the Food and Drug Administration (FDA) recalled most products containing this substance, and on March 22, 1990 a second recall was ordered.

The Center for Disease Control (CDC) defines EMS as a patient having an eosinophil count of at least 1,000 cells/cubic millimeter; generalized myalgia (muscle pain) severe enough to interfere with patient's daily activities; and the absence of any infection or tumor that could account for the first two points.

There have been many milder cases with "flu-like" symptoms that would not satisfy all three points. By September 1, 1991, 1,507 cases of EMS and 31 deaths from EMS had been reported to the CDC. It has been estimated that as many as 5,000 persons have probably been afflicted, with most of these not being reported.

The real cause of EMS is thought to be a contaminant of the L-tryptophan made by a single Japanese manufacturer. However, until that contaminant can be identified and eliminated from the manufacturing process, all brands of this drug should be avoided. Some people with EMS respond to stopping the drug and taking corticosteroids (derivatives of cortisone).

turmeric A remedy made from the perennial plant *Curcuma xanthorrhizia* for the treatment of indigestion, liver and gallbladder complaints and loss of appetite. Turmeric is a widely used culinary spice. In *Advance for Nurses*, April 28, 2003, Mary Ann Hogan, M.S.N., states, "Turmeric, a principal ingredient of curry, may protect cancer patients from the burns and blisters they often face because of radiation therapy, according to researchers from the University of Rochester (NY) Medical Center. . . . Curcumin, which gives turmeric its yellow color, has been shown to have anti-inflammatory benefits. Evidence also suggests it may be able to suppress tumor growth . . . and has long been used to treat burns in India."

See CURCUMA.

tussilago See COLTSFOOT.

tyrosine (oxyphenylaminopropionic acid p-hydroxyphenylalanine) A nonessential amino acid, synthesized from the essential amino acid phenylalanine, which is found in most proteins.

Uses

Tyrosine is required for the formation of thyroid hormones, catecholamines (biochemicals such as the neurotransmitters dopamine, norepinephrine and epinephrine, or adrenaline) and melanin (dark skin pigment). Tyrosine seems to aid cocaine and amphetamine ("speed") users in withdrawing from these drugs.

Deficiency

A dietary lack of phenylalanine for conversion to tyrosine or a problem with the enzyme needed for this reaction to occur may result in a deficit of norepinephrine. An inadequacy of this important neurotransmitter may cause depression.

Phenylketonuria, or PKU, is an inherited disorder in which a defective enzyme fails to convert the phenylalanine to tyrosine. This disease causes brain damage, mental retardation, tremors, spasticity, convulsions, eczema, contorted position of the hands and malodorous sweat and urine. If the disease is not detected at birth by a diagnostic test of the newborn's urine, brain damage may occur within the first three years of life. Expression of the disease may be prevented by rigid dietary restriction.

See also PHENYLKETONURIA.

ubiquinone (coenzyme Q-10 [CoQ]) A substance synthesized by cells throughout the body, or ubiquitous, hence the name "ubiquinone." CoQ acts as a catalyst in the series of chemical reactions called the respiratory chain that create energy from carbohydrates. It is not classified as a vitamin and no deficiencies have been identified. However, levels of CoQ generally decrease with age and have been found to be low in patients with heart disease. CoQ also has antioxidant properties and is structurally similar to vitamin E.

Some studies suggest that CoQ has the potential to protect the myocardium, or heart muscle, during open-heart surgery. CoQ is used in Japan to treat congestive heart failure and has resulted in less shortness of breath and stamina. Exercise tolerance also improved following the compound's use in a group of patients with chronic stable angina.

Dosage

The National Research Council does not consider CoQ an essential nutrient since it is synthesized in the cells, and therefore there is no Recommended Dietary Allowance (RDA). Doses of supplements range from 10 to 300 mg but doses up to 600 mg have been used in clinical trials.

Dietary Sources

Good sources of CoQ include beef heart, sardines, peanuts and spinach. A similar compound is found in plants but does not have the same beneficial properties.

Toxicity

Adverse effects include loss of appetite, nausea and diarrhea, but are unusual.

See also COENZYME Q-10.

ulmus See SLIPPERY ELM.

umeboshi plum A dried species of apricot (*umeboshi* means "dried plum") used as food and medicine in China, Korea and Japan. Ume contains twice the amount of protein, minerals and fat found in other fruits. It also is rich in calcium, iron, phosphorus and organic acids, particularly citric acid and phosphoric acid, which do not break down in the pickling process.

usnea (beard lichen) Common lichens (algae and fungus in symbiotic growth resembling moss) of the *Usnea* genus, such as *U. barbata*, that thrive on tree branches. Usnea is considered by herbalists to be a remedy for fungal, viral and bacterial infections.

uva ursi (bearberry) A trailing evergreen plant, *Arctostaphylos uva-ursi*, of the Ericaceae family, whose leaves are used in herbal medicine as a diuretic, urinary antiseptic and astringent, especially for the treatment of bladder, urethra and kidney inflammation and blood in the urine.

uzara The herb *Xysmalobium undulatum*, native to South Africa, prepared as a dry extract or liquid for the treatment of diarrhea. Its main active ingredient is uzarone, which slows the movement of the bowels and strengthens the heartbeat. Uzara is not recommended for use by individuals taking digitalis or heart medications such as digoxin (Lanoxin).

valerian Perennial herbs of the Valerianaceae family long believed to have medicinal properties, such as *Valeriana officinalis,* named after the Roman province Valeria. In Ayurvedic practice, valerian serves as a nervine, antispasmodic, carminative and sedative. The herb's rhizome is the medicinal part used in preparations for insomnia, stress and anxiety, pain and cramps.

vamsha rochana See BAMBOO.

vanadium A rare metallic element. Although the human body stores about 29 mg, very little is known about requirements for this mineral. If it is essential, it is sufficiently plentiful in food, water and air to satisfy human needs.

There are some reports that vanadium plays a role in cholesterol metabolism and hormone production. Animal studies suggest that vanadium may also play a role in slowing the growth of tumors and protect against breast cancer. Sources of vanadium include whole-grain breads and cereals, nuts, root vegetables, liver, fish and vegetable oils.

Chronic inhalation of vanadium compounds (vanadiumism) may cause pneumonitis, an inflammatory lung condition. It may also cause anemia and inflammation of the eyes.

vanilla bean The fruit of *Vanilla planifolia,* of the Vanilla family, which produces an extract used as a flavoring agent and an aphrodisiac. Vanillin, or artificial vanilla, is synthesized from chemicals called lignins, which are composed of the aromatic polymers conyiferyl, para-coumaryl and sinapyl alcohols. Some plant lignins have anticancer, antibacterial, antifungal and antiviral properties.

varnish tree See RHUS.

vegetarian diets The daily intake of foods and liquids partially or totally devoid of animal sources. Because dietary fats are essential for the absorption of some nutrients, these diets are at risk of being deficient in protein, vitamins B_{12}, D and riboflavin and the minerals iron, selenium, copper, manganese and zinc. Modifications such as lactovegetarian or lacto-ovo vegetarian diets include dairy products in the former, and dairy and eggs in the latter. Essential nutrients, including vitamin B_{12}, can be obtained in the diet that includes dairy products or eggs.

vervain See BLUE VERVAIN.

vetiverian The plant *Andropogon muricatus,* of the Graminaceae family, whose root is used in herbal medicine as an antipyretic and astringent.

vidari-kanda See GINSENG.

viola (violet, sweet violet) The flowering plant *Viola odorata,* of the Violaceae family, made into a syrup for sore throat, cough and dry airways and prepared as an herbal medicine for high blood pressure, tumors and cancerous growths. Violet is also a pot herb. Ayurvedic practitioners use it as an alterative, antiseptic and expectorant.

vision and vitamin A See A, VITAMIN; EYE DISEASES.

vitamin An organic compound that is required in small amounts for normal health, growth and well-being of the organism. Vitamins are not utilized primarily as a source of energy or as a source of structural tissue components, but rather as catalysts. Vitamins are micronutrients that promote physiologic processes necessary for continued life of the organism. There are 13 vitamins; only three of these, vitamins D, biotin and pantothenic acid, are manufactured by the body, and even these may not be sufficient for good health. Therefore vitamins must be supplied by exogenous, or from outside, sources. Vitamin deficiency results in a well-defined disease that is prevented or cured by replacement of that vitamin.

vitamin deficiency A syndrome or disease caused by a lack or an inadequate supply of a substance required by the body for optimal functioning and health. A deficiency is often curable with adequate supplementation of the missing or inadequate substance. According to the American Dietetic Association, most Americans can get adequate nutrition from the United States food supply. However, because of social, cultural or economic factors, several groups may have diets deficient in recommended nutrients. Surveys identify adolescent girls, individuals on limited incomes, pregnant and lactating women and the elderly as the groups most likely to have inadequate intake of the vitamins A, C and folic acid and the minerals calcium, iron and zinc.

vitamin-like substances See PSEUDOVITAMINS.

vitamin metabolism The intake, processing and elimination of vitamins by the human body. Vitamins are ingested orally (or by injection directly into the bloodstream), then absorbed through the intestinal wall into the bloodstream. They are

TABLE 32 CAUSES OF DIETARY VITAMIN DEFICIENCY

- Crop failure
- Improperly stored or prepared foods
- Inadequate oral intake because of poverty, eating disorders, anorexia due to disease or depression, fad and weight-loss diets, nausea of pregnancy or alcoholism
- Decreased absorption (malabsorption) from diseases, malignancies and parasitic infestations
- Increased requirements by increased physical activity, infections, pregnancy and lactation, some drugs, rapid growth, vitamin imbalance
- Increased losses due to excessive sweating or diuresis.

metabolized, or processed, by the liver and then transported through the blood to tissues. Once the vitamin or its metabolites (breakdown products) enter tissue cells, they convert to coenzymes, couple to enzymes, perform metabolic tasks or break down to other metabolites. Finally, the vitamin, and in some cases its by-products, are excreted in urine or feces.

vitis (grape) Vines of the Vitaceae family, found in the northern hemisphere, such as *V. vinifera, thunbergii, amurensis, bryoniaefolia, flexuosa* and *lambrusca,* whose fruit is eaten or made into juice, jellies, jams and wine. As the oldest cultivated fruit of the Ancient Greeks and Romans, grapes and grape root, root bark, and leaf sap also have medicinal value, according to herbalists. Various preparations are made for the treatment of wounds, cancer, lymphatic tuberculosis and urinary problems.

wahoo (spindle tree, arrow wood, bitter ash, burning bush) A North American deciduous fruit-bearing shrub or tree, *Euonymous atropurpureus,* of the Celastraceae family, with bark of medicinal value in the treatment of chest and lung congestion, cardiac irregularities, and other ailments. Other herbalists use wahoo as a purgative, antipyretic and diuretic. Wahoo may cause symptoms of poisoning.

walnut See JUGLANS.

water The combination of hydrogen and oxygen that forms a generally tasteless, colorless, odorless fluid. Constituting about 65 percent of male body weight and 55 percent of female body weight, water is necessary for cellular metabolism and as the agent that transports various substances including, nutrients throughout the body. In addition, water is considered the universal solvent and the basis for all body fluids, including blood, lymph, tissue fluid, secretions such as saliva, bile, sweat and stomach juices, and excretory fluids such as urine.

An excessive intake of water results in water intoxication; an excessive loss or lack of water results in dehydration, which can be life-threatening, especially in infants with severe diarrhea. Symptoms of water intoxication are sodium retention, abdominal cramps, dizziness, lethargy, nausea, vomiting, convulsions and coma. Although a certain amount of moisture may be derived from food, the human body cannot survive very long without water, also responsible for regulating and maintaining a constant body temperature and for providing the base solution for the electrolytes sodium and potassium.

See also WATER INTOXICATION; WATER, HARD; WATER, SOFT.

water, hard Water containing the dissolved salts of the minerals calcium and magnesium.

water intoxication Results when excessive water is ingested, disturbing the electrolyte balance. As intoxication worsens there are subtle changes in mental status, lethargy, confusion and diminished urine output. With progression the individual may lapse into a coma and die. This disorder is rare, but seen occasionally in psychotic individuals.

water, mineral or spring Water that contains dissolved mineral salts sufficient to impart a particular taste or other properties. There is no standardization of commercially available brands.

water, potable Safe drinking water, that is, water free of harmful microorganisms and minerals.

water, purified According to the U.S. Pharmacopeia (USP), mineral-free water as a result of distillation or deionization.

water, pyrogen-free Water free of proteins (specifically, bacteria and their metabolic products) that cause fevers. Sterilized, pyrogen-free water is suitable for hypodermic injection.

water, soft Water containing only a small amount of dissolved magnesium and calcium salts.

watercress (scurvy grass, nasturtium) A European and American perennial, *Nasturtium officinale* or *Rorippa nasturtium,* of the Cruciferae family, that flourishes in clear, cold water. Fresh watercress is eaten as a salad green and has herbal medicinal value in its leaves, roots and young shoots. It is used as a diuretic, purgative, expectorant, stomachic and stimulant. Watercress is rich in vitamin C, hence the name "scurvy grass," and contains minerals including iodine and iron.

Wernicke-Korsakoff syndrome   See BERIBERI; THIAMINE.

wheat   Varieties of grasses cultivated for their grains, which are hulled and ground into flour to make bread that contains minerals, fat, protein and starch. Cereals and pastas are also made from wheat. The milling process removes the bran and germ of the wheat, which results in the loss of B-complex vitamins, vitamin E and phosphorus and iron.

wheat germ   Embryo of the wheat kernel separated during the milling process. It is a source of vitamin E.

See also E, VITAMIN; PROCESSING OF FOODS; WHEAT.

white button mushroom   A type of mushroom rich in the mineral zinc, essential for the maintenance of normal white blood cells and other immune-system functions. This mushroom is reported also to contain a significant amount of the oxygenating element germanium, and it is said to help neutralize toxic residues that form as a result of eating meat.

See also GERMANIUM.

wild Oregon grape   See OREGON GRAPE.

Wilson's disease (hepatolenticular degeneration)
An inherited disorder of autosomal recessive expression in which copper accumulates in the body tissues, especially the red blood cells, kidneys, liver and brain. Treatment with D-penicillamine is usually successful. However, if untreated, this disorder is fatal, with death resulting from liver failure or infection.

See also COPPER.

wintergreen (pyrola, wild lily-of-the-valley)
The plant *Pyrola rotundifolia*, of the Pyrolaceae family, named from the Greek word *pyrus*, or pear, found in Eurasia, Greenland and parts of North America including Quebec, Nova Scotia, and Newfoundland. In Chinese medicine, the fermented plant is used to treat weakness, tuberculosis, anxiety, bloody sputum and rheumatism.

wintersweet   See CHIMONANTHUS.

wormwood   An alternate name for species of Artemisia (see MUGWORT).

xanthium (cocklebur) A Japanese, Chinese, Korean, Taiwanese and European herb, *Xanthium strumarium*, of the Compositae family, whose fruits, stems, roots and hairy leaves are used in Chinese traditional medicine as remedies for the common cold, headache, German measles and other ailments.

xanthosis The yellowing of the skin as a result of eating foods containing excessive amounts of carotenoids, such as carrots, squash, egg yolk, etc. While xanthosis may increase lipochromes in the blood of individuals with thyroid or pancreatic disease, it is usually harmless and reversible by reducing the quantities of yellow or orange foods eaten.

yam See DIOSCOREA.

yarrow (nosebleed, soldier's woundwort, milfoil) The aromatic, flowering herb *Achillea millefolium,* of the Compositae family, found in Eurasia, with herbal medicinal use as an anti-inflammatory, anti-pyretic, astringent, antispasmodic, hemostatic, diaphoretic, carminative and stomachic. Ailments including influenza, the common cold, menstrual cramps, bleeding and hemorrhoids may be treated with yarrow infusion or other preparation.

yellowdock (rumex, garden patience, sour dock, narrow dock) A European, American and southern Canadian perennial, *Rumex crispus,* of the Polygonaceae family, whose root serves as an astringent and tonic in herbal medicine. Considered a "blood purifier" in the 19th century, yellowdock has also been used as a laxative and cholagogue, or agent that promotes the flow and discharge of bile into the small intestine. Yellowdock is a source of organic iron.

yellow wood sorrel See OXALIS.

yerba mate See PARAGUAY COPPER TEA.

yerba santa (bearsweed, holy herb, mountain balm, tarweed, consumptive's weed) A western American evergreen shrub, *Eriodictyon califoricum* or *glutinosum,* of the Hydrophyllaceae family, whose leaves were chewed or smoked by Native Americans with asthma. In contemporary herbal medicine, the aromatic leaves are considered a good expectorant as well as an antispasmodic and tonic. Yerba santa reduces fever and has been prescribed for tuberculosis and rheumatism.

yogurt A milk product with a pudding-like consistency that has been curdled by the *Lactobacillus bulgaricus* and which is claimed to be nutritive and therapeutic, particularly for bowel disorders, when added to the daily diet.
    See ACIDOPHILUS.

yohimbe The extract of the bark of the mature African Coryanthe Yohimbe tree, claimed to be an aphrodisiac and remedy for sexual problems.

yucca (Spanish bayonet) Mostly western American plants of the *Yucca* genus and Liliaceae family. Yuccas have a woody base and rigid, swordlike leaves, and they bear large white flowers. Yucca root is used by herbalists as a remedy for arthritic and rheumatic pain and intestinal cramps.

Z

zea See CORN.

zedoary The plant *Curcuma zedoaria,* from the same family as turmeric, used in folk and Asian medicine as a remedy for indigestion, bloating, nausea, gas and heavy menstrual flow. Not used as a spice for food, zedoary extracts in herbal preparations are said to stimulate digestive juices and act as an antispasmodic in the gastrointestinal tract.

See also CURCUMA; JAVANESE TURMERIC.

zein The maize or corn protein that is lacking in two of the amino acids, lysine and tryptophan.

See also AMINO ACIDS.

zinc A bluish-white metallic element whose salts are often used in pharmaceuticals. First recognized as an element in the early 1500s, it was not considered necessary for animals until 1934 and only in 1956 was it found that human deficiency could occur. In trace amounts, zinc is an essential (required in the diet) mineral as a component of many enzymes, playing a role in protein synthesis and cell division. While not an antioxidant alone, zinc works in conjunction with antioxidant enzymes and is inclined in many antioxidant vitamin and mineral supplements.

Large amounts of zinc are deposited in muscle and bone, but these supplies are not readily available. The freely available zinc pool is small, and deficiencies may become apparent (as demonstrated in laboratory animals) despite the total body zinc content.

Small amounts of dietary zinc are absorbed more efficiently than larger amounts. Individuals who are zinc-poor seem to more readily absorb the mineral. The amount of zinc excreted in the feces is approximately proportional to that ingested in the diet.

Deficiency

Loss of appetite, anemia, growth retardation resulting in short stature and hypogonadism, impaired wound-healing and other signs of impaired immunity, diminished sense of taste and geographia, hair loss, night blindness and photophobia (difficulty tolerating light) and behavioral changes are signs of zinc deficiency. In the Middle East, hypogonadism, a deficiency in sexual growth and development, has been attributed to zinc deficiency. Male infants seem to be more sensitive to zinc deficiency since increasing zinc supplementation results in increased growth rate in male but not female babies.

There may be problems with the metabolism of zinc in diabetics with increased losses of zinc in the urine. Both insulin-dependent and non-insulin-dependent diabetics might benefit from zinc supplements. Alcoholics, those with malabsorption disorders with chronic diarrhea, pregnant and elderly persons and those with chronic infections and AIDS may also benefit from additional zinc in their diets or by supplements.

Dietary Sources

Meat is the principal source of zinc in American diets, supplying approximately 70 percent of intake. Cereals supply most of the balance. The amount in drinking water is negligible. The bioavailability of zinc from meat, especially liver, eggs and seafood such as oysters, is greater than that from whole-grain foods. Zinc in American diets may interact with protein, phosphorus and iron, thereby increasing zinc requirements. But no strong evidence of any clinical significance of suspected interactions exists. In some parts of the world, high dietary fiber and phytate may impair zinc absorption.

Average North American diets supply from 5.5 mg daily for infants to 10 to 15 mg for adults. However, the elderly may only take in 7 to 10 mg.

Recommended Dietary Allowances

The Food and Nutrition Board of the National Research Council estimates that the at least 12 mg of zinc is required to maintain normal zinc status in healthy young men. To allow for a margin of safety, the RDA has been set at 15 mg for adult males and for females during pregnancy, and 12 mg for nonpregnant women. During lactation, mothers require an additional 7 mg for the first six months and 4 mg per day from six through 12 months of age for infants. These RDAs take into account that some individuals may consume diets low in bioavailable zinc on a routine basis. Studies have demonstrated that formula-fed infants supplemented with zinc had better growth rates than those who did not receive the supplements. The zinc RDA established, then, for formula-fed infants is 5 mg per day. Preadolescent children require 10 mg per day.

Toxicity

While as little as 2 mg of zinc as sulfate can cause gastric upset and vomiting, doses of 18.5 to 25 mg have been shown to reduce copper levels, resulting in microcytosis (smaller than normal red blood cells) and neutropenia (diminished number of neutrophillic white blood cells). Megadoses of zinc equivalent to 20 times the RDA for six weeks caused impaired immune responses in a group of healthy adults. Furthermore, doses of 80 to 150 mg daily for as little as several weeks reduced high-density lipoproteins (the so-called good cholesterol) levels.

In vitro (test tube) experiments with zinc and human A-beta, a substance found in the human brain and other body tissues, suggest that zinc may be instrumental in forming plaques in the brains of Alzheimer's patients. Therefore Boston researchers caution against megadoses of zinc.

The chronic ingestion of greater than 15 mg per day of zinc on a daily basis is not recommended without careful medical scrutiny.

zingiber   See GINGER.

ziziphus (Chinese jujube, Chinese date, hong zao, suan ao ren)   A southern Chinese and Indian spiny shrub or tree, *Ziziphus jujuba* and *spinosa*, of the Rhamnaceae family, whose fruits, seeds, bark, root and leaves are used in Chinese traditional medicine to treat anxiety, insomnia, alopecia, night sweats, vertigo, scorpion stings, fever and diarrhea.

Zymain   A nutritional complex of vitamin C; zinc; manganese; the enzymes papain, trypsin, chymotrypsin and bromelain and bioflavonoids formulated to optimize the healing process for acute inflammation. Manufactured by Anabolic Laboratories, in Irvine, California, Zymain also contains beef cartilage and shave grass (a source of silicon).

APPENDIXES

APPENDIX I
FOOD PYRAMID

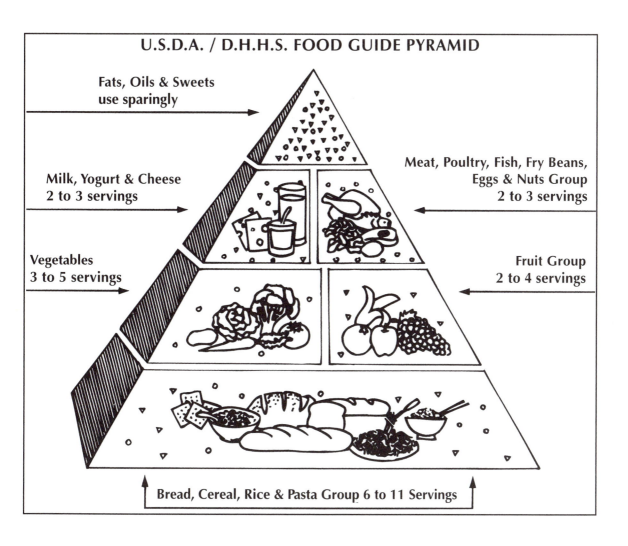

U.S.D.A. / D.H.H.S. FOOD GUIDE PYRAMID

Fats, Oils & Sweets
use sparingly

Milk, Yogurt & Cheese
2 to 3 servings

Meat, Poultry, Fish, Fry Beans,
Eggs & Nuts Group
2 to 3 servings

Vegetables
3 to 5 servings

Fruit Group
2 to 4 servings

Bread, Cereal, Rice & Pasta Group 6 to 11 Servings

APPENDIX II
NUTRITION CHRONOLOGY

The Garden of Eden, in the Old Testament, is the archetypal garden, with a central tree as the life-nourisher.

In Tibetan mythology, the goddess of healing introduced fragrant healing plants and planted gardens of them, called the paradise gardens. The Buddha is also associated with "a cosmic tree" and legendary gardens.

- **5000 B.C.** A Chinese herbal lists rhubarb, poppy and ephedra among the medicinal plants.

  About 4,500 years ago, the ancient Hindu text, the *Rig Veda,* listed more than 1,000 medicinal herbs, including senna and cinnamon.

- **2700 B.C.** Chinese medicine expands to acupuncture and a system of polypharmacy.

- **c. 2697 B.C.** Chinese emperor Shen Nung becomes known as "the divine farmer" and the father of agriculture and herbal medicine.

- **c. 2697–2595 B.C.** Chinese emperor Huang Ti wrote *The Nei Ching,* or *Yellow Emperor's Classic of Internal Medicine.* The book is still used as a medical text in China. The Chinese combined acupuncture, herbs, massage, exercise and diet as therapeutic modalities.

- **2000 B.C.** "Oracle bones," i.e., bones that had the names of plants and diseases etched on them, are considered part of China's prehistoric evidence of herbal medicine.

- **1500 B.C.** The ancient Egyptian Ebers papyrus listed plants, including garlic and the opium poppy, and medicinal formulas made from them. The Arabs were considered the first modern pharmacists. They distilled the first pure alcohol (*al-kohl,* in Arabic, meaning quintessence) in

which to soak medicinal plants. These concentrated extracts are known today as tinctures. Ancient Egyptians are also credited with knowledge of what came to be known as vitamins.

By 1000 B.C., Ayurveda, the Hindu "science of life," is thought to be already highly developed.

- **c. 600 B.C.** King Nebuchadnezzar of Babylon created the Hanging Gardens, one of the seven wonders of the world, for his homesick wife. In the three-acre gardens the king ordered the cultivation of shrubs, trees and flowers that were both beautiful and medicinal.

- **460–377 B.C.** Hippocrates, ancient Greek physician called "the father of medicine," listed 350 plants, including thyme and mint, as useful for cooking and medicine.

  In Greek mythology, famous gardens include the Blessed Isles. There the Hesperides guarded and cultivated golden apples of the sun.

- **c. 1000 A.D.** Europe emerges from the Dark Ages, during which Greek and Roman medicine languished. Renewed trade between Arab countries and Europe brought Arab medical knowledge to the Benedictine monks, who were enthusiastic herbalists praised by Charlemagne. He encouraged the monks' "physic gardens" and their prowess as physicians. In their tinctures, they substituted wine for pure alcohol and invented liqueurs (meant to settle the stomach after dinner).

  In the 1st century A.D., the *Charaka Samhita,* an Indian Vedic medical text, is written, based on the oral tradition dating from preliterate times. The text lists 500 herbal drugs.

  Also in the 1st century A.D., Roman physicians Galen and Dioscorides set forth books on medicine that included information on animal, vegetable and mineral therapies and a system of classifying herbs for medicinal use.

For about 500 years following the 6th century A.D., Anglo-Saxon medicine relied on *The Leech Book of Bald,* authored by a 10th-century monk. The book included many Greek and Roman medical therapies.

- **11th, 12th, and 13th centuries** The Crusades sparked Europe's desire for Asian spices for cooking, perfumes and medicines. The Crusades also introduced Europeans to a new manner of gardening, and eating and celebrating in open, fragrant and lush gardens. In the 1400s, Christopher Columbus reached the West Indies and returned with *kian* (cayenne) pepper from the Caribbean peoples.

  Paracelsus, a Swiss-born alchemist and physician (1493–1541), catalyzed the movement toward mineral medicines and predicted that there were therapeutic substances in plants and minerals.

- **1497** Portuguese navigator Vasco da Gama lost 100 of his 160 men to scurvy, a disease caused by the lack of vitamin C, during the voyage around the Cape of Good Hope.

- **1542** German physician and botanist Leonhard Fuchs wrote a book citing 400 medicinal plants, including American corn and pumpkin. The fuschia was named after him.

- **1597** Surgeon John Gerard published *Herbal,* a book on herbs and their uses.

  Also during the Renaissance, "wise women," as they were called, handed down herbal recipes, cosmetics and medicines to younger generations after a great many years of practice. These women contributed significantly to the survival of herbal knowledge.

- **1640** John Parkinson published his book on herbs.

- **1649** Nicholas Culpeper, a British astrologer/physician, educated at Cambridge University, published *The Complete Herbal.* One of the most revered herbalists of all time, Culpeper refused to participate in other physicians' snobbery evidenced by their much-inflated medical mystique. Rather, he wrote in vernacular (as did Paracelsus) and treated the poor of London with herbal preparations they could afford. Culpeper could aptly be called a grassroots caregiver. More than 41 editions of his book have been published, the latest by Sterling Publishing Company, Inc., New York, in 2002: *Culpeper's Color Herbal,* edited by David Potterton.

- **1754** Scottish naval surgeon James Lind discovered that scurvy could be prevented and cured by lemon and orange juice.

- **1773** The Boston Tea Party: Outraged North American colonists dumped tons of tea into Boston harbor when Parliament threatened a tax. Originally a Chinese stimulant, tea became a catalyst for the American Revolution.

  Concurrently, colonists learned Native American herbalism from the Plains Indians. Old World herbalism blended with Native American practices, among them the use of cascara sagrada (a tree bark) as a laxative, and echinacea to fight colds, flu and infections.

- **1775** Dr. William Withering discovered the benefits of digitalis, from the foxglove plant, in treating angina pectoris (chest pain related to heart disease).

  Also during the 18th century, French chemist Antoine Laurent Lavoisier described the relationship between respiration (the intake of oxygen and output of carbon dioxide) and food metabolism. Lavoisier, known as "the father of nutrition," investigated the calorie and energy values of carbohydrates, proteins and fats.

- **1896** W. O. Atwater, known as "the father of American nutrition," published the first comprehensive table of food values in America, where it had previously been believed that only protein and calories were important.

- **1897** Christiann Eijkman described a beriberi-like disease in pigeons and chickens, which led to the modern concept of vitamins.

- **1906** The federal Food and Drug Administration was established.

- **1909** The American Home Economics Association was established.

- **1912** The original term "vitamine," referring to "vital amine," was coined by Casimir Funk, a chemist of the Lister Institute in London. Funk designated the accessory food factors required for human life. The final "e" was eventually dropped when it was discovered that most vitamins were not amines.

- **1916** Nutritionist E. V. McCollum, who specialized in the field of accessory food factors, gave the public the idea of "protective foods," the best sources of vitamins and minerals. As a result, milk, citrus fruit and green leafy vegetables became more popular in the American diet. Around the same time, calorie expert Graham Lusk emphasized that adolescents required as much food as adults.

- **1917** The American Dietetic Association was established.

- **1929** Sir Alexander Fleming (1881–1955), a British bacteriologist, discovered penicillin in mold.

- **1933** The American Institute of Nutrition was established.

- **1940** The Food and Nutrition Board of the National Research Council was established. As precursor to a new, international approach to nutrition, the council began to study nutrition throughout the world.

- **1941** The first recommended daily dietary allowances were published by the League of Nations as a result of the studies by the National Research Council. Also in 1941 the Nutrition Foundation, which published the monthly *Nutrition Reviews,* was established.

- **1947** Reserpine, an antihypertensive drug, was isolated from the rauwolfia plant by Ciba, a Swiss chemical company. Rauwolfia had been used in Asian Indian folk medicine.

- **1952** The Committee on Therapeutic Nutrition published the amounts of extra nutrients necessary in the event of disease and injury.

- **1954** American chemist Linus Pauling (1901–1994) won the Nobel Prize in chemistry for his research on DNA molecules and the structure of antibodies, proteins and other complex substances.

- **1962** Linus Pauling won the Nobel Prize for peace for his campaign against nuclear weapons.

- **1966** The International Education and Health Act (along with the Foreign Aid Program and the Food for Freedom Program) was established to fight malnutrition. These programs were associated with the Food and Agriculture Organization (FAO), the World Health Organization (WHO) and the United Nations International Children's Emergency Fund, later known as the United Nations Children's Fund, but still called UNICEF.

- **1968** The first set of dietary guidelines in the world appeared in Scandinavia.

- **1969** A White House Conference on Food, Nutrition and Health was held. The purpose of the conference was to improve the nutritional status of pregnant and nursing mothers, children, adolescents, the elderly and the very poor; to develop new technologies for food production; to improve education on nutrition in schools, including nursing and medical schools; and to improve federal programs—school lunches, food stamps and others—that affect nutritional status.

  During the 1970s, hearings were held by the Senate's Poverty Subcommittee and the Select Committee on Nutrition and Human Needs. Hunger and malnutrition in the United States thus became a political issue.

- **1970** American chemist Linus Pauling, of the Linus Pauling Institute of Science and Medicine in Palo Alto, California, published a best-selling book, *Vitamin C and the Common Cold,* which advocated large doses of the vitamin as a preventive and therapeutic measure against colds, cancer and cardiovascular diseases. Although Pauling's theories had many detractors, he received many awards—the National Medal of Science in 1975 and the Priestly Medal from the American Chemical Society in 1984, among them.

- **1974** Four private nutrition agencies, the American Institute of Nutrition, the American Society for Clinical Nutrition, the American Dietetic Association and the Institute of Food Technology, formed the National Nutrition Consortium, Inc. Also in 1974, the first meeting of the United Nations World Food Council was held in Rome.

- **1977** *Dietary Goals for the United States* was published by the government.
- **1987–88** Nutrition survey conducted by the Health and Nutrition Examination Survey (HANES) and the Nationwide Food Consumption survey. One of the factors the survey indicated was that overweight and obesity were not so much caused by overeating as by inactivity.
- **1988** *The Surgeon General's Report on Nutrition and Health* was published.
- **1989** The National Research Council published *Diet and Health: Implications for Reducing Chronic Disease Risk.*
- **1990** *The Dietary Guidelines for Americans* was published.
- **1991** The Nutrition Labeling and Education Act of 1990 was passed into law by Congress and signed by President George Bush.
- **1994** Public Law 103–417, Dietary Supplement Health and Education Act of 1994, was enacted.
- **1988–1994** The third National Health and Nutrition Examination Survey (NHANES III) was conducted by the National Center for Health Statistics of the Centers for Disease Control and Prevention, Atlanta, Georgia.
- **1996** A World Food Summit was conducted by the Food and Agriculture Organization (FAO), November 13–17.
- **1997** In February, the American Nutraceutical Association was established, with a mission to develop and provide educational materials and programs on nutraceuticals and nutrition for healthcare professionals, consumers and sales associates from nutraceutical companies. The ANA now has several thousand members in the United States and in more than 10 other countries.

- **2000** The Great Nutrition Debate, a millennial symposium, was sponsored by the Department of Agriculture on February 24; best-selling diet authors took part and Dietary Guidelines 2000 were issued.

  In November, the U.S. Department of Health and Human Services published *Healthy People 2010,* part of which addresses the nation's issues, trends, objectives, weight status and growth, food and nutrient consumption, iron deficiency and anemia, schools, worksites and nutrition counseling, food security and other topics.

- **2001** The American Nutraceutical Association published *Nutraceuticals: The Complete Encyclopedia of Supplements, Herbs, Vitamins, and Healing Foods.*

- **2002** WHO/FAO Global Expert Consultation on Acrylamide in Foods was announced by the Swedish National Food Authority's report in May; French fries, potato chips and other snack foods were found to have high levels of carcinogenic acrylamide. A World Health Organization Conference was held June 25–27.

  On July 19, the Food Safety Inspection Service issued a recall on hamburger and released new instructions for cooking beef.

  At a November American Heart Association meeting in Chicago, researchers reported that among 74,000 women, those who increased their fruit and vegetable intake over a 12-year study period were 26 percent less likely to become obese than were women who decreased their consumption of these foods.

- **2003** The American Dietetic Association released its new position statements, conducted a public-policy workshop and established a new international membership category.

APPENDIX III
DRUG AND NUTRIENT INTERACTIONS

Many of the interactions listed below are dose-related and some may be clinically important and some are not. If you are taking prescription medications, always ask your physician before adding any supplements to your regimen. Furthermore, the authors make no claims for the completeness of this list.

Drug Causing Vitamin Deficiency	Deficient Fat-Soluble Vitamin
cholestyramine (Questran) colestipol (Colestid) mineral oil neomycin antacids	vitamin A

cholestyramine (Questran)
colestipol (Colestid)
mineral oil
neomycin
antibacterials:
  sulfonamides (Bactrim, Septra, etc.)
  naldixic acid (NegGram)
  tetracyclines
antacids
antituberculars:
  isoniazid (INH)
  rifampin
major tranquilizers:
  thioridazine (Mellaril)
  chlorpromazine (Thorazine)	

trifluoperazine (Stelazine)
haloperidol (Haldol)
anticonvulsants:
  phenytoin (Dilantin)
  primadone (Mysoline)
  phenobarbital
	vitamin D

(continued)

Drug Causing Vitamin Deficiency	Deficient Fat-Soluble Vitamin

thiazide diuretics
  corticosteroids:
  prednisone (Deltasone)
  dexamethasone (Decadron)
methyprednisolone (Medrol)	

cholestyramine (Questran) colestipol E (Colestid) mineral oil	vitamin E
cholestyramine (Questran) colestipol (Colestid) mineral oil neomycin antibacterials (see above) anticonvulsants (see above) laxatives	vitamin K

Drug Causing Vitamin Deficiency	Deficient Water-Soluble Vitamin
antibacterials (see above) oral contraceptives salicylates such as aspirin indomethacin (Indocin) acetaminophen (Tylenol) nicotine (cigarettes) corticosteroids (see above)	ascorbic acid (vitamin C)
antacids antibacterials (see above) oral contraceptives alcohol to excess	thiamine (vitamin B_1)
neomycin oral contraceptives major tranquilizers (see above) tetracycline estrogens (Premarin)	riboflavin (vitamin B_2)
antitubercular drugs (see above) tetracycline	niacin
neomycin oral contraceptives antitubercular drugs (see above) hydralazine (Apresoline) anticonvulsants (see above) penicillamine estrogens (Premarin) corticosteroids (see above)	pyridoxine

Drug Causing Vitamin Deficiency	Deficient Water-Soluble Vitamin
cholestyramine (Questran) colestipol (Colestid) neomycin oral contraceptives major tranquilizers (see above) ascorbic acid (megadoses) methyldopa (Aldomet) estrogens (Premarin)	vitamin B_{12}
cholestyramine (Questran) colestipol (Colestid) antacids antibacterials (see above) anticonvulsants (see above) antitubercular drugs (see above) oral contraceptives salicylates, e.g., aspirin alcohol excess methotrexate tetracycline methyldopa (Aldomet) estrogens (Premarin) corticosteroids (see above)	folic acid

Drug Causing Mineral Deficiency	Deficient Mineral
cholestyramine (Questran) colestipol (Colestid) neomycin oral contraceptives anticonvulsants (see above) tetracycline furosemide (Lasix) digoxin (Lanoxin) corticosteroids (see above)	calcium
penicillamine cholestyramine (Questran) colestipol (Colestid) neomycin antacids salicylates, e.g. aspirin indomethacin (Indocin)	copper iron

oral contraceptives
anticonvulsants (see above)
  tetracycline
thiazide diuretics
cisplatinum
loop diuretics
  e.g., furosamide (Lasix)
	magnesium

(continued)

Drug Causing Mineral Deficiency	Deficient Mineral
digoxin (Lanoxin) estrogens (Premarin)	
hydralazine (Apresoline)	manganese
antacids	phosphate
neomycin thiazide diuretics loop diuretics corticosteroids (see above)	potassium
thiazide diuretics	sodium
penicillamine thiazide diuretics	zinc

Vitamin or Mineral Causing Toxicity	Drug Involved
vitamin D	magnesium-containing antacids (may cause toxicity in kidney dialysis patients)
vitamin D and calcium	digitalis products (Lanoxin and others) High calcium levels may cause heart rhythm disturbances. verapamil (Isoptin, Calan, Veralan) atrial fibrillation
vitamin E niacinamide (in doses larger than those found in multivitamin formulas) potassium digitalis products (see above) may cause heart rhythm disturbances A.C.E. inhibitors, e.g., captopril (Capoten), enalapril (Vasotec) others	warfarin (Coumadin) carbamazapine (Tegretol) primidone (Mysoline)
oral contraceptives	vitamin A
thiazide diuretics + vit D in patients with hypoparathyroidism	calcium
phenytoin and barbiturates	vitamin D
A.C.E. inhibitors (see above)	potassium

Vitamin or Mineral Causing Diminished Effectiveness of Drug	Drug Involved
ascorbic acid	warfarin (Coumadin) [rarely]
niacin	sulfinpyrazone or probenecid
pyridoxine (vitamin B_6	anticonvulsants (monitor blood levels):
	phenobarbital
	phenytoin
	levodopa
folic acid	anticonvulsants (monitor blood levels) (see above)
vitamin K	warfarin (Coumadin)
calcium salts	iron salts
	atenolol (Tenormin)
	tetracyclines
	verapamil (Calan, Isoptin, Veralan)
calcium carbonate	norfloxacin (Norloxin)
iron salts	doxycycline
	penicillamine
	tetracycline
magnesium salts	nitrofurantoin
	tetracycline
	aminoquinolines
	digoxin (Lanoxin)
	penicillamine
zinc	fluoroquinolones
	tetracycline

APPENDIX IV
RECOMMENDED DIETARY ALLOWANCE CHARTS

FOOD AND NUTRITION BOARD, NATIONAL ACADEMY OF SCIENCES—NATIONAL RESEARCH COUNCIL RECOMMENDED DIETARY ALLOWANCES,[a] REVISED 1989

Designed for the maintenance of good nutrition of practically all healthy people in the United States

Category	Age (years) or Condition	Weight[b] (kg)	Weight[b] (lb)	Height[b] (cm)	Height[b] (in)	Protein (g)	Fat-Soluble Vitamins Vitamin A (µg RE)[c]	Vitamin D (µg)[d]	Vitamin E (mg α-TE)[e]	Vitamin K (µg)
Infants	0.0–0.5	6	13	60	24	13	375	7.5	3	5
	0.5–1.0	9	20	71	28	14	375	10	4	10
Children	1–3	13	29	90	35	16	400	10	6	15
	4–6	20	44	112	44	24	500	10	7	20
	7–10	28	62	132	52	28	700	10	7	30
Males	11–14	45	99	157	62	45	1,000	10	10	45
	15–18	66	145	176	69	59	1,000	10	10	65
	19–24	72	160	177	70	58	1,000	10	10	70
	25–50	79	174	176	70	63	1,000	5	10	80
	51+	77	170	173	68	63	1,000	5	10	80
Females	11–14	46	101	157	62	46	800	10	8	45
	15–18	55	120	163	64	44	800	10	8	55
	19–24	58	128	164	65	46	800	10	8	60
	25–50	63	138	163	64	50	800	5	8	65
	51+	65	143	160	63	50	800	5	8	65
Pregnant						60	800	10	10	65
Lactating	1st 6 months					65	1,300	10	12	65
	2nd 6 months					62	1,200	10	11	65

FOOD AND NUTRITION BOARD, NATIONAL ACADEMY OF SCIENCES—NATIONAL RESEARCH COUNCIL RECOMMENDED DIETARY ALLOWANCES,[a] REVISED 1989

Designed for the maintenance of good nutrition of practically all healthy people in the United States

Category	Age (years) or Condition	Weight[b] (kg)	Weight[b] (lb)	Height[b] (cm)	Height[b] (in)	Protein (g)	Vitamin C (mg)	Thiamin (mg)	Riboflavin (mg)	Niacin (mg NE)[f]	Vitamin B6 (mg)	Folate (μg)	Vitamin B12 (μg)
Infants	0.0–0.5	6	13	60	24	13	30	0.3	0.4	5	0.3	25	0.3
	0.5–1.0	9	20	71	28	14	35	0.4	0.5	6	0.6	35	0.5
Children	1–3	13	29	90	35	16	40	0.7	0.8	9	1.0	50	0.7
	4–6	20	44	112	44	24	45	0.9	1.1	12	1.1	75	1.0
	7–10	28	62	132	52	28	45	1.0	1.2	13	1.4	100	1.4
Males	11–14	45	99	157	62	45	50	1.3	1.5	17	1.7	150	2.0
	15–18	66	145	176	69	59	60	1.5	1.8	20	2.0	200	2.0
	19–24	72	160	177	70	58	60	1.5	1.7	19	2.0	200	2.0
	25–50	79	174	176	70	63	60	1.5	1.7	19	2.0	200	2.0
	51+	77	170	173	68	63	60	1.2	1.4	15	2.0	200	2.0
Females	11–14	46	101	157	62	46	50	1.1	1.3	15	1.4	150	2.0
	15–18	55	120	163	64	44	60	1.1	1.3	15	1.5	180	2.0
	19–24	58	128	164	65	46	60	1.1	1.3	15	1.6	180	2.0
	25–50	63	138	163	64	50	60	1.1	1.3	15	1.6	180	2.0
	51+	65	143	160	63	50	60	1.0	1.2	13	1.6	180	2.0
Pregnant						60	70	1.5	1.6	17	2.2	400	2.2
Lactating	1st 6 months					65	95	1.6	1.8	20	2.1	280	2.6
	2nd 6 months					62	90	1.6	1.7	20	2.1	260	2.6

FOOD AND NUTRITION BOARD, NATIONAL ACADEMY OF SCIENCES—NATIONAL RESEARCH COUNCIL RECOMMENDED DIETARY ALLOWANCES,[a] REVISED 1989

Designed for the maintenance of good nutrition of practically all healthy people in the United States

Category	Age (years) or Condition	Weight[b] (kg)	Weight[b] (lb)	Height[b] (cm)	Height[b] (in)	Protein (g)	Minerals Calcium (mg)	Minerals Phosphorus (mg)	Minerals Magnesium (mg)	Minerals Iron (mg)	Minerals Zinc (mg)	Minerals Iodine (µg)	Minerals Selenium (µg)
Infants	0.0–0.5	6	13	60	24	13	400	300	40	6	5	40	10
	0.5–1.0	9	20	71	28	14	600	500	60	10	5	50	15
Children	1–3	13	29	90	35	16	800	800	80	10	10	70	20
	4–6	20	44	112	44	24	800	800	120	10	10	90	20
	7–10	28	62	132	52	28	800	800	170	10	10	120	30
Males	11–14	45	99	157	62	45	1,200	1,200	270	12	15	150	40
	15–18	66	145	176	69	59	1,200	1,200	400	12	15	150	50
	19–24	72	160	177	70	58	1,200	1,200	350	10	15	150	70
	25–50	79	174	176	70	63	800	800	350	10	15	150	70
	51+	77	170	173	68	63	800	800	350	10	15	150	70
Females	11–14	46	101	157	62	46	1,200	1,200	280	15	12	150	45
	15–18	55	120	163	64	44	1,200	1,200	300	15	12	150	50
	19–24	58	128	164	65	46	1,200	1,200	280	15	12	150	55
	25–50	63	138	163	64	50	800	800	280	15	12	150	55
	51+	65	143	160	63	50	800	800	280	10	12	150	55
Pregnant						60	1,200	1,200	300	30	15	175	65
Lactating	1st 6 months					65	1,200	1,200	355	15	19	200	75
	2nd 6 months					62	1,200	1,200	340	15	16	200	75

[a]The allowances, expressed as average daily intakes over time, are intended to provide for individual variations among most normal persons as they live in the United States under usual environmental stresses. Diets should be based on a variety of common foods in order to provide other nutrients for which human requirements have been less well defined. See text for detailed discussion of allowances and of nutrients not tabulated.

[b]Weights and heights of Reference Adults are actual medians for the U.S. population of the designated age, as reported by NHANES II. The median weights and heights of those under 19 years of age were taken from Hamill et al. (1979) (see pages 16–17). The use of these figures does not imply that the height-to-weight ratios are ideal.

[c]Retinol equivalents. 1 retinol equivalent = 1 µg retinol or 6 µg β-carotene.

[d]As cholecalciferol. 10 µg cholecalciferol = 400 IU of vitamin D.

[e]α-Tocopherol equivalents. 1 mg d-α tocopherol = 1 α-TE.

[f]1 NE (niacin equivalent) is equal to 1 mg of niacin or 60 mg of dietary tryptophan.

SUMMARY TABLE
ESTIMATED SAFE AND ADEQUATE DAILY DIETARY INTAKES OF SELECTED VITAMINS AND MINERALS[a]

Category	Age (years)	Vitamins	
		Biotin (µg)	Pantothenic Acid (mg)
Infants	0–0.5	10	2
	0.5–1	15	3
Children and adolescents	1–3	20	3
	4–6	25	3–4
	7–10	30	4–5
	11+	30–100	4–7
Adults	30–100	4–7	

Category	Age (years)	Trace Elements[b]				
		Copper (mg)	Manganese (mg)	Fluoride (mg)	Chromium (µg)	Molybdenum (µg)
Infants	0–0.5	0.4–0.6	0.3–0.6	0.1–0.5	10–40	15–30
	0.5–1	0.6–0.7	0.6–1.0	0.2–1.0	20–60	20–40
Children and adolescents	1–3	0.7–1.0	1.0–1.5	0.5–1.5	20–80	25–50
	4–6	1.0–1.5	1.5–2.0	1.0–2.5	30–120	30–75
	7–10	1.0–2.0	2.0–3.0	1.5–2.5	50–200	50–150
	11+	1.5–2.5	2.0–5.0	1.5–2.5	50–200	75–250
Adults	1.5–3.0	2.0–5.0	1.5–4.0	50–200	75–250	

[a]Because there is less information on which to base allowances, these figures are not given in main table of RDA and are provided here in the form of ranges of recommended intakes.
[b]Since the toxic levels for many trace elements may be only several times usual intakes, the upper levels for the trace elements given in this table should not be habitually exceeded.

APPENDIX V
POSITION OF THE AMERICAN DIETETIC ASSOCIATION: FOOD AND NUTRITION MISINFORMATION

ABSTRACT

It is the position of the American Dietetic Association that food and nutrition misinformation can have harmful effects on the health and economic status of consumers. It is the role of nationally credentialed dietetics professionals to advocate for and promote sound, science-based nutrition information to the public, function as primary nutrition educators to health professionals, and actively counter and correct food and nutrition misinformation. The federal government has recognized the strong link between nutrition and health in recent years. Consumers are taking greater responsibility for self-care and are hungry for food and nutrition information, creating opportunities for nutrition misinformation, health fraud, and quackery to flourish. The media are consumers' leading source of nutrition information, but news reports rarely provide enough context for consumers to interpret the advice given. Promoters turn preliminary findings into sales pitches with baseless claims, often for the sole purpose of economic gain. Effective nutrition communication is consumer focused and presented with sufficient context to allow consumers to weigh the information and determine whether it applies to his or her unique needs. Nationally credentialed dietetics professionals are best prepared to communicate sound advice and scientific advances about nutrition. These dietetics professionals have a responsibility to take an active role in providing accurate, easily understood food and nutrition information, interpreting emerging research for media and consumers and encouraging consumers to look for credentialed dietetics professionals as nutrition experts.

In recent years, the federal government and leading healthcare organizations have begun to acknowledge the link between nutrition and health. Enormous advances have been made in the science of food and nutrition, leading to a fine-tuning of many recommendations about eating healthfully. Despite these positive developments, misinformation about the role of nutrition in health abounds in our society, allowing nutrition-related misbeliefs, health fraud, and quackery to flourish.

Consistent with its vision that members "are the leading source of food and nutrition services," the American Dietetic Association (ADA) recognizes its responsibility to help consumers identify food and nutrition misinformation in the following ways:

- ADA members need to be leaders in providing consumers with sound, science-based nutrition information and helping them to recognize and avoid misinformation.

- ADA members need to be primary resources of sound nutrition information for the media and to inform the media when misinformation is presented, as the electronic and print media are primary sources of nutrition information for consumers (1).

- ADA, the world's largest organization of food and nutrition professionals, must continue to work diligently with other healthcare practitioners, educators, policy makers, and the food and dietary supplement industry to responsibly address the medical and economic effects of food- and nutrition-related misinformation on consumers.

POSITION STATEMENT

It is the position of the American Dietetic Association that food and nutrition misinformation can have harmful effects on the health and economic status of consumers. Nationally credentialed dietetics professionals working in healthcare, academia, public health, nutrition communications, media, and the food industry and serving in policy-making/regulatory roles are uniquely qualified to advocate for and promote sound, science-based nutrition information to the public, function as primary nutrition educators to health professionals, and actively counter and correct food and nutrition misinformation.

TYPES OF NUTRITION MISINFORMATION

The public is bombarded with an overwhelming amount of food and nutrition information. Unfortunately, it is not always clear how to distinguish nutrition facts from nutrition misinformation. Nutrition facts result from application of the scientific method and can withstand replication and peer review. Nutrition misinformation, on the other hand, consists of erroneous information, formulated with or without malicious intent, or misinterprets food and nutrition science. The danger of nutrition misinformation is that it may be harmful to health, or be used to fuel food faddism, quackery, or health fraud.

Food fads involve unreasonable or exaggerated beliefs that foods or supplements or their components may cure disease, convey special health benefits, or offer quick weight loss. Food fads may also involve combining or eliminating certain foods from the diet. The US Surgeon General's Report on Nutrition and Health defines food quackery as "the promotion for profit of special foods, products, processes or appliances with false or misleading health or therapeutic claims" (2). Food quackery is exploitative and entrepreneurial. Nevertheless, many people

who promote quackery schemes may themselves be victims of misinformation or incomplete information and may sincerely believe that they are promoting accurate information. Health fraud shares many of the characteristics of food faddism and food quackery, yet it is always deliberate and done for gain. According to the ADA's *Complete Food and Nutrition Guide*, "Health fraud means promoting for financial gain, a health remedy that doesn't work—or hasn't yet been proven to work" (3).

THE HARMFUL EFFECTS ON THE HEALTH AND ECONOMIC STATUS OF CONSUMERS

The public has seen a shift in the health and nutrition environment that recognizes the link between diet, disease prevention and optimal health. New science has revealed a place for functional foods and the assimilation of some forms of complementary medicine into mainstream healthcare. Consumers are taking greater responsibility for self-care, perhaps as a by-product of an evolving healthcare system, and are hungry for food and nutrition information. With these changes have also come increased opportunities for food and nutrition misinformation to impact the health and economic status of consumers, leaving them perhaps more vulnerable to fraud than ever before. Indeed, nutrition products have been found to be among the most commonly misused (4). This issue becomes even more critical as the population ages, as there is evidence that the majority of victims of healthcare fraud—up to 60%—are older people (5). The population is also becoming more overweight and is spending billions of dollars annually to combat obesity. Americans have spent $33 billion annually on weight-loss foods, products, and services (6). Yet fewer than half of obese patients have reported receiving any advice from healthcare professionals to lose weight (7), suggesting that qualified professionals need to be more proactive in providing sound information about appropriate weight-loss methods and referrals to qualified dietetics professionals. The true cost of health fraud is difficult to calculate, but is likely in the tens of billions of dollars, especially when considering the cost of purchasing products that may do no harm but also provide no benefit, whether purported or not.

Dietary supplements are a particular area of concern because of the rapid expansion of the market and changing federal regulations. No longer limited to vitamins and minerals, a plethora of herbal, botanical and sports supplements, and other products now comprises over half the dietary supplement industry and have helped sales increase by over 60% to $13.9 billion (8). Consumer spending on dietary supplements, natural/organic food, natural personal care products and functional foods totaled $128 billion in 2000 (9). Herbs and botanicals, sports and meal supplements and other specialty products account for slightly more than half of these sales (8) yet only 12% use herbal supplements (1). Many supplements, such as herbs, remain largely uncontrolled and unregulated, so long as their labels contain no health claims. The Dietary Supplement Health Education Act of 1994 established specific guidelines for health claims and the labeling of dietary supplements but also shifted the burden of proving the accuracy of claims, safety, and quality from the manufacturer to the Food and Drug Administration (FDA) (10). This shift towards having to prove harm rather than safety can potentially impact consumers by lending an air of credibility to misinformation or fraud simply because the federal government has not yet discovered or taken action against it. Over 1,000 new dietary supplements are added annually to the already 29,000 already available (8). Monitoring the claims made by marketers of those products creates an overwhelming task for the FDA, further delaying the time when information can be retracted or products removed from the marketplace.

The health consequences of food quackery, faddism, misinformation, or the misuse or misinterpretation of emerging science, may include: delay or failure to seek legitimate medical care or continue essential treatment, undesirable drug-nutrient interactions, the effects of nutrient toxicities or toxic components of products, and interference with sound nutrition education and practices. Economic harm occurs when purported remedies, treatments and cures fail to work and when products are purchased needlessly. With the burden of proof now on the federal government, there are fewer roadblocks to developing costly but useless products. Indirect impact on health and economic

status can occur when the media report conflicting stories or stories that contain information that may be accurate but incomplete.

SOURCES OF NUTRITION MISINFORMATION

Consumers receive nutrition information from a variety of sources. According to the ADA's *Nutrition and You: Trends 2000* survey, the media are consumers' leading source of nutrition information, with television (48%), magazines (47%), and newspapers (18%) cited as the top three information sources. Other sources cited include books (12%), doctors (11%), and family and friends (11%). Dietitians (1%) and nutritionists (1%) were not frequently cited (1).

The Internet is a burgeoning source of health and nutrition information. According to a Harris Interactive poll, an estimated 100 million consumers sought health information on the Internet in the year 2000, up from 70 million in 1999 (*Wall Street Journal*, 12/29/00).

Consumer interest in health and nutrition information is high, and more than four in 10 (43%) consumers say they like to hear about new studies. However, one in five consumers (22%) report being confused by reports giving dietary advice (1). The sheer volume and varying quality of the information received, as well as perceptions that the information is always changing, fuels consumer confusion about who or what to believe.

Specific sources of nutrition misinformation are discussed below.

Misinterpretation of Scientific Studies in the Media

Scientific progress alone does not prevent or eliminate nutrition misinformation. Too often the popular media capitalize on preliminary research data in an effort to enhance audience and readership ratings. Promoters quickly turn legitimate research findings into sales pitches, products, and services. Therefore, universities, research groups, and commercial enterprises that fund a study and release the results to the media must use caution in presenting their findings.

In addition, news reports on food and nutrition rarely provide enough context for consumers to interpret the advice given. Frequently absent are details about how much more or less of a food to eat, how often to eat a food and to whom the advice applies (11). Both the news media and researchers must share responsibility for reporting accurate, balanced, and complete information to the public.

The *New England Journal of Medicine,* concerned about the way scientific articles in their journal are sensationalized by the media, has responded by developing the following four caveats for the media to use when assessing research findings:

- An association between two events is not the same as a cause and effect.

- Demonstrating one link in a postulated chain of events does not mean that the whole chain is proved.

- Probabilities are not the same as certainties.

- The way a scientific result is framed can greatly affect its impact (12).

The evaluation of nutrition information through the media is best done through proper interpretation of scientific studies by qualified dietetics professionals and other credentialed experts. Initiatives such as the ADA's national media spokesperson program have made great strides nationally and locally in relaying accurate food and nutrition information to the public and positioning registered dietitians as the experts. Yet, a competitive field of celebrities, fitness experts, psychologists and others without nutrition credentials are frequent sources for nutrition-related interviews (13).

For their part, researchers must put their own findings into context by explaining the connection with other studies that show different outcomes. Researchers can also lay the groundwork for ensuring that their findings are presented accurately by critically evaluating the supporting documentation used in their research. One model to follow is the rigorous criteria used by the National Research Council in determining what studies to cite in the report *Diet and Health: Implications for Reducing Chronic Disease Risk* (14). The Council first assessed the strengths and weaknesses of each kind of study and then evaluated the total evidence against six criteria: strength of association, dose-response relationship, temporally correct association, consistency of association, specificity of association, and biological plausibility. To properly evaluate reports of scientific studies, such criteria are needed, as well as knowledge of whether the studies were conducted by experienced investigators (15,16).

Dietetics professionals must be trained in critical research skills, including how to interpret research findings and communicate them to the public. They must recognize and communicate the fact that studies done on small, select groups are not applicable to the general population and that a single study should not form the basis for clinical practice. Dietetics professionals also must recognize that scientific studies will always be open to differences of interpretation; a clear scientific consensus on an issue may not emerge for many years.

Challenges from the Internet

The emergence of the Internet as a major source of health and nutrition information reflects the fact that consumers are taking more responsibility for researching and participating in their own health-care decisions. However, consumers must be reminded that the accuracy of information appearing on Web sites is not governed by any regulatory agency (17). Therefore, sites featuring sound science-based content coexist with sites containing questionable, inaccurate or alarming information promoted by individuals and groups espousing unscientific views. Chat rooms, "listservs," and electronic bulletin boards that are not supervised by qualified health professionals can provide a forum for the exchange of inaccurate advice about nutrition and health.

In addition, the popularization of electronic mail has resulted in rapid and widespread dissemination of false nutrition and health-related stories via the Internet. Recent examples of these unfounded "urban health myths" are that bananas from Costa Rica carry flesh-eating bacteria, and that the sweetener aspartame causes numerous ills such as multiple sclerosis and lupus.

Several health organizations are addressing the proliferation of misinformation on the Internet. For example, the American Medical Association has issued guidelines for medical and health information sites on the Internet (18). The Health On the Net Foundation sets ethical standards for Web site developers and strives to guide medical practitioners and consumers to useful and reliable online medical and health information (19).

Influence of Culture and Food Beliefs

Nutrition misinformation and mistaken beliefs flourish to some degree because they often are deeply rooted in our cultural milieu. Throughout history, many cultures have ascribed health promoting powers to certain foods, and many religions have followed specific dietary practices. The Chinese "herbs of immortality" that were a popular fad among the ancient Egyptians (20) have their modern manifestation in Chinese herbs promoted to bodybuilders in health food stores.

An example of a cultural belief is the concept of "hot" and "cold" foods rooted in Hispanic culture. This belief refers to food's influence on health and well-being, not to the temperature or spiciness of foods. "Cold" foods include most vegetables, tropical fruits, dairy products, and inexpensive cuts of meat. "Hot" foods include chili peppers, garlic, onion, most grains, expensive cuts of meat, oils, and alcohol (21). Pregnancy is considered a "hot" condition during which many Latinos typically avoid "hot" foods, believing this will prevent the infant from contracting a "hot" illness, such as a skin rash (22).

In contrast to the Hispanic "hot/cold" beliefs, the Chinese believe that pregnancy is a "cold" condition during which the expectant mother should consume "hot" foods to keep herself in balance for good health (23).

Fundamental to mistaken beliefs about nutrition is the statement "you are what you eat," which implies that everything from mood and behavior to intellectual capacity is determined by diet. "Bee pollen boosts energy," "fish is brain food," and "eating grapefruit burns body fat" are some common mistaken beliefs about food.

Although some food beliefs that are rooted in traditional cultures and religions are unsupported by scientific evidence, they can be respected as long as they do not result in possible harm and economic exploitation to adherents.

Other Sources of Misinformation

Nutrition misinformation is often disseminated by multilevel marketing companies that promote unproven health products such as dietary supplements, weight loss products and herbs. These companies claim that their products can prevent or cure disease. Product literature may contain illegal therapeutic claims or product distributors may supply such information through anecdotes and independently published literature (24).

Testimonials also may spread misinformation. People tend to believe information that is reinforced by sports figures, celebrities, health food store personnel, teachers, coaches, ministers, legislators, healthcare workers, media commentators, health professionals, and other persons they respect. When such public role models give scientifically unfounded testimonials about the benefits of specific nutritional practices, the effects can be far-reaching and potentially harmful to the public. Thus, these role models should carefully examine the accuracy and reliability of any nutrition information they disseminate and sharpen their skills at making appropriate inferences from scientific reports. When they are uncertain about the scientific merit of nutrition products they are asked to endorse, or do not have the scientific expertise to identify nutrition misinformation, role models should seek the advice of a dietetics professional. Dietetics professionals must be aware of the various sources and forms of nutrition misinformation and be prepared to counter them with science-based information.

COMMUNICATING SCIENCE-BASED FOOD AND NUTRITION INFORMATION

Finding effective approaches for disseminating objective, science-based nutrition and health information to the public is challenging. The high volume of media coverage about emerging nutrition science contributes to consumer confusion (16,1), while seemingly conflicting advice causes disenchantment among consumers (25). Nutrition and health professionals, as well as consumer groups, are concerned that promoters of questionable products and services are likely to exaggerate potential benefits while playing down or eliminating information about possible harmful effects.

The impact of nutrition communication on promoting healthful lifestyles depends on how effectively sound nutrition messages are communicated to consumers and how well consumers discern science-based advice (25). Nutrition information must be presented with sufficient context to allow a consumer to weigh the information and determine whether it applies to his or her unique needs (16).

Effective nutrition communication is consumer focused. Focus group research can help guide nutrition professionals in crafting meaningful and effective consumer communications. Well-focused, individualized nutrition and health messages have the most positive impact on consumer behavior. The campaign *It's All About You*™ is the product of an alliance of food industry, health organizations, and the government and is designed to help consumers implement the Dietary Guidelines for Americans. As part of the campaign, several essentials were identified:

- Nutrition experts need to speak in layman's language.
- Communications that make healthful eating and activity fun and easy are more motivating.
- The emphasis should be on improvement, not perfection.
- The benefit to the consumer must be clear.
- Consistency is essential (26).

The Role of Dietetics Professionals

Qualified dietetics professionals and nutrition educators with the expertise to evaluate and communicate balanced, accurate information on nutrition and health to consumers are best prepared to deliver sound advice and news of scientific advances in nutrition. These professionals should be encouraged to take an active role in disseminating accurate nutrition and health information through public information channels (27,28), such as the media and consumer-targeted books. Dietetics professionals have a responsibility to clarify and demystify consumer-targeted nutrition messages, to help interpret emerging research for media and consumers, and to encourage consumers to look to credentialed dietetics professionals as nutrition experts. To be effective, dietetics professionals and

nutrition educators must be aware of diversity and respect cultural beliefs and design food, nutrition, and health messages appropriately. The sidebars [on page 217 and 218] provide some strategies for dietetics professionals to use in interpreting and communicating nutrition information to the public.

The ADA provides support for members through its Knowledge Center, a leading source of scientifically based, objective food and nutrition information for dietetics professionals, the media, other health care providers, and researchers. Practical, positive nutrition information is provided to professionals and consumers by the Knowledge Center through recorded nutrition messages (1-800-366-1655), National Nutrition Month®, publications, and ADA's Web site, http://www.eatright.org, which offers a gateway to government agencies and many allied professional organizations that focus on nutrition and health.

The Role of Allied Health Professionals

Consistent nutrition guidance and messages from all sources reduce consumer confusion and reinforce the credibility of science-based nutrition information. For this reason, allied health professionals are urged to collaborate with qualified dietetics experts to provide consumer-focused health education, train medical and health personnel, and implement community nutrition education outreach. Physicians, nurse practitioners, and other healthcare providers need to seek the knowledge, skills, and services of dietetics professionals. Strategic partnerships between allied health professionals and related scientific and professional organizations and the nutrition community can help ensure the delivery of consistent nutrition and health messages to consumers.

In addition to the services of the American Dietetic Association, credible nutrition information is offered by many other scientific and professional organizations including, but not limited to, the American Academy of Pediatrics, The American Council on Science and Health, American Society for Nutritional Sciences, American Society for Clinical Nutrition, American Medical Association, American Cancer Society, American Diabetes Association, American Heart Association, and the Society for Nutrition Education. WebMD and the Tufts

STRATEGIES FOR COMMUNICATING ACCURATE NUTRITION INFORMATION TO THE PUBLIC (27)

- Keep advice simple to understand and implement.
- Avoid contributing to the public's confusion by being too quick to laud the latest nutrition theory.
- Avoid speaking in nutrition buzzwords.
- React continually to misinformation.
- Keep your nutrition messages positive.
- Stay current with the latest literature.
- Avoid going against the tide. Tie your nutrition message to current lifestyle trends.
- Avoid being an alarmist. If you constantly proclaim danger about food, people will soon believe that nothing is really dangerous.
- Acknowledge possible ethical conflicts.
- Avoid arguing with other health professionals about subjects that have been discussed for years with no conclusion in sight.
- Stay inside your area of expertise.
- Know your subject area.
- Be brief.

University Nutrition Navigator offer gateways that can lead health professionals, media, and consumers to allied health organizations with credible nutrition information: http://www.webmd.com and http://navigator.tufts.edu.

The Food and Nutrition Science Alliance (FANSA) is a partnership of four professional scientific societies whose members have joined forces to speak with one voice on food and nutrition science issues: The American Dietetic Association, American Society for Clinical Nutrition, American Society for Nutritional Sciences, and Institute of Food Technologists. FANSA developed the "Ten Red Flags of Junk Science" [see page 219] (29).

The Role of Government/Regulatory Bodies

Government agencies play regulatory and disseminating roles with respect to nutrition information. Through the FDA's labeling programs, the government regulates nutrition information and health claims on food and dietary supplement labels. Federal agencies provide science-based nutrition, food, and health guidance, including the Dietary Guidelines for Americans and the Food Guide Pyramid, as well as sound nutrition and food safety informa-

tion through publications and Web sites. The Dietary Guidelines for Americans and the Food Guide Pyramid reflect the nutrient recommendations provided in the Dietary Reference Intakes from the Institute of Medicine/National Research Council. Public-private partnerships, such as the *It's All About You*™ and the *5-A-Day for Better Health*™ campaigns, also communicate positive, simple, and consistent messages to help consumers achieve healthful, active lifestyles.

Many federal, state, and local government agencies employ dietetics professionals for their expertise in nutrition, food science, and nutrition education. Qualified dietetics professionals work in or collaborate with government/regulatory bodies to help educate the public, communicating guidance from government agencies to media and the public. Nutrition experts also have a responsibility to share their professional expertise in the shaping of public policy on consumer nutrition and food communication and misinformation. Many states also license qualified nutrition experts.

Government departments and agencies that provide reliable nutrition and health information include the Federal Trade Commission, Department of Health and Human Services, Food and Drug Administration, National Center for Complementary and Alternative Medicine, US Department of Agriculture, State Cooperative Extension Services, National Institutes of Health (National Cancer Institute, National Heart, Lung, and Blood Institute, National Institute on Aging, National Institute of Allergy and Infectious Diseases, National Institute of Diabetes and Digestive and Kidney Diseases, National Library of Medicine and others), and the Centers for Disease Control and Prevention. Nutrition, food and food safety, and health information from US government agencies can be accessed through the Web site http://www.nutrition.gov. Another government Web site that leads to reputable nutrition information is: http://www.healthfinder.gov.

The Role of Media and Journalists

Consumers report that television, newspapers, magazines, radio, as well as Internet media, are their leading sources of information about nutrition (1). Collaboration between dietetics professionals

---

CRAFTING CONSUMER TIPS (26)

- Keep tips positive, short, and simple.
- Be specific; describe an action (where appropriate).
- Don't assume consumers always know the payoff or benefit.
- Make it manageable.
- Don't perpetuate the "good foods/bad foods" myth. Steer clear of labeling foods as "good," "bad," or "can't haves." Show them how all foods fit into a healthy lifestyle.
- Provide concrete, measurable results.
- Don't over promise; show realistic outcomes.
- Include examples of foods and activities that reflect the lifestyle, preferences, and culture of your audience.
- Use humor when possible and appropriate.
- Incorporate timesaving tips whenever possible.

QUESTIONS TO ASK ABOUT A RESEARCH REPORT

- Was the research done by a credible institution? A qualified researcher?
- Is this a preliminary study? Have other studies reached the same conclusions?
- Was the study done with animals or humans?
- Was the research population large enough? Was the study long enough?
- Who paid for the study? Might that affect the findings? Is the science valid despite the funding source?
- Was the report reviewed by peers?
- Does the report avoid absolutes, such as "proves" or "causes"?
- Does the report reflect appropriate context: for example, how the research fits into a broader picture of scientific evidence and consumer lifestyles?
- Do the results apply to a certain group of people? Do they apply to someone your age, gender, and health condition?
- What do follow-up reports from qualified nutrition experts say?

---

and media professionals is key to consumers receiving sound science-based information about nutrition, food and nutrition science, and food safety issues. Through these joint efforts, the dissemination of nutrition misinformation can be minimized or avoided. Additionally, sound nutritional advice on emerging science can minimize the confusion often experienced by the consumer related to reports of new findings (25).

Many qualified nutrition experts work with the media as spokespersons, media hosts, journalist, writers, and expert consultants. The ADA's media spokespersons are trained, experienced resources for credible food and nutrition information. All qualified nutrition experts can make themselves available to media to present sound nutrition messages, offer an expert's perspective on emerging science, and dispel nutrition misinformation.

Public understanding of emerging nutrition science can be improved if journalistic reporting is accurate and balanced, offers a healthy skepticism, provides practical consumer advice, and presents reports that reflect sound scientific principles (16).

The Role of the Food Industry

The American food industry can be the nutrition professional's ally when it comes to providing complete and reliable nutrition information to the public. The food industry can also help consumers understand emerging nutrition issues by providing accurate information and feedback (16). Many food companies employ dietetics professionals for their expertise in nutrition issues, communications, and consumer affairs. Qualified dietetics professionals need to continue to work with the food industry to help shape the public's food choices, knowledge of nutrition and health, and ability to think more critically about food and nutrition issues. Partnerships between the food industry and health-focused associations, such as the *Home Food Safety: It's In Your Hands*™ campaign, also communicate positive, simple, and consistent health messages for consumers.

Industry trade groups and organizations that provide reputable, evidence-based nutrition information to the public include, but are not limited to, the International Food Information Council, National Cattlemen's Beef Association, Food Marketing Institute, National Dairy Council, National Food Processors Association, National Pork Producers Council, Produce for Better Health Foundation, American Egg Board, American Soybean Association, The Sugar Association, Inc., California

Tree Nut Council, and the Wheat Foods Council. Many food industry Web sites can be accessed and evaluated through the Tufts University Nutrition Navigator: http://navigator.tufts.edu.

The Role of Consumers

Self-care is a consumer trend; today's consumers are more proactive in gathering nutrition and health information (16,1). To take responsibility for their personal health behaviors, consumers need to meet the communication process halfway. Consumers need to recognize qualified dietetics professionals as credible resources for nutrition information and for helping consumers make sound decisions that match their personal needs. Knowing how to access credible information through ADA's Web site, the Tufts University Nutrition Navigator, or various US government Web sites, is one important skill. Consumers need to learn how to recognize science-based nutrition and health advice, to critically examine what they read or hear, and to distinguish fact from fiction (25). [Below are] questions that consumers, as well as qualified dietetics professionals, need to ask about research reports.

Ten Red Flags of Junk Science (29)

1. Recommendations that promise a quick fix.
2. Dire warnings of danger from a single product or regimen.
3. Claims that sound too good to be true.
4. Simplistic conclusions drawn from a complex study.
5. Recommendations based on a single study.
6. Dramatic statements that are refuted by reputable scientific organizations.
7. Lists of "good" and "bad" foods.
8. Recommendations made to help sell a product.
9. Recommendations based on studies published without peer review.
10. Recommendations from studies that ignore differences among individuals or groups.

Food and Nutrition Science Alliance (FANSA). *10 Red Flags to Spot Junk Science.* Available at: http://www.eatright.org/pr/pr4.html. Accessed 2/8/01.

Many consumers may not even be aware that misinformation exits. To avoid being lured by misinformation, consumers need to:

- question the qualifications of authors, presenters, and other nutrition advocates, as well as the evidence for any claims or advice;
- take steps to evaluate nutrition reports or promotions before they become victims of the ploys, by becoming more aware of the many ways misinformation, food fraud, and quackery are conveyed.
- think critically about food and nutrition messages used to promote the sale of a products or services;
- ask a qualified nutrition expert for help in evaluating a statement, product, or service;
- inquire at the medical or nutrition department of a nearby university or college, or at the food and nutrition department of a local hospital/medical center, to obtain current and accurate information and to find nutrition services for the public; or
- check with the American Dietetic Association—http://www.eatright.org (go to "Find a Dietitian") or the Consumer Nutrition Hotline at 1-800-366-1655—for a referral to a qualified nutrition expert.

ADA's Consumer Nutrition Hotline and Web site not only offer consumers a referral service to registered dietitians, but also provide sound nutrition information on timely issues. Reputable consumer organizations that deal with consumer fraud include the Better Business Bureau, Consumers Union, and National Council Against Health Fraud, American Council for Science and Health, and their Web sites.

SUMMARY

Food and nutrition misinformation can be a serious barrier to public health. Misinformed consumers may not only have a false sense of security about their health and well-being, but they also may delay appropriate, effective healthcare or replace it with products, services, or behaviors that may be harmful to their health or, at best, do no good or harm. Misinformation also may result in unnecessary financial expenditure.

The ADA encourages its members take an active role in providing consumers with objective, science-based nutrition information and in helping them recognize and avoid following misinformation. Qualified dietetics professionals can positively shape the food choices of Americans in many ways:

- collaborate with the media to communicate science-based nutrition information to consumers and to counter misinformation;

- write letters to the editors of newspapers and magazines and the producers of electronic media to offer sound information that counters inaccurate and biased articles;

- call television and radio shows that interview nutrition extremists and purveyors of misinformation to express their professional concerns;

- provide positive reinforcement; contact broadcast and print media to recognize accurate nutrition messages, especially when challenging topics are presented;

- direct media and consumers to responsible sources of nutrition information;

- encourage researchers to present their results with a balanced and contextual perspective;

- collaborate with the food industry to provide reliable nutrition information; and

- cooperate with other health practitioners to expose emerging misinformation, misbeliefs, frauds, and quackery before they are widely accepted.

The challenge of dealing with food and nutrition misinformation is long-standing and persistent. Nationally credentialed dietetics professional, in partnership with other members of the health-care team, educators, and representatives of the food industry, can be a forceful voice against food and nutrition misinformation while positively shaping food choices.

REFERENCES

1. *Nutrition and You—Trends 2000 Final Report.* American Dietetic Association: October 1999.

2. *US Surgeon General's Report on Nutrition and Health* Washington, DC: US Department of Health and Human Services; 1988: DHHS Publication 88–50210, p696.

3. Duyff RL. *The American Dietetic Association's Complete Food & Nutrition Guide.* 2nd ed. New York: John Wiley; 2002, in chapter 24. (in press)

4. Louis Harris and Associates. *Health, Information and the Use of Questionable Treatments: A Study of the American Public.* Washington, DC: US Department of Health and Human Services; 1987.

5. National Institute on Aging. *Health Quackery.* Available at: http://www.nih.gov/nia/health/agepages/healthqy.htm. Accessed January 31, 2001.

6. Colditz GA. Economic costs of obesity. *Am J Clin Nutr.* 1992; 55:503–507s.

7. Galuska DA, Will JC, Serdula MK, Ford ES. Are health care professionals advising obese patients to lose weight? *JAMA.* 1999:282; 1576–1578.

8. Sarubin A. *The Health Professional's Guide to Popular Dietary Supplements.* Chicago, IL: The American Dietetic Association; 2000.

9. *Nutrition Business Journal.* Available at: www.nutritionbusiness.com. Accessed May 14, 2001.

10. The Dietary Supplement Health and Education Act of 1994; Pub L No. 103–417 (S784) (codified at 42 USC 287C–11).

11. International Food Information Council. *Food for Thought III—A Quantitative and Qualitative Content Analysis of Diet, Nutrition and Food Safety Reporting.* February 2000: p.v.

12. Angell M, Kassuer JP. Clinical research—what should the public believe? [editorial] *N Engl J Med.* 1994; 331:189–190.

13. MacLaren T. Messages for the masses: Food and nutrition issues on television. *J Am Diet Assoc.* 1997; 97:733–734.

14. National Research Council. *Diet and Health: Implications for Reducing Chronic Disease Risk.* Washington, DC: National Academy Press; 1989.

15. Larkin T. Evidence vs. nonsense: a guide to the scientific method. *FDA Consumer.* 1985; 19:27–31.

16. Harper AE. Nutrition: from myth and magic to science. *Nutrition Today.* 1988; 23(1):8–17.

17. Vozenilek G. The wheat from the chaff: Sorting out nutrition information on the Internet. *J Am Diet Assoc.* 1998; 98:1270–1272.

18. Winker MA, Flanagin A, Chi-Lum B, White J, Andrews K, Kennett RL, DeAngelis CD, Musacchio RA. Guidelines for Medical and Health Information Sites on the Internet: Principles Governing AMA Web Sites. *JAMA.* 2000; 283:1600–1606. Also available at: http://jama.ama-assn.org/issues/v283n12/ffull/jsc00054.html. Accessed February 8, 2001.

19. Health on the Net Foundation home page. Available at: http://www.hon.ch. Accessed February 8, 2001.

20. Mahdihassan S. A comparative study of Greek and Chinese alchemy. *Am J Chinese Med.* 1979; 7:171–181.

21. Mahan LK, Escott-Stump S, eds. *Krause's Food, Nutrition & Diet Therapy.* Philadelphia, PA: WB Saunders Company; 2000, p. 349.

22. American Public Health Association. Available at: http://www.apha.org/ppp/red/labeliefs.htm. Accessed November 25, 2001.

23. American Public Health Association. Available at: http://www.apha.org/ppp/red/asiabeliefs.htm. Accessed November 25, 2001.

24. Coleman E. *Nutrition Quackery.* Eureka, CA: Nutrition Dimension; 1998.

25. Goldberg JP. Nutrition Communication in the 21st Century: What Are the Challenges and How Can We Meet Them? *Nutrition.* 2000; 16:644–646.

26. The Dietary Guidelines Alliance. *Reaching Consumers with Meaningful Health Messages;* 1996.

27. Short SH. Health quackery: Our role as professionals. *J Am Diet Assoc.* 1994; 94:607–661.

28. Brown H, Cassileth BR, Lewis JP, Renner JH. Alternative medicine—or quackery? *Patient Care.* 1994; 28(11):80–97.

29. Food and Nutrition Science Alliance (FANSA). *10 red flags to spot junk science.* Available at: http://www.eatright.org/pr/pr4.html. Accessed February 8, 2001.

ADA Position adopted by the House of Delegates on October 16, 1994. The original ADA Position was approved by the House of Delegates on August 26, 1988, and reaffirmed on September 12, 1999. This position is in effect until December 2004. The American Dietetic Association authorizes republication of the position statement/support paper, in its entirety, provided full and proper credit is given. Requests to use portions of the position must be directed to ADA Headquarters at 800/877-1600, ext 4835 or ppapers@eatright.org.

Recognition is given to the following for their contributions:

Authors:

Keith-Thomas Ayoob, EdD, RD, FADA (Rose F. Kennedy Children's Evaluation and Rehabilitation Center, Albert Einstein College of Medicine, Bronx, NY); Roberta L. Duyff, MS, RD, FADA (Duyff Associates, St. Louis MO); Diane Quagliani, MBA, RD (Quagliani Communications, Inc., Western Springs, IL)

Reviewers:

Dietitians in Business and Communication dietetic practice group: Lisa Poggas, RD (Alterra Healthcare Corp., Denver, CO);

Cathy Kapica, PhD, RD (The Quaker Oats Company, Barrington, IL);

Bettye Nowlin, MPH, RD, FADA (Dairy Council, Culver City, CA);

Nutrition in Complementary Care dietetic practice group: Lisa Fieber, MS, RD (Health Information Services, Inc. Grayville, IL);

Nutrition Education for the Public dietetic practice group: Tab Forgac, MS, RD (National Dairy Council, Rosemont, IL); and William D. Evers, PhD, RD (Purdue University, West Lafayette, IN);

Public Health Nutrition dietetic practice group: Kathleen Leger, MS, RD (Ira Greene Positive Pace Clinic, San Jose, CA); and Margaret F. Lewis, MHE, RD (Tennessee Department of Health, Columbia, TN);

Chris Rosenbloom, PhD, RD (Georgia State University, Atlanta, GA);

Nancy E. Schwartz, PhD, RD (Nutrition Consultant, Oakville, Ontario, Canada)

Members of the Association Positions Committee Workgroup:

Sylvia Escott-Stump, MA, RD (Workgroup chair); Barbara Baron, MS, RD; Mary Marian, MS, RD; Nancy Cotugna, DrPH, RD (content advisor)

POSITION OF THE AMERICAN DIETETIC ASSOCIATION AND DIETITIANS OF CANADA: VEGETARIAN DIETS

It is the position of the American Dietetic Association and Dietitians of Canada that appropriately planned vegetarian diets are healthful, nutritionally adequate, and provide health benefits in the prevention and treatment of certain diseases. Approximately 2.5% of adults in the United States and 4% of adults in Canada follow vegetarian diets. A vegetarian diet is defined as one that does not include meat, fish, or fowl. Interest in vegetarianism appears to be increasing, with many restaurants and college foodservices offering vegetarian meals routinely. Substantial growth in sales of foods attractive to vegetarians has occurred, and these foods appear in many supermarkets. This position paper reviews the current scientific data related to key nutrients for vegetarians, including protein, iron, zinc, calcium, vitamin D, riboflavin, vitamin B-12, vitamin A, n-3 fatty acids, and iodine. A vegetarian, including vegan, diet can meet current recommendations for all of these nutrients. In some cases, use of fortified foods or supplements can be helpful in meeting recommendations for individual nutrients. Well-planned vegan and other types of vegetarian diets are appropriate for all stages of the life cycle, including during pregnancy, lactation, infancy, childhood, and adolescence. Vegetarian diets offer a number of nutritional benefits, including lower levels of saturated fat, cholesterol, and animal protein as well as higher levels of carbohydrates, fiber, magnesium, potassium, folate, and antioxidants such as vitamins C and E and phytochemicals. Vegetarians have been reported to have lower body mass indices than nonvegetarians, as well as lower rates of death from ischemic heart disease; vegetarians also show lower blood cholesterol levels; lower blood pressure; and lower rates of hypertension, type 2 diabetes, and prostate and colon cancer. Although a number of federally funded and institutional feeding programs can accommodate vegetarians, few have foods suitable for vegans at this time. Because of the variability of dietary practices among vegetarians, individual assessment of dietary intakes of vegetarians is required. Dietetics professionals have a responsibility to support and encourage those who express an interest in consuming a vegetarian diet. They can play key roles in educating vegetarian clients about food sources of specific nutrients, food purchase and preparation, and any dietary modifications that may be necessary to meet individual needs. Menu planning for vegetarians can be simplified by use of a food guide that specifies food groups and serving sizes. *J Am Diet Assoc. 2003; 103:748–765.*

POSITION STATEMENT

It is the position of the American Dietetic Association and Dietitians of Canada that appropriately planned vegetarian diets are healthful, nutritionally adequate, and provide health benefits in the prevention and treatment of certain diseases.

VEGETARIANISM IN PERSPECTIVE

A vegetarian is a person who does not eat meat, fish, or fowl or products containing these foods. The eating patterns of vegetarians may vary considerably. The lacto-ovo-vegetarian eating pattern is based on grains, vegetables, fruits, legumes, seeds, nuts, dairy products, and eggs but excludes meat, fish, and fowl. The lacto-vegetarian excludes eggs as well as meat, fish, and fowl. The vegan, or total vegetarian, eating pattern is similar to the lacto-vegetarian pattern, with the additional exclusion of dairy and other animal products. Even within these patterns, considerable variation may exist in the extent to which animal products are avoided.

People choosing macrobiotic diets are frequently identified as following a vegetarian diet. The macrobiotic diet is based largely on grains, legumes, and vegetables. Fruits, nuts, and seeds are used to a lesser extent. Some people following a macrobiotic diet are not truly vegetarian because they use limited amounts of fish. Some "self-described" vegetarians, who are not vegetarians at all, will eat fish, chicken, or even meat (1,2). Some research studies have identified these "self-described" vegetarians as semivegetarians and have defined semivegetarian as occasional meat eaters who predominately practice a vegetarian diet (3) or those who eat fish and poultry but less than 1 time per week (4). Individual assessment is required to accurately evaluate the nutritional quality of the diet of a vegetarian or someone who says that they are vegetarian.

Common reasons for choosing a vegetarian diet include health considerations, concern for the environment, and animal welfare factors (5,6). Vegetarians also cite economic reasons, ethical considerations, world hunger issues, and religious beliefs as their reasons for following their chosen eating pattern.

CONSUMER TRENDS

In 2000, approximately 2.5% of the US adult population (4.8 million people) consistently followed a vegetarian diet and affirmed that they never ate meat, fish, or poultry (7). Slightly less than 1% of those polled were vegans (7). According to this poll, vegetarians are most likely to live on the east or west coast, in large cities, and to be female. Approximately 2% of 6- to 17-year-old children and adolescents in the United States are vegetarians, and around 0.5% of this age group are vegan (8). According to a 2002 survey (9), about 4% of Canadian adults are vegetarian; this represents an estimated 900,000 people. Factors that may affect the number of vegetarians in the United States and Canada in the future include an increased interest in vegetarianism and the arrival of immigrants from countries where vegetarianism is commonly practiced (10). Twenty to 25% of adults in the United States report that they eat 4 or more meatless meals weekly or "usually or sometimes maintain a vegetarian diet," suggesting an interest in vegetarianism (11). Additional evidence for the increased interest in vegetarianism includes the emergence of animal rights/ethics courses on college and university campuses; the proliferation of Web sites, magazines and newsletters, and cookbooks with a vegetarian theme; and the public's attitude toward ordering a vegetarian meal when eating away from home. More than 5% of those surveyed in 1999 said they always order a vegetarian meal when they eat out; close to 60% "sometimes, often, or always" order a vegetarian item at a restaurant (12).

Restaurants have responded to this interest in vegetarianism. The National Restaurant Association reports that 8 out of 10 restaurants in the United States with table service offer vegetarian entrees (13). Fast-food restaurants are beginning to offer salads, veggie burgers, and other vegetarian options. Many college students consider themselves vegetarians. In response to this, most university foodservices offer vegetarian options (14).

There has also been a growth in professional interest in vegetarian nutrition; the number of articles in the scientific literature related to vegetarianism has increased from less than 10 articles per year in the late 1960s to 76 articles per year in the 1990s (15). In addition, the main focus of the articles is changing. Twenty-five or more years ago, articles primarily had themes questioning the nutritional adequacy of vegetarian diets. More recently, the theme has been the use of vegetarian diets in the prevention and treatment of disease.

More articles feature epidemiological studies, and fewer reports are case studies and letters to the editor (15).

There is a growing appreciation for the benefits of plant-based diets, defined as diets that include generous amounts of plant foods and limited amounts of animal foods. The American Institute for Cancer Research and the World Cancer Research Fund call for choosing predominantly plant-based diets rich in a variety of vegetables and fruits, legumes, and minimally processed starchy staple foods and limiting red meat consumption, if red meat is eaten at all (16). The American Cancer Society recommends choosing most food from plant sources (17). The American Heart Association recommends choosing a balanced diet with an emphasis on vegetables, grains, and fruits (18), and the Heart and Stroke Foundation of Canada recommends using grains and vegetables instead of meat as the centerpiece of meals (19). The Unified Dietary Guidelines developed by the American Cancer Society, the American Heart Association, the National Institutes of Health, and the American Academy of Pediatrics call for a diet based on a variety of plant foods, including grain products, vegetables, and fruits to reduce risk of major chronic diseases (20).

New Product Availability

The US market for vegetarian foods (foods like meat analogs, nondairy milks, and vegetarian entrees that directly replace meat or other animal products) was estimated to be $1.5 billion in 2002, up from $310 million in 1996 (21). This market is expected to nearly double by 2006 to $2.8 billion (21). Canadian sales of meat analogs more than tripled between 1997 and 2001 (22).

The ready availability of new products, including fortified foods and convenience foods would be expected to have a marked impact on nutrient intake of vegetarians. Fortified foods such as soymilks, meat analogs, juices, and breakfast cereals can add substantially to vegetarians' intakes of calcium, iron, zinc, vitamin B-12, vitamin D, and riboflavin. Vegetarian convenience foods including veggie burgers and veggie dogs, frozen entrees, meals in a cup, and soymilk can make it much simpler to be a vegetarian today than in the past.

Vegetarian foods are readily available, both in supermarkets and in natural foods stores. About half of vegetarian foods volume is sold through supermarkets and about half through natural foods stores (12). Three-fourths of soymilk sales take place in supermarkets (21).

Public Policy Statements and Vegetarian Diets

The United States Dietary Guidelines (23) state, "Vegetarian diets can be consistent with the *Dietary Guidelines for Americans,* and meet Recommended Dietary Allowances for nutrients." They give recommendations on meeting nutrient requirements for those who choose to avoid all or most animal products. Some have said that implementation of the Dietary Guidelines can best be achieved by use of vegetarian and plant-rich diets (24). National food guides include some vegetarian options. Foods commonly eaten by vegetarians such as legumes, tofu, soyburgers, and soymilk with added calcium are included in a table accompanying the USDA's Food Guide Pyramid (23). Canada's Food Guide to Healthy Eating can be used by lacto and lacto-ovo-vegetarians (25). Health Canada has stated that well-planned vegetarian diets are supportive of good nutritional status and health (26).

HEALTH IMPLICATIONS OF VEGETARIANISM

Vegetarian diets offer a number of advantages, including lower levels of saturated fat, cholesterol, and animal protein and higher levels of carbohydrates, fiber, magnesium, boron, folate, antioxidants such as vitamins C and E, carotenoids, and phytochemicals (27–30). Some vegans may have intakes for vitamin B-12, vitamin D, calcium, zinc, and occasionally riboflavin that are lower than recommended (27,29,31).

NUTRITION CONSIDERATIONS FOR VEGETARIANS

Protein

Plant protein can meet requirements when a variety of plant foods is consumed and energy needs are met. Research indicates that an assortment of plant foods eaten over the course of a day can provide all essential amino acids and ensure adequate nitrogen retention and use in healthy adults, thus complementary proteins do not need to be consumed at the same meal (32).

Estimates of protein requirements of vegans vary, depending to some degree on diet choices (33). A recent metaanalysis of nitrogen balance studies found no significant difference in protein needs due to the source of dietary protein (34,35). Based primarily on the lower digestibility of plant proteins, other groups have suggested that protein requirements of vegans may be increased by 30% to 35% for infants up to the age of 2 years, 20% to 30% for 2- to 6-year-old children, and 15% to 20% for those 6 years and older, in comparison with those of nonvegetarians (36).

The quality of plant proteins varies. Based on the protein digestibility corrected amino acid score (PDCAAS), which is the standard method for determining protein quality, isolated soy protein can meet protein needs as effectively as animal protein, whereas wheat protein eaten alone, for example, may be 50% less usable than animal protein (37). Nutrition care professionals should be aware that protein needs might be higher than the RDA in vegetarians whose dietary protein sources are mainly those that are less well digested, such as some cereals and legumes.

Cereals tend to be low in lysine, an essential amino acid. This may be relevant when evaluating diets of individuals who do not consume animal protein sources and are relatively low in protein (35). Dietary adjustments such as the use of more beans and soy products in place of other protein sources that are lower in lysine or an increase in dietary protein from all sources can ensure an adequate intake of lysine.

Although some vegan women have protein intakes that are marginal, typical protein intakes of lacto-ovo-vegetarians and of vegans appear to meet and exceed requirements (29). Athletes can also meet their protein needs on plant-based diets (38,39).

Iron

Plant foods contain only nonheme iron, which is more sensitive than heme iron to both inhibitors and enhancers of iron absorption. Inhibitors of iron absorption include phytate; calcium; teas, including some herb teas; coffee; cocoa; some spices; and fiber (40). Vitamin C and other organic acids found in fruits and vegetables can enhance iron absorption and can help to reduce effects of phytate (41–43). Studies show that iron absorption would be significantly reduced if a diet were to be high in inhibitors and low in enhancers. Recommended iron intakes for vegetarians are 1.8 times those of nonvegetarians because of lower bioavailability of iron from a vegetarian diet (44).

The main inhibitor of iron absorption in vegetarian diets is phytate. Because iron intake increases as phytate intake increases, effects on iron status are somewhat less than might be expected. Fiber appears to have a minor effect on iron absorption (45,46). Vitamin C, consumed at the same time as the iron source, can help to reduce the inhibitory effects of phytate (42,43), and some research links high vitamin C intake to improved iron status (47,48). The same is true for organic acids in fruits and vegetables (41). The higher intakes of vitamin C and of vegetables and fruits by vegetarians can favorably impact iron absorption (2). Some food preparation techniques such as soaking and sprouting beans, grains, and seeds can hydrolyze phytate (49–51) and may improve iron absorption (42,51,52). Leavening of breads hydrolyzes phytate and enhances iron absorption (49–51,53,54). Other fermentation processes, such as those used to make soy foods like miso and tempeh, may also make iron more available (55), although not all research supports this. Whereas many studies of iron absorption have been short term, there is evidence that adaptation to low intakes takes place over the longer term and involves both increased absorption and decreased losses (56,57). It is likely that iron needs will depend on the make up of the overall diet and be significantly lower for some vegetarians than for others.

Studies typically show iron intake by vegans to be higher than that of lacto-ovo-vegetarians and of nonvegetarians, and most studies show iron intake by lacto-ovo-vegetarians to be higher than that of nonvegetarians (29). Iron sources are shown in the Table. Incidence of iron deficiency anemia among vegetarians is similar to that of nonvegetarians (29,31,58). Although vegetarian adults have lower iron stores than nonvegetarians, their serum ferritin levels are usually within the normal range (58–62).

Zinc

Because phytate binds zinc, and animal protein is believed to enhance zinc absorption, total zinc bioavailability appears to be lower on vegetarian diets (63). Also, some vegetarians have diets that are significantly below recommended intakes for zinc (27,29,64,65). Although overt zinc deficiency has not been seen in Western vegetarians, the effects of marginal intakes are poorly understood (66). Zinc requirements for vegetarians whose diets are high in phytate may exceed the RDA (44). Zinc sources are shown in the Table.

Compensatory mechanisms may help vegetarians adapt to lower intakes of zinc (65,67). Some food preparation techniques, such as soaking and sprouting beans, grains, and seeds as well as leavening bread, can reduce binding of zinc by phytate and increase zinc bioavailability (49,50,68).

Calcium

Calcium is present in many plant foods and fortified foods (see Table). Low-oxalate greens (bok choy, broccoli, Chinese/Napa cabbage, collards, kale, okra, turnip greens) provide calcium with high bioavailability (49% to 61%), in comparison with calcium-set tofu, fortified fruit juices, and cow's milk (bioavailability in the range of 31% to 32%) and with fortified soymilk, sesame seeds, almonds, and red and white beans (bioavailability of 21% to 24%) (69–71). Figs and soy foods such as cooked soybeans, soy nuts, and tempeh provide additional calcium. Calcium-fortified foods include fruit juices, tomato juice, and breakfast cereals. Thus, various food groups contribute dietary calcium (72,73). Oxalates present in some foods can greatly reduce calcium absorption, so vegetables that are very high in these compounds, such as spinach, beet greens, and Swiss chard, are not good sources of usable calcium despite their high calcium content. Phytate may also inhibit calcium absorption. However, some foods with high contents of both phytate and oxalate, such as soy foods, still provide well-absorbed calcium (71). Factors that enhance calcium absorption include adequate vitamin D and protein.

VEGETARIAN FOOD SOURCES OF NUTRIENTS

Nutrient	Amount Per Serving
Iron	← mg →
Soyfoods	
Soybeans, cooked, 1/2 c (125 mL)	4.4.
Soybeans, dry roasted, (soy nuts), 1/4 c (60 mL)	1.7
Soymilk 1/2 c (125 mL)	0.4–1.0
Tempeh, 1/2 c (83 g)	2.2
Tofu, firm, 1/2 c (126 g)	6.6
Veggie "meats," fortified, 1 oz (28 g)	0.5–1.9
Legumes (cooked, 1/2 c/125 mL)	
Adzuki beans	2.3
Baked beans, canned, vegetarian	1.7
Black beans	1.8
Chickpeas, garbanzo beans	2.4
Great northern beans	1.9
Kidney beans	2.6
Lentils	3.3
Lima beans	2.2
Navy beans	2.3
Pinto beans	2.2
Nuts, peanuts, seeds, and their butters	
Almonds, 1/4 c (60 mL)	1.5
Cashews, 1/4 c (60 mL)	2.1
Peanut butter, 2 tbsp (30 mL)	0.6
Peanuts, dry roast, 1/4 c (60 mL)	0.8
Pumpkin and squash seeds, dried, 1/4 c (60 mL)	5.2
Sesame tahini, 2 tbsp (30 mL)	2.7
Sunflower seeds, toasted, 1/4 c (60 mL)	2.3
Breads, cereals, and grains	
Barley, pearled, cooked, 1/2 c (125 mL)	1.0
Cereal, ready-to-eat, fortified, 1 oz (28 g)	2.1–18
Cream of Wheat, cooked, 1/2 c (125 mL)	5.1
Oatmeal, instant, fortified, cooked, 1/2 c (125 mL)	4.2
Oatmeal, regular, quick or instant, cooked, 1/2 c (125 mL)	1.6
Quinoa, cooked, 1/2 c (125 mL)	2.1
Wheat germ, 2 tbsp (14 g)	0.9
Whole wheat or white enriched bread, 1 slice (28 g)	0.9
Fruits (dried, 1/4 c/60 mL)	
Apricots	1.5
Currants	1.2
Figs	1.1
Prunes	1.1
Raisins	1.1

Nutrient	Amount Per Serving
Iron	← mg →
Vegetables (cooked, 1/2 c/125 mL unless indicated otherwise)	
Bok choy (Chinese cabbage, pak choi)	0.9
Broccoli	0.7
Green or yellow beans	0.8
Kale	0.6
Mung bean sprouts	0.8
Mushrooms	1.4
Potato, baked, with skin, 1 medium (173 g)	2.3
Tomato juice	0.7
Turnip greens	0.6
Other foods	
Blackstrap molasses, 1 tbsp (15 mL)	3.5
Zinc	
Soyfoods	
Soybeans, cooked, 1/2 c (125 mL)	1.0
Soybeans, dry roasted, 1/2 c (60 mL)	2.1
Soymilk, 1/2 c (125 mL)	0.3
Soymilk, fortified, 1/2 c (125 mL)	0.5–1.0
Tempeh, 1/2 c (83 g)	0.9
Tofu, firm, 1/2 c (126 g)	1.0
Veggie "meats," fortified, 1 oz (28 g)	1.2–2.3
Legumes (cooked, 1/2 c/125 mL)	
Adzuki beans	2.0
Baked beans, canned, vegetarian	1.8
Black beans	1.0
Chickpeas, garbanzo beans	1.3
Great northern beans	0.8
Kidney beans	0.9
Lima beans	0.9
Lentils	1.2
Navy beans	2.3
Nuts, peanuts, seeds, and their butters	
Almonds, 1/4 c (60 mL)	1.2
Cashews, 1/4 c (60 mL)	1.9
Peanut butter, 2 tbsp (30 mL)	0.9
Peanuts, dry roast, 1/4 c (60 mL)	1.2
Pumpkin and squash seeds, dried, 1/4 c (60 mL)	2.6
Sesame tahini, 2 tbsp (30 mL)	1.4
Sunflower seeds, toasted, 1/4 c (60 mL)	1.8
Breads, cereals, and gains	
Barley, pearled, cooked, 1/2 c (125 mL)	0.6
Cereal, ready-to-eat, fortified, 1 oz (28 g)	0.7–15
Quinoa, cooked, 1/2 c (125 mL)	0.8
Wheat germ, 2 tbsp (14 g)	1.8
Whole wheat bread, 1 slice (28 g)	0.5

Nutrient	Amount Per Serving
Zinc	
Vegetables (cooked, 1/2 cup/125 mL)	
Mushrooms	0.7
Peas	1.0
Dairy foods and eggs	
Cow's milk, 1/2 c (125 mL)	0.5
Cheddar cheese, 3/4 oz (21 g)	0.7
Egg, large, 1 (50 g)	0.5
Yogurt, 1/2 c (125 mL)	0.8–1.1
Calcium	
Soyfoods	
Cultured soy yogurt, fortified, 1/2 c (125 mL)	367
Soybeans, cooked, 1/2 c (125 mL)	88
Soybeans, dry roasted, (soy nuts), 1/4 c (60 mL)	60
Soybeans, green, 1/2 c (125 mL)	130
Soymilk, fortified, 1/2 c (125 mL)	100–159
Tofu, firm, calcium-set, 1/2 c (126 g)	120–430
Tempeh, 1/2 c (83 g)	92
Legumes (cooked, 1/2 c/125 mL)	
Black beans	46
Chickpeas, garbanzo beans	40
Great northern or navy beans	60–64
Pinto beans	41
Vegetarian baked beans	64
Nuts, seeds and their butters	
Almonds, 1/4 c (60 mL)	88
Almond butter, 2 tbsp (30 mL)	86
Sesame tahini, 2 tbsp (30 mL)	128
Breads, cereals, and grains	
Cereal, ready-to-eat, fortified, 1 oz (28 g)	55–315
Fruits	
Figs, dried, 5	137
Orange, 1 large	74
Orange juice, fortified, 1/2 c (125 mL)	150
Vegetables (cooked, 1 c/250 mL)	
Bok choy (Chinese cabbage, pak choi)	167–188
Broccoli	79
Collard greens	239
Kale	99
Kale, Scotch	181
Mustard greens	109
Okra	107
Turnip greens	208

Nutrient	Amount Per Serving
Calcium	
Other foods	
Blackstrap molasses, 1 tbsp (15 mL)	172
Dairy products	
Cow's milk, 1/2 c (125 mL)	137–158
Cheddar cheese, 3/4 oz (21 g)	153
Yogurt, plain, 1/2 c (125 mL)	137–230
Vitamin D	←mcg→
Cereals, ready-to-eat, fortified, 1 oz (28 g)	0.5–1
Egg yolk, large, 1 (17 g)	0.6
Cow's milk, fortified, 1/2 c (125 mL)	1.2–1.3
Soymilk or other nondairy milk, fortified, 1/2 c (125 mL)	0.5–1.5
Riboflavin	←mg→
Almonds, 1/4 c (60 mL)	0.3
Cereal, ready-to-eat, fortified, 1 oz (28 g)	0.2–1.7
Cow's milk, whole, 2% or skim, 1/2 c (125 mL)	0.2
Yogurt, 1/2 c (125 mL)	0.3
Egg, large, 1 (50 g)	0.6
Mushrooms, cooked, 1/2 c (125 mL)	0.2
Nutritional yeast miniflakes, 1 tbsp (3 g)	1.9
Soymilk, fortified, 1/2 c (125 mL)	0.2
Vitamin B-12	←mcg→
Cereals, ready-to-eat, fortified, 1 oz (28 g)	0.6–6.0
Cow's milk, 1/2 c (125 mL)	0.4–0.5
Egg, large, 1 (50 g)	0.5
Nutritional yeast (Red Star Vegetarian Support Formula), miniflakes, 1 tbsp (3 g)	1.5
Soymilk or other nondairy milks, fortified, 1/2 c (125 mL)	0.4–1.6
Veggie "meats," fortified, 1 oz (28 g)	0.5–1.2
Linolenic acid	←g→
Canola oil, 1 tbsp (15 mL)	1.3–1.6
Flaxseed, ground, 1 tbsp (15 mL)	1.9–2.2
Flaxseed oil, 1 tsp (5 mL)	2.7
Soybean oil, 1 tbsp (15 mL)	0.9
Soybeans, cooked, 1/2 c (125 mL)	1.0
Tofu, 1/2 c (126 g)	0.7
Walnuts, 1/4 c (60 mL)	2.7
Walnut oil, 1 tbsp (15 mL)	1.4–1.7

Sources: Package information and data from US Department of Agriculture, Agricultural Research Service, 2002; USDA Nutrient Database for Standard Reference, Release 15; Nutrient Data Laboratory Home Page, http://www.nal.usda.gov/fnic/foodcomp; Bhatty RS. Nutrient composition of whole flaxseed and flaxseed meal. In: Cunnane SC, Thompson LU, eds. Flaxseed and Human Nutrition. Champaign, IL: AOCS Press; 1995:22–42.

Calcium intakes of lacto-vegetarians are comparable with or higher than those of nonvegetarians (74,75), whereas intakes of vegans tend to be lower than both groups and often below recommended intakes (27,31,71,75). Diets high in sulfur-containing amino acids may increase losses of calcium from bone. Foods with a relatively high ratio of sulfur-containing amino acids to protein include eggs, meat, fish, poultry, dairy products, nuts, and many grains. There is some evidence that the impact of sulfur-containing amino acids is only important with low calcium intakes. Excessive sodium intake may also promote calcium losses. In addition, some studies show that the ratio of dietary calcium to protein is more predictive of bone health than calcium intake alone. Typically, this ratio is high in lacto-ovo-vegetarian diets and favors bone health, whereas vegans have a calcium to protein ratio that is similar to or lower than that of nonvegetarians (71,76).

All vegetarians should meet the recommended intakes for calcium, established for their age group by the Institute of Medicine (77). This can be accomplished, in nonpregnant, nonlactating adults, by consuming at least 8 servings per day of foods that provide 10% to 15% of the Adequate Intake (AI) for calcium, as indicated in the Vegetarian Food Guide Pyramid and Vegetarian Food Guide Rainbow (72,73). Adjustments for other stages of the life cycle are available (72,73). Many vegans may find that it is easier to meet needs if fortified foods or supplements are included (69–71,78).

Vitamin D

Vitamin D status depends on sunlight exposure and intake of vitamin D fortified foods or supplements. Sun exposure to the face, hands, and forearms for 5 to 15 minutes per day during the summer at the 42nd latitude (Boston) is believed to provide sufficient amounts of vitamin D for light-skinned people (79). Those with dark skin require longer exposure (79). Sun exposure may be inadequate for those living in Canada and at northern latitudes in the United States, especially in winter months, for those in smoggy regions, and for those whose sun exposure is limited. Furthermore, infants, children, and older adults synthesize vitamin D less efficiently (77,79,80). Sunscreen can interfere with vitamin D synthesis,

although reports are inconsistent and may depend on amount of sunscreen applied (79,81,82). Low vitamin D levels and reduced bone mass have been observed in some vegan populations at northern latitudes who did not use supplements or fortified foods, particularly children following macrobiotic diets and adult Asian vegetarians (29,83–85).

Foods that are fortified with vitamin D include cow's milk, some brands of soymilk and rice milk, and some breakfast cereals and margarines (see Table). Vitamin D3 (cholecalciferol) is of animal origin, whereas vitamin D2 (ergocalciferol) is a form acceptable to vegans. Vitamin D2 may be less bioavailable than vitamin D3, which could raise the requirements of vegetarians who depend on D2 supplements to meet vitamin D needs (86). If sun exposure and intake of fortified foods are insufficient, vitamin D supplements are recommended.

Riboflavin

Some studies have shown vegans to have lower intakes of riboflavin, compared with nonvegetarians; however, clinical riboflavin deficiency has not been observed (27,29,31). In addition to foods shown in the Table, foods that provide about 1 mg of riboflavin per serving are asparagus, bananas, beans, broccoli, figs, kale, lentils, peas, seeds, sesame tahini, sweet potatoes, tofu, tempeh, wheat germ, and enriched bread (87).

Vitamin B-12

Sources of vitamin B-12 that are not derived from animals include B-12 fortified foods (such as some brands of soymilk, breakfast cereals, and nutritional yeast) or supplements (see Table). Unless fortified, no plant food contains significant amounts of active vitamin B-12. Foods such as sea vegetables and spirulina may contain vitamin B-12 analogs; neither these nor fermented soy products can be counted on as reliable sources of active vitamin B-12 (29,88). Lacto-ovo-vegetarians can get adequate vitamin B-12 from dairy foods and eggs if these foods are consumed regularly.

Vegetarian diets are typically high in folic acid, which can mask the hematological symptoms of vitamin B-12 deficiency. Therefore, some cases of deficiency may not be detected until after the onset of neurological symptoms (89). If there are concerns about vitamin B-12 status, serum homocysteine, methylmalonic acid, and holotranscobalamin II should be measured (90).

A regular source of vitamin B-12 is crucial for pregnant and lactating women and for breastfed infants if the mother's diet is not supplemented. Infants born to vegan mothers whose diets lack reliable sources of this vitamin are at especially high risk of deficiency. Maternal vitamin B-12 intake and absorption during pregnancy appear to have a more important influence on vitamin B-12 status of the infant than do maternal vitamin B-12 stores (91). Because 10% to 30% of those over the age of 50 years, regardless of the type of diet they follow, lose their ability to digest the protein-bound form of the vitamin that is present in eggs, dairy, and other animal products, all people over the age of 50 should use vitamin B-12 supplements or fortified foods (92).

Studies indicate that some vegans and other vegetarians do not regularly consume reliable sources of vitamin B-12 and that this is reflected in less than adequate vitamin B-12 status (27,29,88, 89,93–95). It is essential that all vegetarians use a supplement, fortified food, dairy products, or eggs to meet recommended intakes of vitamin B-12 (see Table).

Absorption is most efficient when small amounts of vitamin B-12 are consumed at frequent intervals. This could be achieved through use of fortified foods. When less than 5 µg of crystalline vitamin B-12 is consumed at one time, approximately 60% is absorbed, whereas ≤1% of a dose of 500 µg or higher of vitamin B-12 is absorbed (92).

Vitamin A/Beta Carotene

Because preformed vitamin A is found only in animal foods, vegans get all of their vitamin A from conversion of dietary carotenoids, particularly beta carotene. Research suggests that absorption of beta carotene from plant foods is less efficient than previously believed (44,96). This suggests that vegans intake of vitamin A is about half of what previous studies have suggested, and intake by lacto-ovo-vegetarians may be 25% lower than previously shown. Despite this, vegetarians have been reported to have higher serum carotenoid levels

than nonvegetarians (29). Vitamin A requirements can be met with the inclusion of three servings per day of deeply yellow or orange vegetables, leafy green vegetables, or fruits that are rich in beta carotene (apricots, cantaloupe, mango, pumpkin). Cooking increases beta carotene absorption, as does the addition of small amounts of fat to meals (97). Chopping and pureeing vegetables may also increase bioavailability (98,99).

N-3 Fatty Acids

Whereas vegetarian diets are generally rich in n-6 fatty acids (especifically linoleic acid), these diets can be low in n-3 fatty acids, resulting in an imbalance that can inhibit production of the physiologically active long chain n-3 fatty acids, eicosapentaenoic acid (EPA), and docosahexaenoic acid (DHA). Diets that do not include fish, eggs, or generous amounts of sea vegetables generally lack direct sources of EPA and DHA. Recently, vegan sources of DHA derived from microalgae have become available as supplements in nongelatin capsules. Algae sources of DHA have been shown to positively affect blood levels of DHA and of EPA through retroconversion (100).

Most studies show vegetarians, and particularly vegans, to have lower blood levels of EPA and DHA than nonvegetarians (101–104). The new Dietary Reference Intakes recommend intakes of 1.6 and 1.1 grams of α-linolenic acid per day for men and women, respectively. These are designated as AIs rather than RDAs. These recommendations assume some intake of long-chain n-3 fatty acids and may not be optimal for vegetarians who consume little if any DHA and EPA (35). The Joint World Health Organization/Food Agriculture Organization (WHO/FAO) Expert Consultation on Diet, Nutrition and the Prevention of Chronic Diseases (105) recommends 5% to 8% of calories from n-6 fatty acids and 1% to 2% of calories from n-3 fatty acids. Based on an energy intake of 2,000 kcal per day, this would suggest a daily intake of 2.2 to 4.4 grams of n-3 fatty acids. Those who do not receive a preformed source of EPA and DHA require increased amounts of n-3 fatty acids. The recommended ratio of n-6 to n-3 fatty acids is in the range of 2:1 to 4:1 (106–109).

It is recommended that vegetarians include good sources of α-linolenic acid in their diet

(106,110). These would include foods like flaxseed and flaxseed oil (see Table). Those with increased requirements (eg, pregnant and lactating women or those with diseases associated with poor essential fatty acid status) or those at risk for poor conversion (eg, people with diabetes) may benefit from direct sources of long-chain n-3 fatty acids, such as DHA-rich microalgae (100,106,111).

Iodine

Some studies suggest that vegans who do not consume iodized salt may be at risk for iodine deficiency; this appears to be particularly true for those living in iodine-poor areas (29,112,113). Bread can be a source of iodine because some dough stabilizers contain iodine. In the United States, about 50% of the general population uses iodized salt, whereas, in Canada, all table salt is fortified with iodine. Sea salt and kosher salt are generally not iodized nor are salty seasonings such as tamari. Concern has been raised about vegetarian diets that include foods, such as soybeans, cruciferous vegetables, and sweet potatoes, that contain natural goitrogens. However, these foods have not been associated with thyroid insufficiency in healthy people provided iodine intake is adequate. The adult RDA for iodine is easily met by one-half teaspoon of iodized salt daily (44). Some vegetarians may have very high intakes of iodine because of consumption of sea vegetables.

VEGETARIANISM THROUGHOUT THE LIFE CYCLE

Well-planned vegan, lacto-vegetarian, and lacto-ovo-vegetarian diets are appropriate for all stages of the life cycle, including pregnancy and lactation. Appropriately planned vegan, lacto-vegetarian, and lacto-ovo-vegetarian diets satisfy nutrient needs of infants, children, and adolescents and promote normal growth (36,114,115). Vegetarian diets in childhood and adolescence can aid in the establishment of lifelong healthy eating patterns and can offer some important nutritional advantages. Vegetarian children and adolescents have lower intakes of cholesterol, saturated fat, and total fat and higher intakes of fruits, vegetables, and fiber than nonvegetarians (2,116–118). Vegetarian children have also been reported to be

leaner and to have lower serum cholesterol levels (119–121).

Infants

When vegetarian infants receive adequate amounts of breast milk or commercial infant formula and their diets contain good sources of energy and nutrients such as iron, vitamin B-12, and vitamin D, growth throughout infancy is normal. Extremely restrictive diets such as fruitarian and raw foods diets have been associated with impaired growth and therefore cannot be recommended for infants and children (29).

Many vegetarian women choose to breastfeed their infants (122), and this practice should be encouraged and supported. The breast milk of vegetarian women is similar in composition to that of nonvegetarians and is nutritionally adequate. Commercial infant formulas should be used if infants are not breastfed or are weaned before 1 year of age. Soy formula is the only option for vegan infants who are not being breastfed.

Soymilk, rice milk, homemade formulas, cow's milk, and goat's milk should not be used to replace breast milk or commercial infant formula during the first year because these foods do not contain the proper ratio of macronutrients nor do they have appropriate micronutrient levels for the young infant.

Guidelines for the introduction of solid foods are the same for vegetarian and nonvegetarian infants (115). When it is time for protein-rich foods to be introduced, vegetarian infants can have mashed or pureed tofu, legumes (pureed and strained if necessary), soy or dairy yogurt, cooked egg yolks, and cottage cheese. Later, foods such as cubes of tofu, cheese or soy cheese, and bite-size pieces of soy burger can be started. Commercial, full-fat, fortified soymilk, or cow's milk can be used as a primary beverage starting at age 1 year or older for a child who is growing normally and is eating a variety of foods (115). Foods that are rich in energy and nutrients such as legume spreads, tofu, and mashed avocado should be used when the infant is being weaned. Dietary fat should not be restricted in children younger than 2 years.

Breastfed infants whose mothers do not consume dairy products, foods fortified with vitamin

B-12, or B-12 supplements regularly will need vitamin B-12 supplements (115). Guidelines for the use of iron and vitamin D supplements in vegetarian infants do not differ from guidelines for nonvegetarian infants. Zinc supplements are not routinely recommended for vegetarian infants because zinc deficiency is rarely seen (123). Zinc intake should be individually assessed and zinc supplements or zinc-fortified foods used during the time when complementary foods are being introduced if the diet is low in zinc or mainly consists of foods with low zinc bioavailability (124,125).

Children

Lacto-ovo-vegetarian children exhibit growth similar to that of their nonvegetarian peers (114,119,126). Little information about the growth of nonmacrobiotic vegan children is available, although findings suggest that children tend to be slightly smaller but within the normal ranges of the standards for weight and height (114 ,122). Poor growth in children has been seen primarily in those on very restricted diets (127).

Frequent meals and snacks and the use of some refined foods (such as fortified breakfast cereals, breads, and pasta) and foods higher in unsaturated fat can help vegetarian children meet energy and nutrient needs. Average protein intake of vegetarian children (lacto-ovo, vegan, and macrobiotic) generally meets or exceeds recommendations, although vegetarian children may consume less protein than nonvegetarian children (116,128). Vegan children may have protein needs that are slightly higher than those of nonvegan children because of differences in protein digestibility and amino acid composition of plant food proteins (36,129), but these protein needs are generally met when diets contain adequate energy and a variety of plant foods (35). Good sources of calcium, iron, and zinc should be emphasized for vegetarian children along with dietary practices enhance absorption of zinc and iron from plant foods. A reliable source of vitamin B-12 is important for vegan children. If there is concern about vitamin D synthesis owing to limited sunlight exposure, skin tone, season, or sunscreen use, vitamin D supplements or fortified foods should be used. The Table provides information about food sources of nutrients. Food guides for vegetarian children under 4 years of age

(36,130) and for older children (72,73) have been published elsewhere.

Adolescents

There are limited data available on the growth of vegetarian adolescents, although studies suggest there is little difference between vegetarians and nonvegetarians (131). In the West, vegetarian girls tend to reach menarche at a slightly later age than nonvegetarians (132,133), although not all research supports this finding (134,135). If slightly later menarche does occur, it may offer health advantages, including lower risk of developing breast cancer and obesity (136,137). Vegetarian diets appear to offer some nutritional advantages for adolescents. Vegetarian adolescents are reported to consume more fiber, iron, folate, vitamin A, and vitamin C than nonvegetarians (2,60). Vegetarian adolescents also consume more fruits and vegetables and few sweets, fast foods, and salty snacks compared with nonvegetarian adolescents (2,118). Key nutrients for adolescent vegetarians include calcium, vitamin D, iron, zinc, and vitamin B-12.

Vegetarian diets are somewhat more common among adolescents with eating disorders than in the general adolescent population; therefore, dietetics professionals should be aware of young clients who greatly limit food choices and who exhibit symptoms of eating disorders (138,139). However, recent data suggest that adopting a vegetarian diet does not lead to eating disorders, rather that vegetarian diets may be selected to camouflage an existing eating disorder (27,140,141). With guidance in meal planning, vegetarian diets are appropriate and healthful choices for adolescents.

Pregnant and Lactating Women

Lacto-ovo-vegetarian and vegan diets can meet the nutrient and energy needs of pregnant women. Infants of vegetarian mothers generally have birth weights that are similar to those of infants born to nonvegetarians and to birth weight norms (122,142,143). Diets of pregnant and lactating vegans should contain reliable sources of vitamin B-12 daily. If there is concern about vitamin D synthesis because of limited sunlight exposure, skin tone, season, or sunscreen use, pregnant and lactating women should use vitamin D supplements or fortified foods. Iron supplements may be needed to prevent or treat iron-deficiency anemia, which is commonly seen during pregnancy. Women capable of becoming pregnant and women in the periconceptional period are advised to consume 400 μg of folate daily from supplements, fortified foods, or both in addition to consuming food folate from a varied diet (92).

Infants of vegetarian mothers have been reported to have lower cord and plasma DHA than do infants of nonvegetarians, although the functional significance of this is not known (104,143). Breast milk DHA levels in vegan and lacto-ovo-vegetarian women appear to be lower than levels in nonvegetarians (144). Because DHA seems to play a role in the development of the brain and the eye and because a dietary supply of DHA may be important for the fetus and newborn, pregnant and lactating vegans and vegetarians (unless eggs are eaten regularly) should include sources of the DHA precursor linolenic acid in their diet (ground flaxseed, flaxseed oil, canola oil, soybean oil) or use a vegetarian DHA supplement (from microalgae). Foods containing linoleic acid (corn, safflower, and sunflower oil) and *trans*-fatty acids (stick margarine, foods with hydrogenated fats) should be limited because these fatty acids can inhibit DHA production from linolenic acid (145).

Older Adults

Studies indicate that most older vegetarians have dietary intakes that are similar to nonvegetarians (146,147). With aging, energy needs decrease, but recommendations for several nutrients, including calcium, vitamin D, vitamin B6, and possibly protein, are higher. Sunlight exposure is often limited, and vitamin D synthesis is decreased in older adults so that dietary or supplemental sources of vitamin D are especially important.

Older adults may have difficulty with vitamin B-12 absorption from food so vitamin B-12 fortified foods or supplements should be used because the vitamin B-12 in fortified foods and supplements is usually well absorbed (92). Protein requirements for older adults are controversial. The current DRIs do not recommend additional protein for older adults (35). A metaanalysis of nitrogen balance studies concluded that there is not enough evidence to recommend different pro-

tein intakes for older adults but pointed out that the data are limited and contradictory (34). Others have concluded that protein requirements of older adults may be around 1 to 1.25 g/kg body weight (148,149). Older adults can easily meet protein needs on a vegetarian diet if a variety of protein-rich plant foods, including legumes and soy products, are eaten daily.

Vegetarian diets, which are high in fiber, may be beneficial for older adults with constipation. Older vegetarians may benefit from nutritional counseling on foods that are easy to chew, require minimal preparation, or are appropriate for therapeutic diets.

Athletes

Vegetarian diets can also meet the needs of competitive athletes. Nutrition recommendations for vegetarian athletes should be formulated with consideration of the effects of both vegetarianism and exercise. The position of the American Dietetic Association and Dietitians of Canada on nutrition and athletic performance (39) provides appropriate dietary guidance for athletes, although some modification may be needed to address vegetarians' needs. Protein recommendations for endurance athletes are 1.2 to 1.4 g/kg body weight, whereas resistance and strength-trained athletes may need as much as 1.6 to 1.7 g/kg body weight (39). Not all groups support an increased protein need for athletes (35). Vegetarian diets that meet energy needs and contain a variety of plant-based protein foods, such as soy products, other legumes, grains, nuts, and seeds, can provide adequate protein without the use of special foods or supplements (150). For adolescent athletes, special attention should be given to meeting energy, protein, calcium, and iron needs. Amenorrhea may be more common among vegetarian than nonvegetarian athletes, although not all research supports this finding (151,152). Female vegetarian athletes may benefit from diets that include adequate energy, higher levels of fat, and generous amounts of calcium and iron.

VEGETARIAN DIETS AND CHRONIC DISEASE

Obesity

Among Seventh-day Adventists (SDA), 40% of whom follow a meatless diet, vegetarian eating patterns have been associated with lower body mass index (BMI). In the Adventist Health Study, which compared vegetarians and nonvegetarians within the Adventist population, BMI increased as the frequency of meat consumption increased in both men and women (4). In the Oxford Vegetarian Study, BMI values were higher in nonvegetarians compared with vegetarians in all age groups and for both men and women (112).

In a study of 4,000 men and women in England comparing the relationship between meat consumption and obesity among meat eaters, fish eaters, lacto-ovo-vegetarians, and vegans, mean BMI was highest in the meat eaters and lowest in the vegans (153). BMI was lowest in those lacto-ovo-vegetarians and vegans who had adhered to their diet for 5 years or longer.

Factors that may help to explain the lower BMI among vegetarians include differences in macronutrient content (lower protein, fat, and animal fat intake), higher fiber consumption, decreased alcohol intake, and greater consumption of vegetables.

Cardiovascular Disease

An analysis of five prospective studies involving more than 76,000 subjects showed that death from ischemic heart disease was 31% lower among vegetarian men compared with nonvegetarian men and 20% lower among vegetarian women compared with nonvegetarian women (154). Death rates were also lower for vegetarian men and women compared with semivegetarians, those who ate fish only or ate meat less than once per week. Among SDA, vegetarian men had a 37% reduction in risk of developing ischemic heart disease compared with nonvegetarian men (4). In the only study to include vegan subjects, risk for developing heart disease was even lower among SDA vegan men than in the SDA lacto-ovo-vegetarians (155).

The lower rates of heart disease among vegetarians are explained in part by their lower blood cholesterol levels. A review of 9 studies found that, in comparison to nonvegetarians, lacto-ovo-vegetarians and vegans had mean blood cholesterol levels that were 14% and 35% lower, respectively (156). Although the lower average BMI of vegetarians may help to explain this, Sacks and colleagues found that, even when vegetarian subjects were heavier than nonvegetarian subjects, the vegetari-

ans had markedly lower plasma lipoprotein values (157), and Thorogood and colleagues found that differences in plasma lipids in vegetarians, vegans, and meat eaters persisted, even following adjustment for BMI (158). Some, but not all, studies have shown lower high-density lipoprotein (HDL) levels in vegetarian subjects (29). Lower HDL levels may be due to the type or amount of dietary fat or to lower alcohol intake. This may help to explain the smaller differences in heart disease rates between vegetarian and nonvegetarian women because HDL may be a more important risk factor than LDL levels for women (159). Average triglyceride levels tend to be similar in vegetarians and nonvegetarians.

A number of factors in vegetarian diets may affect cholesterol levels. Although studies show that most vegetarians do not typically consume low-fat diets, saturated fat intake is considerably lower among vegetarians than nonvegetarians, and vegans have a lower ratio of saturated to unsaturated fat in their diets (29). Vegetarians also consume less cholesterol than nonvegetarians, although the range of intake varies considerably across studies. Vegan diets are free of cholesterol.

Vegetarians consume between 50% and 100% more fiber than nonvegetarians, and vegans have higher intakes than lacto-ovo-vegetarians (29). Soluble fiber may lower risk for cardiovascular disease by reducing blood cholesterol levels (160). Limited research suggests that animal protein is directly associated with higher serum cholesterol levels even when other dietary factors are controlled (161). Lacto-ovo-vegetarians consume less animal protein than nonvegetarians, and vegans consume no animal protein. Research shows that consumption of at least 25 g per day of soy protein, either in place of animal protein or in addition to the usual diet, reduces cholesterol levels in people with hypercholesterolemia (162). Soy protein may also raise HDL levels (162). Vegetarians are likely to consume more soy protein than the general population.

Other factors in vegetarian diets may impact cardiovascular disease risk independent of effects on cholesterol levels. Vegetarians have higher intakes of the vitamin antioxidants vitamins C and E, which may reduce oxidation of LDL cholesterol. Isoflavones, which are phytoestrogens found in soy foods, may also have antioxidant properties (163) as well as enhancing endothelial function and arterial compliance (164). Although there is limited information available about intake of specific phytochemicals among population groups, vegetarians appear to consume more phytochemicals than nonvegetarians because a greater percentage of their energy comes from plant foods. Some phytochemicals may affect plaque formation through effects on signal transduction and cell proliferation (165) and may exert antiinflammatory effects (166). Research from Taiwan found that vegetarians had significantly better vasodilation responses, which correlated directly with years on a vegetarian diet, suggesting a direct beneficial effect of vegetarian diet on vascular endothelial function (167).

Not all aspects of vegetarian diets are associated with reduced risk for heart disease. Some (89,103,168–171) but not all (62,172) studies have found higher serum homocysteine levels in vegetarians compared to nonvegetarians. Homocysteine is believed to be an independent risk factor for heart disease. Inadequate intake of vitamin B-12 may be the explanation. Vitamin B-12 injections lowered homocysteine levels in vegetarians, many of whom had low B-12 levels and high serum homocysteine (173). In addition, low intakes of n-3 fatty acids and a high ratio of n-6 to n-3 fatty acids in the diet may raise risk of heart disease among some vegetarians (173).

There are only limited data on the role of vegetarian diets as intervention for heart disease. Vegetarian diets used in these studies have usually been very low in fat. Because these diets have been used along with other lifestyle changes and they have produced weight loss, it has not been possible to ascertain any direct effect of adoption of vegetarian diet on risk factors for heart disease or mortality. Vegetarian diets can be planned to conform to standard recommendations for the treatment of hypercholesterolemia.

Hypertension

Many studies show that vegetarians have both lower systolic and diastolic pressures with differences between vegetarians and nonvegetarians generally falling between 5 and 10 mm Hg (29). In the Hypertension Detection and Follow-Up Program, blood pressure reduction of just 4 mm Hg caused marked reduction in mortality from all causes (174).

In addition to having lower blood pressures in general, vegetarians have markedly lower rates of hypertension than meat eaters (175,176). In one study, 42% of nonvegetarians had hypertension (defined as 140/90 mm Hg) compared with only 13% of vegetarians. Even semivegetarians are 50% more likely to have hypertension than vegetarians (4). Even when body weights were similar between subjects, vegetarians had lower blood pressures. Placing nonvegetarian subjects on a vegetarian diet led to reduced blood pressure in normotensive (177) and hypertensive subjects (178).

A number of studies have controlled for various factors that might help to explain the lower blood pressures of vegetarians and the hypotensive effects of changing to a vegetarian diet. The lower blood pressures do not appear to be due to lower BMI (175), exercise habits (179), absence of meat (180), milk protein (181), fat content of diet (182), fiber (183) or differences in potassium, magnesium, or calcium intakes (184). Because sodium intake of vegetarians is comparable or only modestly lower than that of nonvegetarians, sodium does not explain the differences either. Suggested explanations include a difference in blood glucose-insulin response because of a lower glycemic index of vegetarian diets (185) or a collective effect of beneficial compounds from plant foods (186).

Diabetes

Vegetarian diets can meet guidelines for the treatment of diabetes (187), and some research suggests that diets that are more plant-based reduce risk for type 2 diabetes. Rates of self-reported diabetes among Seventh-day Adventists (SDA) were less than half those of the general population, and, among SDA, vegetarians had lower rates of diabetes than nonvegetarians (188). In the Adventist Health Study, age-adjusted risk for developing diabetes for vegetarian, semivegetarian, and nonvegetarian men was 1.00, 1.35, and 1.97, respectively, and, for women, it was 1.00, 1.08, and 1.93 (4). Among the possible explanations for a protective effect of vegetarian diet are the lower BMI of vegetarians and higher fiber intake, both of which improve insulin sensitivity. However, among men in the Adventist Health Study, risk for diabetes was still 80% higher in nonvegetarian men after adjustment for weight. In men, meat consumption was directly associated with increased risk of diabetes. Among women, risk increased only when meat consumption exceeded five servings per week (188).

Cancer

Vegetarians have an overall lower cancer rate compared with the general population, but it is not clear to what extent this is due to diet. When nondietary cancer risk factors are controlled for, differences in overall cancer rates between vegetarians and nonvegetarians are greatly reduced, although marked differences remain in rates of certain cancers. An analysis from the Adventist Health Study that controlled for age, sex, and smoking found no differences between vegetarians and nonvegetarians for lung, breast, uterine, or stomach cancer but did find that nonvegetarians had a 54% increased risk for prostate cancer and an 88% increased risk for colorectal cancer (4). Other research has shown lower rates of colon cell proliferation in vegetarians compared with nonvegetarians (189) and lower levels of serum insulin-like growth factor-I, thought to be involved in the etiology of several cancers in vegans compared with both nonvegetarians and lacto-ovo-vegetarians (190). Both red and white meat have been independently linked to increased risk for colon cancer (4). Observational studies have found an association between high intake of dairy foods and calcium with increased risk for prostate cancer (191–193), although not all studies support this finding (194). A pooled analysis of 8 observational studies found no link between meat or dairy consumption and breast cancer (195).

Research suggests that a number of factors in vegetarian diets may impact cancer risk. Vegetarian diets come closer to matching the dietary guidelines issued by the National Cancer Institute than do nonvegetarian diets, particularly in regard to fat and fiber intakes (196). Although data on fruit and vegetable intake of vegetarians are limited, a recent study found that intake was considerably higher among vegans compared with nonvegetarians

(62). High lifetime exposure to estrogen has been linked to increased breast cancer risk. Some research shows that vegetarians have lower serum and urinary estrogen levels (197). There is also some evidence that vegetarian girls begin menstruation at a later age, which may reduce cancer risk because of lower lifetime estrogen exposure (132,133). High fiber intake is believed to protect against colon cancer, although not all research supports this (198,199). The environment of the colon of vegetarians is strikingly different from that of nonvegetarians. Vegetarians have a lower concentration of potentially carcinogenic bile acids (200) and fewer intestinal bacteria that convert the primary bile acids into carcinogenic secondary bile acids (201). More frequent elimination and the levels of certain enzymes in the colon enhance elimination of potential colon carcinogens (200,202). Most research shows that vegetarians have lower levels of fecal mutagens (203).

Vegetarians do not consume heme iron, which has been shown to lead to the formation of highly cytotoxic factors in the colon increasing colon cancer risk (204). Finally, vegetarians most likely have higher intakes of phytochemicals, many of which have anticancer activity. Isoflavones in soy foods have been shown to have anticancer effects, particularly in regard to breast and prostate cancer, although this is not supported by all research (205,206).

Osteoporosis

Osteoporosis is a complex disease affected by a variety of lifestyle, dietary, and genetic factors. Although some data indicate that osteoporosis is less common in developing countries with a mostly plant-based diet, these studies have relied on hip fracture data, which has been found to be unreliable for comparing bone health across cultures. There is little evidence to suggest that bone mineral density differs between western nonvegetarians and lacto-ovo-vegetarians.

A number of studies have shown that high protein intake, from animal foods in particular, causes increased excretion of calcium and raises calcium needs (207–209). The effect is believed to be due to the increased acid load from metabolism of sulfur-containing amino acids (SAA). However, grains are also high in these amino acids, and some research shows that SAA intake was similar between non-vegetarians and vegetarians (210). Despite this, there is some evidence that postmenopausal women with diets high in animal protein and low in plant protein had a high rate of bone loss and a greatly increased risk of hip fracture (211). Although excessive protein intake may compromise bone health, there is evidence that low protein intakes could raise risk for poorer bone health (212). Although there are very little reliable data on bone health of vegans, some studies suggest that bone density is lower among vegans compared with nonvegetarians (213–215). Vegan women, like other women, may have low calcium intakes despite the availability of nondairy sources of well-absorbed calcium. Some vegan women may also have protein intakes that are marginal, and vitamin D status has shown to be compromised in some vegans (216–218). The lower serum estrogen levels of vegetarians may be a risk factor for osteoporosis. In contrast, short-term clinical studies suggest that soy protein rich in isoflavones decreases spinal bone loss in postmenopausal women (219). Higher intake of potassium and vitamin K among vegetarians may also help to protect bone health. However, the data suggest that a vegetarian diet does not necessarily protect against osteoporosis despite lower animal protein content.

Renal Disease

High intake of dietary protein may worsen existing kidney disease or increase risk for those who are susceptible to this disease because protein intake is associated with a higher glomerular filtration rate (GFR) (220). The GFR of healthy vegetarians is lower than that of nonvegetarians and even lower in vegans (221). The type of protein consumed may also have an effect, with plant foods having a more beneficial effect on GFR than animal protein (222,223). GFR was 16% higher in healthy subjects after eating a meal containing animal protein compared with a meal with soy protein (222). Because the pathology of renal disease is similar to that of atherosclerosis, the lower serum cholesterol levels and reduced cholesterol oxidation resulting from a vegetarian diet may be beneficial for those with kidney disease.

Dementia

Although rates of dementia differ markedly throughout the world, differences in diagnostic criteria make cross-cultural comparisons difficult. In the United States, among [Seventh-day Adventists], those who ate meat were more than twice as likely to develop dementia (224). Those who had eaten meat for many years were more than three times as likely to develop signs of dementia. Diets high in antioxidants have been found to protect cognitive function (225–227). The lower blood pressure of vegetarians may also be protective. There is also some evidence that lower blood cholesterol protects against dementia (228). Higher homocysteine levels are linked to increased risk of dementia, and this may present one risk factor for vegetarians who do not get adequate vitamin B-12 (229–232). Although one observational study found an increased rate of dementia among Japanese American men who ate tofu regularly (233), the study had a number of methodological limitations, and other research has not supported these findings (234).

Other Health Effects of Vegetarian Diets

Diverticular disease Gear and colleagues found that both male and female vegetarians aged 45 to 59 years were 50% as likely to have diverticulitis compared with nonvegetarians (235). Although fiber is believed to be the most important reason for this difference, other factors may have an effect as well. High-fat diets, independent of fiber intake, have been associated with increased risk of diverticulitis (236). Meat intake may also increase risk (236). Older research suggests that meat consumption may promote growth of bacteria that produce a toxic metabolite that weakens the wall of the colon (237).

Gallstones In a study of 800 women aged 40 to 69 years, nonvegetarians were more than twice as likely as vegetarians to suffer from gallstones (238). The relationship held even after controlling for the three known risk factors for gallstones: obesity, gender, and aging.

Rheumatoid arthritis Rheumatoid arthritis (RA), believed to be an autoimmune disease, involves inflammation of the joints. Several studies from one group of researchers in Finland suggest that fasting, followed by vegan diet, may be useful in treatment of RA (239,240).

Although data are very limited and more follow-up is needed before conclusions can be drawn, some studies suggest that a mostly raw foods vegan diet reduces symptoms of fibromyalgia (241) and that a vegetarian diet may reduce symptoms of topical dermatitis (242).

PROGRAMS AND AUDIENCES IMPACTED

Special Supplemental Nutrition Program for Women, Infants, and Children

In the United States, the Special Supplemental Nutrition Program for Women, Infants, and Children (WIC) is a federal grant program that serves pregnant, postpartum, and breastfeeding women and infants and children up to 5 years of age who are documented as being at nutritional risk and with family income below state standards. This program provides checks or coupons to purchase some foods suitable for vegetarians, including infant formula, iron-fortified infant cereal, vitamin C-rich fruit or vegetable juice, carrots, cow's milk, cheese, eggs, iron-fortified ready-to-eat cereal, dried beans or peas, and peanut butter. Individual state agencies are allowed to submit a plan to USDA's Food and Nutrition Service for substitution of foods to allow for different cultural eating patterns, provided the proposed substitute food is nutritionally equivalent or superior to the food it replaces, is widely available, and does not cost more than the food it is to replace (243). This provision could possibly allow more foods suitable for vegans to be purchased.

Canada Prenatal Nutrition Program (CPNP), federally funded by Health Canada, and perinatal community programs provide vouchers, coupons, or groceries to those who meet the income and nutritional risk criteria for the program. Vouchers can be used for some foods acceptable to vegetarians, including milk, juice, cheese, eggs, fortified soymilk, and other foods (244).

Child Nutrition Programs

In the United States, the National School Lunch Program (NSLP) allows nonmeat protein products, including certain soy products, cheese, eggs, cooked dried beans or peas, yogurt, peanut butter, other nut or seed butters, peanuts, tree nuts, and seeds to be used (245,246). USDA information for school foodservice personnel includes several vegetarian and vegan quantity recipes (247). Few public schools regularly feature vegetarian menu items. School lunches are not adequate for vegans even when some vegan options are available because soymilk can only be served as part of school lunch in cases of documented lactose intolerance.

In Canada, school lunch, breakfast, and snack programs; food selection standards; and provision for vegetarian meals vary from one region to another. Nationally, the Canadian Living Foundation's Breakfast for Learning program is developing Best Practice Program Standards for breakfast, snack, and lunch programs. Vegetarian meals based on Canada's Food Guide to Healthy Eating fit within this framework (248).

Feeding Programs for the Elderly

The federal Elderly Nutrition Program (ENP) distributes funds to states, territories, and tribal organizations for a national network of programs that provide congregate and home-delivered meals (often known as Meals on Wheels) for older Americans. Meals served under this program must provide at least one-third of the RDAs (249). Meals are often provided by local Meals on Wheels agencies. A 4-week set of vegetarian menus has been developed for use by the National Meals on Wheels Foundation (250,251).

Correction Facilities

Court rulings in the United States and Canada have granted prison inmates the right to have vegetarian meals for religious and medical reasons (and in Canada, by choice, as well) (252,253). Federal institutions and those for many states and provinces provide vegetarian options for meals. The Canadian federal court has ruled that prison inmates who are opposed to eating meat have a constitutional right to be served vegetarian meals. The Freedom of Conscience provisions in the Charter of Rights allow prisoners to demand vegetarian fare for moral reasons, just as other inmates may request special meals on religious or medical grounds (252).

Military/Armed Forces

The US Army's Combat Feeding Program, which oversees all food regulations, provides a choice of vegetarian menus (254). Canadian Forces Food Services offers one or more vegetarian options at every meal (255). An estimated 10% to 15% of Canadian Forces members choose vegetarian meals for combat rations (individual meal packs) (256).

Other Institutions and Quantity Food Service Organizations

Other institutions, including colleges, universities, hospitals, restaurants, and publicly funded museums and parks offer varying amounts and types of vegetarian selections. Resources are available for vegetarian quantity food preparation . . . . As interest in vegetarianism grows and because of the nutritional and health benefits of choosing a vegetarian diet, increased provision of vegetarian meals on a daily basis should be encouraged.

ROLE OF DIETETICS PROFESSIONALS

Vegetarian clients may seek nutrition counseling services for a specific clinical condition or for assistance in planning healthful vegetarian diets. They may sometimes be referred because of problems related to poor diet choices. Dietetics professionals have an important role in supporting clients who express an interest in adopting vegetarian diets or who already eat a vegetarian diet. It is important for dietetics professionals to support any client who chooses this style of eating and to be able to give current accurate information about vegetarian nutrition. Information should be individualized depending on type of vegetarian diet, age of the client, food preparation skills, and activity level. It is important to listen to the client's own description of his or her diet to ascertain which foods can play a role in meal planning. [The sidebar on this page] provides a listing of Web resources on vegetarianism. [The sidebar on page 239] includes meal planning tips.

Qualified dietetics professionals can help vegetarian clients in the following ways:

- provide information about meeting requirements for vitamin B-12, calcium, vitamin D, zinc, iron, and n-3 fatty acids because poorly planned vegetarian diets may sometimes fall short of these nutrients;

- give specific guidelines for planning balanced lacto-ovo-vegetarian or vegan meals for all stages of the life cycle;

- adapt guidelines for planning balanced lacto-ovo-vegetarian or vegan meals for clients with special dietary needs because of allergies or chronic disease or other restrictions;

USEFUL WEB SITES

General Vegetarian Nutrition:
Food and Nutrition Information Center, USDA
http://www.nal.usda.gov/fnic/etext/000058.html
*http://www.nal.usda.gov/fnic/pubs/bibs/gen/
    vegetarian.htm*

Loma Linda University Vegetarian Nutrition & Health Letter
http://www.llu.edu/llu/vegetarian/vegnews.htm

Seventh-day Adventist Dietetic Association
http://www.sdada.org/facts&fiction.htm

Vegan Outreach
http://www.veganoutreach.org/whyvegan/health.html;
*http://www.veganoutreach.org/health/stayinghealthy.
    html*

The Vegan Society (vitamin B-12)
www.vegansociety.come/html/info/b12sheet.htm

Vegetarian Nutrition Dietetic Practice Group
http://www.vegetariannutrition.net/

Vegetarian Resource Group
http://www.vrg.org/

The Vegetarian Society of the United Kingdom
http://www.vegsoc.org/health/

VegRD
http://vegrd.vegan.com/

Travel:
Happy Cow's Global Guide to Vegetarian Restaurants
www.happycow.net/

VegDining.com
www.vegdining.com/Home.cfm

Vegetarian Resource Group
www.vrg.org/travel/

Quantity Food Preparation:
Vegetarian Resource Group
http://www.vrg.org/fsupdate/

MEAL PLANNING

A variety of menu planning approaches can provide adequate nutrition for vegetarians. The Vegetarian Food Guide Pyramid and Vegetarian Food Guide Rainbow (72,73) suggest one approach. In addition, the following guidelines can help vegetarians plan healthful diets:

- Choose a variety of foods including whole grains, vegetables, fruits, legumes, nuts, seeds, and if desired, dairy products, and eggs.
- Choose whole, unrefined foods often and minimize the intake of highly sweetened, fatty and heavily refined foods.
- Choose a variety of fruits and vegetables.
- If animal foods such as dairy products and eggs are used, choose lower-fat dairy products and use both eggs and dairy products in moderation.
- Use a regular source of vitamin B-12 and, if sunlight exposure is limited, of vitamin D.

- be familiar with vegetarian options at local restaurants;
- provide ideas for planning optimal vegetarian meals while traveling;
- instruct clients about the preparation and use of foods that frequently are part of vegetarian diets; the growing selection of products aimed at vegetarians may make it impossible to be knowledgeable about all such products. However, practitioners working with vegetarian clients should have a basic knowledge of preparation, use, and nutrient content of variety of grains, beans, soy products, meat analogs and fortified foods.
- be familiar with local sources for purchase of vegetarian foods. In some communities, mail order sources may be necessary.
- work with family members, particularly the parents of vegetarian children, to help provide the best possible environment for meeting nutrient needs on a vegetarian diet; and,
- if a practitioner is unfamiliar with vegetarian nutrition, he/she should assist the individual in finding someone who is qualified to advise the client or should direct the client to reliable resources.

CONCLUSIONS

Appropriately planned vegetarian diets have been shown to be healthful, nutritionally adequate, and beneficial in the prevention and treatment of certain diseases. Vegetarian diets are appropriate for all stages of the life cycle. There are many reasons for the rising interest in vegetarianism. The number of vegetarians in the United States and Canada is expected to increase over the next decade. Dietetics professionals can assist vegetarian clients by providing current, accurate information about vegetarian nutrition, foods, and resources.

REFERENCES

1. Barr SI, Chapman GE. Perceptions and practices of self-defined current vegetarian, former vegetarian, and nonvegetarian women. *J Am Diet Assoc.* 2002;102:354–360.
2. Perry CL, McGuire MT, Neumark-Sztainer D, Story M. Adolescent vegetarians. How well do their dietary patterns meet the Healthy People 2010 objectives? *Arch Pediatr Adolesc Med.* 2002;156:431–437.
3. Sabate J, Ratzin-Turner RA, Brown JE. Vegetarian diets: descriptions and trends. In: Sabate J, ed. *Vegetarian Nutrition.* Boca Raton, FL: CRC Press; 2001: 3–17.
4. Fraser GE. Associations between diet and cancer, ischemic heart disease, and all-cause mortality in non-Hispanic white California Seventh-day Adventists. *Am J Clin Nutr.* 1999;70:532S–538S.
5. White RF, Seymour J, Frank E. Vegetarianism among US women physicians. *J Am Diet Assoc.* 1999;99:595–598.
6. Lea E, Worsley A. The cognitive contexts of beliefs about the healthiness of meat. *Public Health Nutr.* 2002;5:37–45.
7. The Vegetarian Resource Group. How many vegetarians are there? Available at: http://www.vrg.org/nutshell/poll2000.htm. Accessed February 10, 2003.
8. The Vegetarian Resource Group. How many teens are vegetarian? How many kids don't eat meat? Available at: http://www.vrg.org/journal/vj2001jan/2001janteen.htm. Accessed February 10, 2003.
9. National Institute of Nutrition. Tracking Nutrition Trends IV: An Update on Canadians' Nutrition-Related Attitudes, Knowledge and Actions, 2001. Available at: www.nin.ca/public_html/EN/consumer_trends.html. Accessed February 10, 2003.
10. Raj S, Ganganna P, Bowering J. Dietary habits of Asian Indians in relation to length of residence in

the United States. *J Am Diet Assoc.* 1999;99: 1106–1108.

11. Ginsberg C, Ostrowski A. The market for vegetarian foods. *Vegetarian J.* 2002;4:25–29.

12. The Vegetarian Resource Group. How many people order vegetarian foods when eating out? Available at: http://www.vrg.org/journal/vj99sep/999scientific.htm. Accessed February 10, 2003.

13. National Restaurant Association. *Tableservice Restaurant Trends,* 2001. Washington, DC: 2001.

14. Crosby M. College and university foodservice operations get high marks from students; 1999. Available at: http://www.restaurant.org/rusa/magArticle.cfm?ArticleID=327. Accessed February 10, 2003.

15. Sabate J, Duk A, Lee CL. Publication trends of vegetarian nutrition articles in biomedical literature; 1966–1995. *Am J Clin Nutr.* 1999; 70(suppl): 601S–607S.

16. World Cancer Research Fund/AICR. *Food, Nutrition, and the Prevention of Cancer: A Global Perspective.* Washington, DC: AICR; 1997.

17. Byers T, Nestle M, McTiernan A, Doyle C, Currie-Williams A, Gansler T, Thun M. American Cancer Society 2001 Nutrition and Physical Activity Guidelines Advisory Committee. American Cancer Society guidelines on nutrition and physical activity for cancer prevention: Reducing the risk of cancer with healthy food choices and physical activity. *CA Cancer J Clin.* 2002;52:92–119.

18. Nutrition Committee of the American Heart Association. AHA Dietary Guidelines Revision 2000: A Statement for Healthcare Professionals From the Nutrition Committee of the American Heart Association. *Circulation.* 2000;102:2296–2311.

19. Heart and Stroke Foundation of Canada. Healthy Eating. Available at: http://ww2.heartandstroke.ca/Page.asp?PageID=33&ArticleID=551&Src=living&From=SubCategory. Accessed February 10, 2003.

20. Deckelbaum RJ, Fisher EA, Winston M, Kumanyika, Lauer RM, Pi-Sunyer FX, St. Jeor, S, Schaefer EJ, Weinstein IB. Summary of a scientific conference on preventive nutrition: Pediatrics to geriatrics. *Circulation.* 1999;100:450–456.

21. Mintel International Group Limited. *The Vegetarian Food Market—US Report.* Chicago, IL: Mintel International Group Limited; 2001.

22. AC Nielsen. *Market Track for 1997 to 2001.* New York, NY: AC Nielsen; 2001.

23. US Department of Agriculture. *Dietary Guidelines for Americans,* 5th ed. Washington, DC: US Government Printing Office; 2000.

24. Haddad EH. Vegetarian diets and dietary guidelines for chronic disease prevention: How meatless diets conform to current recommendations for healthy eating. In: Sabate J, ed. *Vegetarian Nutrition.* Boca Raton, FL: CRC Press; 2001:371–409.

25. Dietitians of Canada. Celebrating the pleasure of vegetarian eating. Available at: http://www.dietitians.ca/english/factsheets/e1995_02.html. Accessed February 10, 2003.

26. Health Canada. *Nutrition for a Healthy Pregnancy: National Guidelines for the Childbearing Years.* Ottawa: Minister of Public Works and Government Services Canada: 1999.

27. Janelle KC, Barr SI. Nutrient intakes and eating behavior scores of vegetarian and nonvegetarian women. *J Am Diet Assoc.* 1995; 95:180–189.

28. Jacob RA, Burri BJ. Oxidative damage and defense. *Am J Clin Nutr.* 1996;63:985S–990S.

29. Messina MJ, Messina VL. *The Dietitian's Guide to Vegetarian Diets: Issues and Applications.* Gaithersburg, MD: Aspen Publishers; 1996.

30. Rainey CJ, Nyquist LA, Christensen RE, Strong PL, Culver BD, Coughlin JR. Daily boron intake from the American diet. *J Am Diet Assoc.* 1999;99:335–340.

31. Larsson CL, Johansson GK. Dietary intake and nutritional status of young vegans and omnivores in Sweden. *Am J Clin Nutr.* 2002;76:100–106.

32. Young VR, Pellett PL. Plant proteins in relation to human protein and amino acid nutrition. *Am J Clin Nutr.* 1994;59:1203S–1212S.

33. Joint FAO/WHO Expert Consultation. *Protein Quality Evaluation.* FAO Food and Nutrition Paper 51. Rome; 1991.

34. Rand WM, Pellett PL, Young VR. Meta-analysis of nitrogen balance studies for estimating protein requirements in healthy adults. *Am J Clin Nutr.* 2003;77:109–127.

35. Food and Nutrition Board, Institute of Medicine. *Dietary Reference Intakes for Energy, Carbohydrate, Fiber, Fat, Fatty Acids, Cholesterol, Protein, and Amino Acids.* Washington, DC: National Academy Press; 2002.

36. Messina V, Mangels AR. Considerations in planning vegan diets: Children. *J Am Diet Assoc.* 2001;101: 661–669.

37. Young VR, Fajardo L, Murray E, Rand WM, Scrimshaw NS. Protein requirements of man: Comparative nitrogen balance response within the submaintenance-to-maintenance range of intakes of wheat and beef proteins. *J Nutr.* 1975;105:534–542.

38. Nieman DC. Physical fitness and vegetarian diets: Is there a relation? *Am J Clin Nutr.* 1999;70: 570S–575S.

39. American Dietetic Association, Dietitians of Canada, the American College of Sports Medicine.

Nutrition and athletic performance—Position of the American Dietetic Association, Dietitians of Canada, and the American College of Sports Medicine. *J Am Diet Assoc.* 2000;100:1543–1556.

40. Hurrell RF, Reddy M, Cook JD. Inhibition of nonhaem iron absorption in man by polyphenolic-containing beverages. *Br J Nutr.* 1999;81:289–295.

41. Gillooly M, Bothwell TH, Torrance JD, MacPhail AP, Derman DP, Bezwoda WR, Mills W, Charlton RW. The effects of organic acids, phytates, and polyphenols on the absorption of iron from vegetables. *Br J Nutr.* 1983;49:331–342.

42. Hallberg L, Hulthen L. Prediction of dietary iron absorption: An algorithm for calculating absorption and bioavailability of dietary iron. *Am J Clin Nutr.* 2000;71:1147–1160.

43. Sandstrom B. Micronutrient interactions: Effects on absorption and bioavailability. *Br J Nutr.* 2001;85 (suppl 2):S181–S185.

44. Food and Nutrition Board, Institute of Medicine. *Dietary Reference Intakes for Vitamin A, Vitamin K, Arsenic, Boron, Chromium, Copper, Iodine, Iron, Manganese, Molybdenum, Nickel, Silicon, Vanadium, and Zinc.* Washington, DC: National Academy Press; 2001.

45. Brune M, Rossander-Hulten L, Hallberg L, Gleerup A, Sandberg AS. Iron absorption from bread in humans: Inhibiting effects of cereal fiber, phytate and inositol phosphates with different numbers of phosphate groups. *J Nutr.* 1992;122:442–449.

46. Coudray C, Bellanger J, Castiglia-Delavaud C, Remesy C, Vermorel M, Rayssignuier Y. Effect of soluble or partly soluble dietary fibres supplementation on absorption and balance of calcium, magnesium, iron and zinc in healthy young men. *Eur J Clin Nutr.* 1997;51:375–380.

47. Backstrand JR, Allen LH, Black AK, De Mata M, Pelto GH. Diet and iron status of nonpregnant women in rural Central Mexico. *Am J Clin Nutr.* 2002;76:156–164.

48. Fleming DJ, Jacques PF, Dallal GE, Tucker KL, Wilson PW, Wood RJ. Dietary determinants of iron stores in a free-living elderly population: The Framingham Heart Study. *Am J Clin Nutr.* 1998;67:722–733.

49. Frolich W. Chelating properties of dietary fiber and phytate: The role for mineral availability: In: Furda I, Brine CJ, eds. *New Developments in Dietary Fiber.* New York, NY: Plenum Press; 1990.

50. Harland BF, Morris ER. Phytate a good or bad food component. *Nutr Res.* 1995;15:733–754.

51. Sandberg AS, Brune M, Carlsson NG, Hallberg L, Skoglund E. Rossander-Hulthen L. Inositol phosphates with different numbers of phosphate groups influence iron absorption in humans. *Am J Clin Nutr.* 1999;70:240–246.

52. Manary MJ, Krebs NF, Gibson RS, Broadhead RL, Hambidge KM. Community-based dietary phytate reduction and its effect on iron status in Malawian children. *Ann Trop Paediatr.* 2002;22:133–136.

53. Bhatia A, Khetarpaul N. Development, acceptability and nutritional evaluation of "Doli Ki Roti"—an indigenously fermented bread. *Nutr Health.* 2001;115:113–120.

54. El-Guindi M, Lynch SR, Cook JD. Iron absorption from fortified flat breads. *Br J Nutr.* 1988;59:205–213.

55. Macfarlane BJ, van der Riet WB, Bothwell TH, Baynes RD, Siegenberg D, Schmidt U, Tol A, Taylor JRN, Mayet F. Effect of traditional Oriental soy products on iron absorption. *Am J Clin Nutr.* 1990;51:873–880.

56. Hunt JR, Roughead ZK. Nonheme-iron absorption, fecal ferritin excretion, and blood indexes of iron status in women consuming controlled lactoovovegetarian diets for 8 wk. *Am J Clin Nutr.* 1999;69:944–952.

57. Hunt JR, Roughead ZK. Adaptation of iron absorption in men consuming diets with high or low iron bioavailability. *Am J Clin Nutr.* 2000;71:94–102.

58. Ball MJ, Bartlett MA. Dietary intake and iron status of Australian vegetarian women. *Am J Clin Nutr.* 1999;70:353–358.

59. Alexander D, Ball MJ, Mann J. Nutrient intake and haematological status of vegetarians and age-sex matched omnivores. *Eur J Clin Nutr.* 1994;48:538–546.

60. Donovan UM, Gibson RS. Iron and zinc status of young women aged 14 to 19 years consuming vegetarian and omnivorous diets. *J Am Coll Nutr.* 1995;14:463–472.

61. Harman, SK, Parnell, WR. The nutritional health of New Zealand vegetarian and non-vegetarian Seventh-day Adventists: Selected vitamin, mineral and lipid levels. *N Z Med J.* 1998;111:91–94.

62. Haddad EH, Berk LS, Kettering JD, Gubbard RW, Peters WR. Dietary intake and biochemical, hematologic, and immune status of vegans compared with nonvegetarians. *Am J Clin Nutr.* 1999;70:586S–593S.

63. Hunt JR, Matthys LA, Johnson LK. Zinc absorption, mineral balanced, and blood lipids in women consuming controlled lactoovovegetarian and omnivorous diets for 8 weeks. *Am J Clin Nutr.* 1998;67:421–430.

64. Ball MJ, Ackland ML. Zinc intake and status in Australian vegetarians. *Br J Nutr.* 2000;83:27–33.

65. Gibson RS. Content and bioavailability of trace elements in vegetarian diets. *Am J Clin Nutr.* 1994;59:1223S–1232S.

66. Hunt JR. Moving toward a plant-based diet: Are iron and zinc at risk? *Nutr Rev.* 2002;60:127–134.

67. Lei S, Mingyan X, Miller LV, Tong L, Krebs NF, Hambidge KM. Zinc absorption and intestinal losses of endogenous zinc in young Chinese women with marginal zinc intakes. *Am J Clin Nutr.* 1996;63:348–353.

68. Gibson RS, Hotz C. Dietary diversification/modification strategies to enhance micronutrient content and bioavailability of diets in developing countries. *Br J Nutr.* 2001; 85(suppl 2):S159–S166.

69. Heaney R, Dowell M, Rafferty K, Bierman J. Bioavailability of the calcium in fortified soy imitation milk, with some observations on method. *Am J Clin Nutr.* 2000;71:1166–1169.

70. Weaver C, Plawecki K. Dietary calcium: Adequacy of a vegetarian diet. *Am J Clin Nutr.* 1994;59:1238S–1241S.

71. Weaver C, Proulx W, Heaney R. Choices for achieving adequate dietary calcium with a vegetarian diet. *Am J Clin Nutr.* 1999; 70:543S–548S.

72. Messina V, Melina V, Mangels AR. A new food guide for North American vegetarians. *J Am Diet Assoc.* 2003;103:771–775.

73. Messina V, Melina V, Mangels AR. A new food guide for North American vegetarians. *Can J Diet Pract Res.* 2003; 64(2).

74. Slattery ML, Jacobs DR Jr, Hilner JE, Caan BJ, Van Horn L, Bragg C, Manolio TA, Kushi LH, Liu KA. Meat consumption and its associations with other diet and health factors in young adults: The CARDIA study. *Am J Clin Nutr.* 1991; 54:930–935.

75. Tesar R, Notelovitz M, Shim E, Dauwell G, Brown J. Axial and peripheral bone density and nutrient intakes of postmenopausal vegetarian and omnivorous women. *Am J Clin Nutr.* 1992; 56:699–704.

76. Remer T. Influence of diet on acid-base balance. *Semin Dial.* 2000;13:221–226.

77. Food and Nutrition Board, Institute of Medicine. *Dietary Reference Intakes for Calcium, Phosphorus, Magnesium, Vitamin D and Fluoride.* Washington, DC: National Academy Press; 1997.

78. Heaney RP, Dowell SD, Bierman J, Hale CA, Bendich A. Absorbability and cost effectiveness in calcium supplementation. *J Am Coll Nutr.* 2001;20:239–246.

79. Holick MF. Vitamin D and bone health. *J Nutr.* 1996;126:1159S–1164S.

80. Lee LT, Drake WM, Kendler DL. Intake of calcium and vitamin D in 3 Canadian long-term care facilities. *J Am Diet Assoc.* 2002;102:244–247.

81. Moloney FJ, Collins S, Murphy GM. Sunscreens: Safety, efficacy and appropriate use. *Am J Clin Dermatol.* 2002;3:185–191.

82. Weinstock MA. Do sunscreens increase or decrease melanoma risk: An epidemiologic evaluation. *J Investig Dermatol Symp Proc.* 1999; 4:97–100.

83. Dagnelie PC, Vergote FJ, van Staveren WA, van den Berg H, Dingjan PG, Hautvast JG. High prevalence of rickets in infants on macrobiotic diets. *Am J Clin Nutr.* 1990; 51:202–208.

84. Parsons TJ, van Dusseldorp M, van der Vliet M, van de Werken K, Schaafsma G, van Staveren WA. Reduced bone mass in Dutch adolescents fed a macrobiotic diet in early life. *J Bone Miner Res.* 1997;12:1486–1494.

85. Fonseca V, Agnew JE, Nag D, Dandona P. Bone density and cortical thickness in nutritional vitamin D deficiency: Effect of secondary hyperparathyroidism. *Ann Clin Biochem.* 1988; 25:271–274.

86. Trang HM, Cole DE, Rubin LA, Pierratos A, Siu S, Vieth R. Evidence that vitamin D-3 increases serum 25-hydroxyvitamin D more efficiently than does vitamin D-2. *Am J Clin Nutr.* 1998;68:854–858.

87. US Department of Agriculture, Agricultural Research Service, 2002. USDA Nutrient Database for Standard Reference, Release 15. Nutrient data laboratory home page. Available at: http://www.nal.usda.gov/fnic/foodcomp. Accessed February 10, 2003.

88. Donaldson MS. Metabolic vitamin B12 status on a mostly raw vegan diet with follow-up using tablets, nutritional yeast, or probiotic supplements. *Ann Nutr Metab.* 2000;44:229–234.

89. Herrmann W, Schorr H, Purschwitz K, Rassoul F, Richter V. Total homocysteine, vitamin B12, and total antioxidant status in vegetarians. *Clin Chem.* 2001;47:1094–1101.

90. Herrmann W, Geisel J. Vegetarian lifestyle and monitoring of vitamin B-12 status. *Clin Chim Acta.* 2002;326:47–59.

91. Luhby AL, Cooperman JM, Donnenfeld AM, Herman JM, Teller DN, Week JB. Observations on transfer of vitamin B_{12} from mother to fetus and newborn. *Am J Dis Child.* 1958;96:532–533.

92. Food and Nutrition Board, Institute of Medicine. *Dietary Reference Intakes for Thiamin, Riboflavin, Niacin, Vitamin B_6, Folate, Vitamin B_{12}, Pantothenic Acid, Biotin, and Choline.* Washington, DC: National Academy Press; 1998.

93. Barr SI, Broughton TM. Relative weight, weight loss efforts and nutrient intakes among health-conscious vegetarian, past vegetarian and nonvegetarian women ages 18 to 50. *J Am Coll Nutr.* 2000;19:781–788.

94. Herbert V. Staging vitamin B_{12} (cobalamin) status in vegetarians. *Am J Clin Nutr.* 1994;59:1213S–1222S.

95. Hokin BD, Butler T. Cyanocobalamin (vitamin B-12) status in Seventh-day Adventist ministers in Australia. *Am J Clin Nutr.* 1999;70:576S–578S.

96. van het Hof KH, Brouwer IA, West CE, Haddeman E, Steegers-Theunissen RP, von Dussledorp M, Weststrate JA, Ekes TK, Hautvast JG. Bioavailability of lutein from vegetables is five times higher than that of beta carotene. *Am J Clin Nutr.* 1999;70: 261–268.

97. Hedren E, Diaz V, Svanberg U. Estimation of carotenoid accessibility from carrots determined by an in vitro digestion method. *Eur J Clin Nutr* 2002;56:425–430.

98. Castenmiller JJ, West CE, Linssen JP, van het Hof KH, Voragen AG. The food matrix of spinach is a limiting factor in determining the bioavailability of beta carotene and to a lesser extent of lutein in humans. *J Nutr.* 1999;129:349–355.

99. Ribaya-Mercado JD. Influence of dietary fat on beta carotene absorption and bioconversion into vitamin A. *Nutr Rev.* 2002; 60:104–110.

100. Conquer JA, Holub BJ. Supplementation with an algae source of docosahexaenoic acid increases (n-3) fatty acid status and alters selected risk factors for heart disease in vegetarian subjects. *J Nutr.* 1996;126:3032–3039.

101. Ågren JJ, Tormala ML, Nenonen MT, Hanninen OO. Fatty acid composition of erythrocyte, platelet, and serum lipids in strict vegans. *Lipids.* 1995;30:365–369.

102. Krajcovicova-Kudlackova M, Simoncic R, Babinska K, Bederova A. Levels of lipid peroxidation and antioxidants in vegetarians. *Eur J Epidemiol.* 1995;11:207–211.

103. Mezzano D, Munoz X, Marinez C, Cuevas A, Panes O, Aranda E, Guasch V, Strobel P, Munoz B, Rodriguez S, Pereira J, Leighton F. Vegetarians and cardiovascular risk factors: Hemostasis, inflammatory markers and plasma homocysteine. *Thromb Haemost.* 1999; 81:913–917.

104. Reddy S, Sanders TA, Obeid O. The influence of maternal vegetarian diet on essential fatty acid status of the newborn. *Eur J Clin Nutr.* 1994;48:358–368.

105. Joint WHO/FAO Expert Consultation on Diet, Nutrition and the Prevention of Chronic Diseases. *Diet, Nutrition and the Prevention of Chronic Diseases.* Draft. Geneva, Switzerland. Jan 28 to Feb 1, 2002. Available at: http://www.who.int/hpr/nutrition/26Aprildraftrev1.pdf. Accessed February 10, 2003.

106. Davis B, Kris-Etherton P. Achieving optimal essential fatty acid status in vegetarians: Current knowledge and practical implications. *Am J Clin Nutr.* In press.

107. Kris-Etherton PM, Taylor DS, Yu-Poth S, Huth P, Moriarty K, Fishell V, Hargrove RL, Zhao G, Etherton TD. Polyunsaturated fatty acids in the food chain in the United States. *Am J Clin Nutr.* 2000; 71:179S–188S.

108. Indu, M and Ghafoorunissa, N-3 fatty acids in Indian diets—comparison of the effects of precursor (alpha-linolenic acid) vs. product (long chain n-3 polyunsaturated fatty acids). *Nutr Res.* 1992;12: 569–582.

109. Masters C. Omega-3 fatty acids and the peroxisome. *Mol Cell Biochem.* 1996;165:83–93.

110. Pereira C, Li D, Sinclair AJ. The alpha-linolenic acid content of green vegetables commonly available in Australia. *Int J Vitam Nutr Res.* 2001; 71:223–228.

111. Burdge GC, Jones AE, Wooton SA. Eicosapentaenoic and docosapentaenoic acids are the principal products of alpha-linolenic acid metabolism in young men. *Br J Nutr.* 2002;88:355–363.

112. Appleby PN, Thorogood M, Mann JI, Key TJ. The Oxford Vegetarian Study: An overview. *Am J Clin Nutr.* 1999;70:525S–531S.

113. Remer T, Neubert A, Manz F. Increased risk of iodine deficiency with vegetarian nutrition. *Br J Nutr.* 1999;81:45–49.

114. Hebbelinck M, Clarys P. Physical growth and development of vegetarian children and adolescents. In: Sabate J, ed. *Vegetarian Nutrition.* Boca Raton, Fl: CRC Press; 2001:173–193.

115. Mangels AR, Messina V. Considerations in planning vegan diets: infants. *J Am Diet Assoc.* 2001;101: 670–677.

116. Sanders TAB, Manning J. The growth and development of vegan children. *J Hum Nutr Diet.* 1992; 5:11–21.

117. Fulton JR, Hutton CW, Stitt KR. Preschool vegetarian children. *J Am Diet Assoc.* 1980;76:360–365.

118. Neumark-Sztainer D, Story M, Resnick MD. Blum RW. Adolescent vegetarians: A behavioural profile of a school-based population in Minnesota. *Arch Pediatr Adolesc Med.* 1997;151:833–838.

119. Sabate J, Linsted KD, Harris RD, Johnston PK. Anthropometric parameters of school children with different life-styles. *Am J Dis Child.* 1990;144: 1159–1163.

120. Ruys J, Hickie JB. Serum cholesterol and triglyceride levels in Australian adolescent vegetarians. *Br Med J.* 1976;2:87.

121. Krajcovicova-Kudlackova M, Simoncic R, Bederova A, Grancicova E, Megalova T. Influence of vegetarian and mixed nutrition on selected

haematological and biochemical parameters in children. *Nahrung.* 1997;41:311–314.

122. O'Connell JM, Dibley MJ, Sierra J, Wallace B, Marks JS, Yip R. Growth of vegetarian children. The Farm study. *Pediatrics.* 1989;84:475–481.

123. Committee on Nutrition, American Academy of Pediatrics. *Pediatric Nutrition Handbook.* 4th ed. Elk Grove Village, IL: AAP; 1998.

124. Allen LH. Zinc and micronutrient supplements for children. *Am J Clin Nutr.* 1998;68(suppl): 495S–498S.

125. Krebs NF. Zinc supplementation during lactation. *Am J Clin Nutr.* 1998;68(suppl):509S–512S.

126. Nathan I, Hackett AF, Kirby S. A longitudinal study of the growth of matched pairs of vegetarian and omnivorous children, aged 7-11 years, in the north-west of England. *Eur J Clin Nutr.* 1997;51: 20–25.

127. van Dusseldorp M, Arts ICW, Bergsma JS, De Jong N, Dagnelie PC, Van Staveren WA. Catch-up growth in children fed a macrobiotic diet in early childhood. *J Nutr.* 1996;126:2977–2983.

128. Nathan I, Hackett AF, Kirby S. The dietary intake of a group of vegetarian children aged 7-11 years compared with matched omnivores. *Br J Nutr.* 1996;75:533–544.

129. Millward DJ. The nutritional value of plant-based diets in relation to human amino acid and protein requirements. *Proc Nutr Soc.* 1999;58:249–260.

130. Mangels AR. Nutrition management of the vegetarian child. In: Nevin-Folino N, ed. *Pediatric Manual of Clinical Dietetics,* 2nd ed. Chicago, IL: American Dietetic Association, 2003.

131. Sabate J, Linsted KD, Harris RD, Sanchez A. Attained height of lacto-ovo-vegetarian children and adolescents. *Eur J Clin Nutr.* 1991;45:51–58.

132. Sanchez A, Kissinger DG, Phillips RI. A hypothesis on the etiological role of diet on age of menarch. *Med Hypotheses.* 1981;7:1339–1345.

133. Kissinger DG, Sanchez A. The association of dietary factors with the age of menarche. *Nutr Res.* 1987;7: 471–479.

134. Barr SI. Women's reproductive function. In: Sabate J, ed. *Vegetarian Nutrition.* Boca Raton, Fl: CRC Press;2001:221–249.

135. Hebbelinck M, Clarys P, De Malsche A. Growth, development, and physical fitness of Flemish vegetarian children, adolescents, and young adults. *Am J Clin Nutr.* 1999;70(suppl):579S–585S.

136. van Lenthe FJ, Kemper HCG, van Mechelen W. Rapid maturation in adolescence results in greater obesity in adulthood: The Amsterdam Growth and Health Study. *Am J Clin Nutr.* 1996;64:18–24.

137. Berkey CS, Frazier AL, Gardner JD, Colditz GA. Adolescence and breast carcinoma risk. *Cancer.* 1999;85:2400–2409.

138. O'Connor AM, Touyz WS, Dunn SM, Beumont PJ. Vegetarianism in anorexia nervosa? A review of 116 consecutive cases. *Med J Aust.* 1987;147: 540–542.

139. Perry CL, McGuire MT, Newmark-Sztainer D, Story M. Characteristics of vegetarian adolescents in a multiethnic urban population. *J Adolesc Health.* 2001;29:406–416.

140. Martins Y, Pliner P, O'Connor R. Restrained eating among vegetarians: Does a vegetarian eating style mask concerns about weight? *Appetite.* 1999;32: 145–154.

141. Barr SI. Vegetarianism and menstrual cycle disturbances: Is there an association? *Am J Clin Nutr.* 1999;70(suppl):549S–554S.

142. Drake R, Reddy S, Davies J. Nutrient intake during pregnancy and pregnancy outcome of lacto-ovo-vegetarians, fish-eaters and non-vegetarians. *Veg Nutr.* 1998;2:45–52.

143. Lakin V, Haggarty P, Abramovich DR. Dietary intake and tissue concentrations of fatty acids in omnivore, vegetarian, and diabetic pregnancy. *Prost Leuk Ess Fatty Acids.* 1998;58:209–220.

144. Sanders TAB, Reddy S. The influence of a vegetarian diet on the fatty acid composition of human milk and the essential fatty acid status of the infant. *J Pediatr.* 1992;120:S71–S77.

145. Hornstra G. Essential fatty acids in mothers and their neonates. *Am J Clin Nutr.* 2000;71(suppl): 1262S–1269S.

146. Marsh AG, Christiansen DK, Sanchez TV, Mickelsen O, Chaffee FL. Nutrient similarities and differences of older lacto-ovo-vegetarian and omnivorous women. *Nutr Rep Int.* 1989;39:19–24.

147. Brants HAM, Lowik MRH, Westenbrink S, Hulshof KFAM, Kistemaker C. Adequacy of a vegetarian diet at old age (Dutch Nutrition Surveillance System). *J Am Coll Nutr.* 1990;9:292–302.

148. Campbell WW, Evans WJ. Protein requirements of elderly people. *Eur J Clin Nutr.* 1996;50 (suppl): S180–S183.

149. American Dietetic Association. Nutrition, aging, and the continuum of care—Position of ADA. *J Am Diet Assoc.* 2000;100:580–595.

150. Larson DE. Vegetarian athletes. In: Rosenbloom CA, ed. *Sports Nutrition. A Guide for the Professional Working with Active People,* 3rd ed. Chicago, IL: American Dietetic Association, Sports, Cardiovascular, and Wellness Dietetic Practice Group; 2000:405–425.

151. Kaiserauer S, Snyder AC, Sleeper M, Zierath J. Nutritional, physiological, and menstrual status of distance runners. *Med Sci Sports Exerc.* 1989;21: 120–125.

152. Slavin J, Lutter J, Cushman S. Amenorrhea in vegetarian athletes. *Lancet.* 1984;1:1974–1975.

153. Key T, Davey G. Prevalence of obesity is low in people who do not eat meat (letter). *Br Med J.* 1996;313:816–817.

154. Key TJ, Fraser GE, Thorogood M, Appleby PN, Beral V, Reeves G, Burr ML, Chang-Claude J, Frentzel-Beyme R, Kuzma JW, Mann J, McPherson K. Mortality in vegetarians and nonvegetarians: Detailed findings from a collaborative analysis of 5 prospective studies. *Am J Clin Nutr.* 1999;70: 516S–524S.

155. Phillips RL, Lemon FR, Beeson L, Kuzma JW. Coronary heart disease mortality among Seventh-Day Adventists with differing dietary habits: A preliminary report. *Am J Clin Nutr.* 1978;31:S191–S198.

156. Resnicow K, Barone J, Engle A, Miller S, Haley NJ, Fleming D, Wynder E. Diet and serum lipids in vegan vegetarians: A model for risk reduction. *J Am Diet Assoc.* 1991;91:447–453.

157. Sacks FM, Castelli WP, Donner A, Kass EH. Plasma lipids and lipoproteins in vegetarians and controls. *N Engl J Med.* 1975;292:1148–1151.

158. Thorogood M, McPherson K, Mann J. Relationship of body mass index, weight, and height to plasma lipid levels in people with different diets in Britain. *Community Med.* 1989;11:230–233.

159. Mosca L, Grundy SM, Judelson D, King K, Limacher M, Oparil S, Pasternak R, Pearson TA, Redberg RF, Smith SC, Winston M, Zinberg S. AHA/ACC Scientific Statement: Consensus Panel Statement: Guide to Preventive Cardiology for Women. *Circulation.* 1999;99:2480–2484.

160. Brown L, Rosner B, Willett WW, Sacks FM. Cholesterol-lowering effects of dietary fiber: A meta-analysis. *Am J Clin Nutr.* 1999;69:30–42.

161. Smit E, Nieto FJ, Crespo CJ. Blood cholesterol and apolipoprotein B levels in relation to intakes of animal and plant proteins in US adults. *Br J Nutr.* 1999;82:193–201.

162. Anderson JW, Johnstone BM, Cook-Newell ME. Meta-analysis of the effects of soy protein intake on serum lipids. *N Engl J Med.* 1995;333:276–282.

163. Wiseman H, O'Reilly JD, Adlercreutz H, Mallet AI, Bowey EA, Rowland IR, Sanders TA. Isoflavone phytoestrogens consumed in soy decrease F(2)-isoprostane concentrations and increase resistance of low-density lipoprotein to oxidation in humans. *Am J Clin Nutr.* 2000;72:395–400.

164. Simons PC, Algra A, Bots ML, Grobbee DE, van der Graaf Y. Common carotid intima-media thickness and arterial stiffness: Indicators of cardiovascular risk in high-risk patients. The SMART Study (Secondary Manifestations of ARTerial disease). *Circulation.* 1999;100:951–957.

165. Dubey RK, Gillespie DG, Imthurn B, Rosselli M, Jackson EK, Keller PJ. Phytoestrogens inhibit growth and MAP kinase activity in human - aortic smooth muscle cells. *Hypertension.* 1999;33:177–182.

166. Chan MM, Ho CT, Huang HI. Effects of three dietary phytochemicals from tea, rosemary, and turmeric on inflammation-induced nitrite production. *Cancer Lett.* 1995;96:23–29.

167. Lin CL, Fang TC, Gueng MK. Vascular dilatory functions of ovo-lacto-vegetarians compared with omnivores. *Atherosclerosis.* 2001;158:247–251.

168. Mann NJ, Li D, Sinclair AJ, Dudman NP, Guo XW, Elsworth GR, Wilson AK, Kelly FD. The effect of diet on plasma homocysteine concentrations in healthy male subjects. *Eur J Clin Nutr.* 1999;53:895–899.

169. Krajcovicova-Kudlackova M, Blazicek P, Kopcova J, Bederova A, Babinska K. Homocysteine levels in vegetarians versus omnivores. *Ann Nutr Metab.* 2000;44:135–138.

170. Hung CJ, Huang PC, Lu SC, Li YH, Huang HB, Lin BF, Chang SJ, Chou HF. Plasma homocysteine levels in Taiwanese vegetarians are higher than those of omnivores. *J Nutr.* 2002;132:152–158.

171. Bissoli L, DiFrancesco V, Ballarin A, Mandragona R, Trespidi R, Brocco G, Caruso B, Bosello O, Zamboni M. Effect of vegetarian diet on homocysteine levels. *Ann Nutr Metab.* 2002;46:73–79.

172. Houghton LA, Green TJ, Donovan UM, Gibson RS, Stephen AM, O'Connor DL. Association between dietary fiber intake and the folate status of a group of female adolescents. *Am J Clin Nutr.* 1997;66: 1414–1421.

173. Mezzano D, Kosiel K, Martinez C, Cuevas A, Panes O, Aranda E, Strobel P, Perez DD, Pereira J, Rozowski J, Leighton F. Cardiovascular risk factors in vegetarians. Normalization of hyperhomocysteinemia with vitamin B(12) and reduction of platelet aggregation with n-3 fatty acids. *Thromb Res.* 2000;100:153–160.

174. Hypertension Detection and Follow-up Program Cooperative Group. Five-year findings of the hypertension detection and follow-up program. I. Reduction in mortality of person with high blood pressure, including mild hypertension. *J Am Med Assoc.* 1979;242:2562–2571.

175. Ophir O, Peer G, Gilad J, Blum M, Aviram A. Low blood pressure in vegetarians: The possible roles of potassium. *Am J Clin Nutr.* 1983;37:755–762.

176. Melby CL, Hyner GC, Zoog B. Blood pressure in vegetarians and non-vegetarians: A cross-sectional analysis. *Nutr Res.* 1985;5:1077–1082.

177. Sciarrone SE, Strahan MT, Beilin LJ, Burke V, Rogers P, Rouse IL. Biochemical and neurohormonal responses to the introduction of a lacto-ovovegetarian diet. *J Hypertens.* 1993;11:849–860.

178. Rouse IL, Beilin LJ, Mahoney DP, Margetts BM, Armstrong BK, Record SJ, Vandongen R, Barden A. Nutrient intake, blood pressure, serum and urinary prostaglandins and serum thromboxane B2 in a controlled trial with a lacto-ovo-vegetarian diet. *J Hypertens.* 1986;4:241–250.

179. Rouse IL, Armstrong BK, Beilin LJ. The relationship of blood pressure to diet and lifestyle in two religious populations. *J Hypertens.* 1983;1:65–71.

180. Prescott SL, Jenner DA, Beilin LJ, Margetts BM, Vandongen R. A randomized controlled trial of the effect on blood pressure of dietary nonmeat protein versus meat protein in normotensive omnivores. *Clin Sci.* 1988;74:665–672.

181. Brussard JH, Van Raaij JM, Stasse-Wolthuis M, Katan MB, Hautvast JG. Blood pressure and diet in normotensive volunteers: Absence of an effect of dietary fiber, protein, or fat. *Am J Clin Nutr.* 1981;34:2023–2029.

182. Sacks FM, Rouse IL, Stampfer MJ, Bishop LM, Lenherr CF, Walther RJ. Effect of dietary fats and carbohydrate on blood pressure of mildly hypertensive patients. *Hypertension.* 1987;10:452–460.

183. Margetts BM, Beilin LJ, Vandongen R, Armstrong BK. A randomized controlled trial of the effect of dietary fiber on blood pressure. *Clin Sci.* 1987;72:343–350.

184. Rouse IL, Beilin LJ, Armstrong BK, Vandongen R. Blood pressure lowering effect of a vegetarian diet: Controlled trial in normotensive subjects. *Lancet.* 1983;1:5–10.

185. Landsberg L, Young JB. The role of the sympathetic nervous system and catecholamines in the regulation of energy metabolism. *Am J Clin Nutr.* 1983;38:1018–1024.

186. Sacks FM, Kass EH. Low blood pressure in vegetarians: Effects of specific foods and nutrients. *Am J Clin Nutr.* 1988;48:795–800.

187. American Diabetes Association Position Statement: Evidence-based nutrition principles and recommendations for the treatment and prevention of diabetes and related complications. *J Am Diet Assoc.* 2002;102:109–118.

188. Snowdon DA, Phillips RL. Does a vegetarian diet reduce the occurrence of diabetes? *Am J Public Health.* 1985;75:507–512.

189. Lipkin M, Uehara K, Winawer S, Sanchez A, Bauer C, Phillips R, Lynch HT, Blattner WA, Fraumeni JF Jr. Seventh-day Adventist vegetarians have a quiescent proliferative activity in colonic mucosa. *Cancer Lett.* 1985;26:139–144.

190. Allen NE, Appleby PN, Davey GK, Key TJ. Hormones and diet: Low insulin-like growth factor-I but normal bioavailable androgens in vegan men. *Br J Cancer.* 2000;83:95–97.

191. Giovannucci E, Rimm EB, Wolk A, Ascherio A, Stampfer MJ, Colditz GA, Willett WC. Calcium and fructose intake in relation to risk of prostate cancer. *Cancer Res.* 1998;58:442–447.

192. Chan JM, Giovannucci E, Andersson SO, Yuen J, Adami HO, Wolk A. Dairy products, calcium, phosphorus, vitamin D, and risk of prostate cancer. *Cancer Causes Control.* 1998;9:559–566.

193. Chan JM, Stampfer MJ, Ma J, Gann PH, Garziano JM, Giovannucci EL. Dairy products, calcium, and prostate cancer risk in the Physician's Health Study. *Am J Clin Nutr.* 2001;74:549–554.

194. Tavani A, Gallus S, Franceschi S, La Vecchia C. Calcium, dairy products, and the risk of prostate cancer. *Prostate.* 2001;48:118–121.

195. Missmer SA, Smith-Warner SA, Spiegelman D, Yaun SS, Adami HO, Beeson WL, van der Brandt PA, Fraser GE, Frendenheim JL, Goldbohm RA, Graham S, Kushi LH, Miller AB, Potter JD, Rohan TE, Speizer FE, Toniolo P, Willet WC, Wolk A, Zeleniuch-Jacquotte A, Hunter DJ. Meat and dairy food consumption and breast cancer: a pooled analysis of cohort studies. *Int J Epidemiol.* 2002;31:78–85.

196. Butrum RR, Clifford CK, Lanza E. National Cancer Institute dietary guidelines: rationale. *Am J Clin Nutr.* 1988;48:888–895.

197. Barbosa JC, Shultz TD, Filley SJ, Nieman DC. The relationship among adiposity, diet, and hormone concentrations in vegetarian and nonvegetarian postmenopausal women. *Am J Clin Nutr.* 1990;51:798–803.

198. Howe GR, Benito E, Castellato R, Cornee J, Esteve J, Gallagher RP, Iscovich JM, Deng-ao J, Kaaks R, Kune GA. Dietary intake of fiber and decreased risk of cancers of the colon and rectum: evidence from the combined analysis of 13 case-control studies. *J Nat Canc Inst.* 1992;84:1887–1896.

199. Alberts DS, Martinez ME, Roe DJ, Guillen-Rodriguez JM, Marshall JR, van Leeuwen JB, Reid ME, Ritenbaugh C, Vargas PA, Bhattacharyya

AB, Earnest DL, Sampliner RE. Lack of effect of a high-fiber cereal supplement on the recurrence of colorectal adenomas. Phoenix Colon Cancer Prevention Physicians' Network. *N Engl J Med.* 2000; 342:1156–1162.

200. van Faassen A, Hazen JM, van den Brandt PA, van den Bogaard AE, Hermus RJ, Janknegt RA. Bile acids and pH values in total feces and in fecal water from habitually omnivorous and vegetarian subjects. *Am J Clin Nutr.* 1993;58:917–922.

201. Finegold SM, Sutter VL, Sugihara PT, Elder HA, Lehmann SM, Phillips RL. Fecal microbial flora in Seventh Day Adventist populations and control subjects. *Am J Clin Nutr.* 1977;30:1781–1792.

202. Davies GJ, Crowder M, Reid B, Dickerson JW. Bowel function measurements of individuals with different eating patterns. *Gut.* 1986;27:164–169.

203. Nader CJ, Potter JD, Weller RA. Diet and DNA-modifying activity in human fecal extracts. *Nutr Rep Int.* 1981;23:113–117.

204. Sesink AL, Termont DS, Kleibeuker JH, van der Meer R. Red meat and colon cancer: The cytotoxic and hyperproliferative effects of dietary heme. *Cancer Res.* 1999;59:5704–5709.

205. Griffiths K. Estrogens and prostatic disease. International Prostate Health Council Study Group. *Prostate.* 2000;45:87–100.

206. Messina MJ, Loprinzi CL. Soy for breast cancer survivors: A critical review of the literature. *J Nutr.* 2001;131:3095S–3108S.

207. Linkswiler HM, Zemel MB, Hegsted M, Schuette S. Protein induced hypercalciuria. *Fred Proc.* 1981;40:2429–2433.

208. Kerstetter JE, Allen LH. Dietary protein increases urinary calcium. *J Nutr.* 1990;120:134–136.

209. Itoh R, Nishiyama N, Suyama Y. Dietary protein intake and urinary excretion of calcium: A cross-sectional study in a healthy Japanese population. *Am J Clin Nutr.* 1998;67:438–444.

210. Kunkel ME, Beauchene RE. Protein intake and urinary excretion of protein-derived metabolites in aging female vegetarians and nonvegetarians. *J Am Coll Nutr.* 1991;10:308–314.

211. Sellmeyer DE, Stone KL, Sebastian A, Cummings SR. A high ratio of dietary animal to vegetable protein increases the rate of bone loss and the risk of fracture in postmenopausal women. *Am J Clin Nutr.* 2001;73:118–122.

212. Kerstetter JE, Svastisalee CM, Caseria DM, Mitnick ME, Insogna KL. A threshold for low-protein diet-induced elevations in parathyroid hormone. *Am J Clin Nutr.* 2000;72:168–173.

213. Marsh AG, Sanchez TV, Michelsen O, Chaffee FL, Fagal SM. Vegetarian lifestyle and bone mineral density. *Am J Clin Nutr.* 1988;48:837–841.

214. Chiu JF, Lan SJ, Yang CY, Wang PW, Yao WJ, Su LH, Hsieh CC. Long term vegetarian diet and bone mineral density in postmenopausal Taiwanese women. *Calcif Tissue Int.* 1997;60:245–249.

215. Hu JF, Zhao XH, Jia JB, Parpia B, Campbell TC. Dietary calcium and bone density among middle aged and elderly women in China. *Am J Clin Nutr.* 1993;58:219–227.

216. Outila TA, Karkkainen MU, Seppanen RH, Lamberg-Allardt CJ. Dietary intake of vitamin D in premenopausal, healthy vegans was insufficient to maintain concentrations of serum 25-hydroxyvitamin D and intact parathyroid hormone within normal ranges during the winter in Finland. *J Am Diet Assoc.* 2000;100:434–441.

217. Outila TA, Lamberg-Allardt CJ. Ergocalciferol supplementation may positively affect lumbar spine bone mineral density of vegans (letter). *J Am Diet Assoc.* 2000;100:629.

218. Lamberg-Allardt C, Karkkainen M, Seppanen R, Bistrom H. Low serum 25-hydroxyvitamin D concentrations and secondary hyperparathyroidism in middle-aged white strict vegetarians. *Am J Clin Nutr.* 1993;58:684–689.

219. Arjmandi BH, Smith BJ. Soy isoflavones' osteo-protective role in postmenopausal women: Mechanism of action. *J Nutr Biochem.* 2002;13:130–137.

220. Bosch JP, Saccaggi A, Lauer A, Ronco C, Belledonne M, Glabman S. Renal functional reserve in humans. Effect of protein intake on glomerular filtration rate. *Am J Med.* 1983;75:943–950.

221. Wiseman MJ, Hunt R, Goodwin A, Gross JL, Keen H, Viberti GC. Dietary composition and renal function in healthy subjects. *Nephron.* 1987;46:37–42.

222. Kontessis P, Jones S, Dodds R, Trevisan R, Nosadini R, Fioretto P, Borsato M, Sacerdoti D, Viberti G. Renal, metabolic and hormonal responses to ingestion of animal and vegetable proteins. *Kidney Int.* 1990;38:136–144.

223. Kontessis PA, Bossinakou I, Sarika L, Iliopoulou E, Papantoniou A, Trevisan R, Roussi D, Stipsanelli K, Grigorakis S, Souvatzoglou A. Renal, metabolic, and hormonal responses to proteins of different origin in normotensive, nonproteinuric type 1 diabetic patients. *Diabetes Care.* 1995;18:1233.

224. Geim P, Beeson WL, Fraser GE. The incidence of dementia and intake of animal products: Preliminary findings from the Adventist Health Study. *Neuroepidemiology.* 1993;12:28–36.

225. Riedel WJ, Jorissen BL. Nutrients, age and cognitive function. *Curr Opin Clin Nutr Metab Care.* 1998;1:579–585.

226. Olson DA. Association of vitamin E and C supplement use with cognitive function and dementia in elderly men. *Neurology.* 2000;55:901–902.

227. Ross GW, Petrovitch H, White LR, Masaki KH, Li CY, Curb JD, Yano K, Rodriguez BL, Foley DJ, Blanchette PL, Havlik R. Characterization of risk factors for vascular dementia: The Honolulu-Asia Aging Study. *Neurology.* 1999;53:337–343.

228. Wolozin B, Kellman W, Ruosseau P, Celesia GG, Siegel G. Decreased prevalence of Alzheimer's Disease associated with 3-hydrozy-3-methylglutaryl coenzyme A reductase inhibitors. *Arch Neurol.* 2000;57:1439–1443.

229. Snowdon DA, Tully CL, Smith CD, Riley KP, Markesbery WR. Serum folate and the severity of atrophy of the neocortex in Alzheimer's disease: Findings from the Nun Study. *Am J Clin Nutr.* 2000;71:993–998.

230. Nourhashemi F, Gillette-Guyonnet S, Andrieu S, Ghisolfi A, Ousset PJ, Grandjean H, Grand A, Pous J, Vellas B, Albarede JL. Alzheimer's Disease: Protective factors. *Am J Clin Nutr.* 2000;71:643S–649S.

231. Nilsson K, Gustafson L, Hultberg B. The plasma homocysteine concentration is better than that of serum methylmalonic acid as a marker for sociopsychological performance in a psychogeriatric population. *Clin Chem.* 2000;46:691–696.

232. Delport R. Hyperhomocyst(e)inemia: Related vitamins and dementias. *J Nutr Health Aging.* 2000;4:195–196.

233. White LR, Petrovitch H, Ross GW, Masaki K, Hardman J, Nelson J, Davis D, Markesbery W. Brain aging and midlife tofu consumption. *J Am Coll Nutr.* 2000;19:242–255.

234. Rice MM, Graves AB, McCurry SM, Gibbons L, Bowen J, McCormick W, Larson EB. Tofu consumption and cognition in older Japanese American men and women. *J Nutr.* 2000;130(suppl 3):676S.

235. Gear JS, Ware A, Fursdon P, Mann JI, Nolan DJ, Broadribb AJ, Vessey MP. Symptomless diverticular disease and intake of dietary fibre. *Lancet.* 1979;1:511–514.

236. Aldoori WH, Giovannucci EL, Rimm EB, Wing AL, Trichopoulos DV, Willett WC, A prospective study of diet and the risk of symptomatic diverticular disease in men. *Am J Clin Nutr.* 1994;60:757–764.

237. Heaton KW. Diet and diverticulosis: New leads (editorial). *Gut.* 1985;26:541–543.

238. Pixley F, Wilson D, McPherson K, Mann J. Effect of vegetarianism on development of gall stones in women. *Br Med J (Clin Res Ed).* 1985;291:11–12.

239. Kjeldsen-Kragh J. Rheumatoid arthritis treated with vegetarian diets. *Am J Clin Nutr.* 1999;70:594S–600S.

240. Muller H, de Toledo FW, Resch KL. Fasting followed by vegetarian diet in patients with rheumatoid arthritis: A systematic review. *Scand J Rheumatol.* 2001;30:1–10.

241. Donaldson MS, Speight N, Loomis S. Fibromyalgia syndrome improved using a mostly raw vegetarian diet: An Observational study. *BMC Complement Altern Med.* 2001;1:7.

242. Tanaka T, Kouda K, Kotani M, Takeuchi A, Tabei T, Masamoto Y, Nakamura H, Takigawa M, Suemura M, Takeuchi H, Kouda M. Vegetarian diet ameliorates symptoms of atopic dermatitis through reduction of the number of peripheral eosinophisl and of PGE2 synthesis by monocytes. *J Physiol Anthropol Appl Human Sci.* 2001;20:353–361.

243. Special Supplemental Nutrition Program for Women, Infants and Children (1–1–02 edition). Federal Register, Code of Federal Regulations, 7CFR, Part 246; 2002.

244. Canada Prenatal Nutrition Program. Projects directory online. Available at: www.ssjs.hc-sc.gc.ca/cpnp. Accessed February 10, 2003.

245. Modification of the "Vegetable Protein Products" requirements for the National School Lunch Program, School Breakfast Program, Summer Food Service Program and Child And Adult Care Food Program. (7 CFR 210, 215, 220, 225, 226) Federal Register. March 9, 2000;65:12429–12442.

246. US Department of Agriculutre. Menu planning in the National School Lunch Program. Available at: http://www.fns.usda.gov/cnd/MenuPlanning/menu.planning.approaches.for.lunch es.doc. Accessed February 10, 2003.

247. US Department of Agriculture. A Toolkit for Healthy School Meals: Recipes and Training Materials. Available at: http://www.nal.usda.gov/fnic/schoolmeals/Training/train.html. Accessed February 10, 2003.

248. Canadian Living Foundation. Breakfast for learning. Available at: www.breakfastforlearning.ca. Accessed February 10, 2003.

249. Administration on Aging. The Elderly Nutrition Program. Available at: http://www.aoa.gov/factsheets/enp.html. Accessed February 10, 2003.

250. The Vegetarian Resource Group. 4-week Vegetarian Menu Set for Meals on Wheels Sites. Available at: http://www.vrg.org/fsupdate/fsu974/fsu974menu.htm. Accessed February 10, 2003.

251. Havala S, Abate T. The National Meals on Wheels Foundation Vegetarian Initiative: A unique collaboration. *J Nutr Elderly.* 1997;17:45–50.

252. Docket T-1487-99, September 29, 2000 and January 21, 2002, between Jack Maurice and Attorney General of Canada, Federal Court of Canada Trial Division.

253. Ogden A, Rebein P. Do Prison Inmates Have a Right to Vegetarian Meals? Vegetarian Journal Mar/Apr 2001. Available at: http://www.vrg.org/journal/vj2001mar/2001marprison.htm. Accessed February 10, 2003.

254. US Department of Defense. DOD Combat Feeding Program. Available at: http://www.sbccom.army.mil/programs/food/. Accessed February 10, 2003.

255. Department of National Defence. *Food Services Direction & Guidance Manual,* Chapter 2. Ottawa, ON, Canada; 2003.

256. Canadian Forces Food Services. Maple Leaf. 2000; Volume 3, Issue 39, page 14–15 and Issue 37, pages 14–15. Available at: www.forces.gc.ca/site/community/mapleleaf/html_files/html_view_e.asp. Accessed February 10, 2003.

ADA Position adopted by the House of Delegates on October 18, 1987, and reaffirmed on September 12, 1992, September 6, 1996 and June 22, 2000. This position was developed collaboratively between the American Dietetic Association and Dietitians of Canada. This position will be in effect until December 31, 2007. ADA authorizes republication of the position statement/support paper, in its entirety, provided full and proper credit is given. Requests to use portions of the position must be directed to ADA Headquarters at 800/877-1600, ext 4835, or ppapers@eatright.org Recognition is given to the following for their contributions:

Authors:

Ann Reed Mangels, PhD, RD, FADA (The Vegetarian Resource Group, Baltimore, MD);
Virginia Messina, MPH, RD (Nutrition Matters, Inc., Port Townsend, WA);
Vesanto Melina, MS, RD (NUTRISPEAK.COM, Langley, BC, Canada).

American Dietetic Association Reviewers:

Judith G. Dausch, PhD, RD (American Dietetic Association Government Relations, Washington, DC);
Sharon Denny, MS, RD (American Dietetic Association Knowledge Center, Chicago, IL);
Elaine K. Fleming, MPH, RD (Loma Linda University, Loma Linda, CA);
Food and Culinary Professionals DPG (Robin Kline, MS, RD, CCP, Savvy Food Communications, Des Moines, IA; Sylvia E. Klinger, MS, RD, Hispanic Food Communications, La Grange, IL);
D. Enette Larson-Meyer, PhD, RD (Pennington Biomedical Research Center, Baton Rouge, LA);
Nutrition in Complementary Care DPG (Dennis Gordon, MEd, RD, Saint Joseph Mercy Health System, Ann Arbor, MI; Rita Batheja, MS, RD, Private Practice, Long Island, NY);
Pediatric Nutrition DPG (Maria Hanna, MS, RD, Children's Hospital of Philadelphia, Philadelphia, PA; Cristine M. Trahms, MS, RD, FADA, University of Washington, Seattle, WA; Tamara Schryver, MS, RD, University of Minnesota, St. Paul, MN);
Sports, Cardiovascular, and Wellness Nutritionist DPG (Gita B. Patel, MS, RD, Alice Peck Day Memorial Hospital, Lebanon, NH; Pamela J. Edwards, MS, RD, University of Nebraska Lincoln, Lincoln, NE);
Vegetarian Nutrition DPG (Winston J. Craig, PhD, RD, Andrews University, Berrien Springs, MI; Catherine Conway, MS, RD, Private Practice, New York, NY);
Women and Reproductive Nutrition DPG (Judith B. Roepke, PhD, RD, Ball State University, Muncie, IN).

Dietitians of Canada Reviewers:

Karen Birkenhead, RD, (Group Health Centre, Sault Ste Marie, ON);
Samara Felesky Hunt (Consulting Dietitian, Calgary AB);
Susie Langley MS, RD (Nutrition Consultant in Private Practice, Toronto, ON);
Pam Lynch, MHE, RD (Nutrition Counselling Services, Halifax, NS);
Shefali Raja (Vancouver Coastal Health Authority, Vancouver BC);
Marilyn Rabin PDt (Douglas Hospital, Verdun, PQ);
Laura Toews, RD (St. Boniface General Hospital, Winnipeg, MB).

Members of the Association Positions Committee Workgroup:

Barbara Emison Gaffield, MS, RD (chair), Barbara Baron, MS, RD; Suzanne Havala Hobbs, DrPH, RD, FADA (content advisor).

A NEW FOOD GUIDE FOR NORTH AMERICAN VEGETARIANS

Virginia Messina, MPH, RD; Vesanto Melina, MS, RD; Ann Reed Mangels, PhD, RD, FADA

The first North American food guide was published by the US Department of Agriculture

(USDA) in 1916. It was not until the 1940s, however, when wartime shortages, indications of malnutrition among citizens, and the release of the first recommended dietary allowances focused greater attention on nutrient requirements, that food guides became a familiar meal-planning tool in the United States (1). The Canadian government released its first food guide at this time, in 1942 (2). Until 1992, when the USDA's Food Guide Pyramid (3) and Canada's Food Guide to Healthy Eating (CFGHE) (2) with its rainbow design were introduced, the emphasis of food guides was largely placed on meeting nutrient needs.

The 1992 guides were the first to consider the harmful effects of overnutrition. They were also the first guides to visually emphasize the importance of plant foods in the diet. However, they did not include sufficient guidelines for planning vegetarian diets. USDA publications noted that vegetarians needed special guidance in planning healthful diets, implying that the USDA's food guide was not appropriate for vegetarians (4).

Over the past several decades, a number of meal-planning tools have been developed specifically for vegetarians (5,6). The majority of these have used the pyramid format or the rainbow design, and many have been revised versions of the USDA's Food Guide Pyramid and CFGHE. However, because vegetarian diets differ in many ways from nonvegetarian diets, the USDA Food Guide Pyramid and CFGHE are not necessarily the most useful starting point when considering guidelines for vegetarians. It is particularly difficult to manipulate these tools when attempting to provide adequate and practical guidelines for vegans (vegans are vegetarians who exclude all animal products).

In designing a new food guide for vegetarians, we aimed to achieve the following goals:

- To establish a guide that would meet the needs of people following different types of vegetarian diets;

- To help vegetarians choose diets that would meet the most recent recommendations established by the Institute of Medicine;

TIPS FOR MEAL PLANNING

1. Choose a variety of foods.
2. The number of servings in each group is for minimum daily intakes. Choose more foods from any of the groups to meet energy needs.
3. A serving from the calcium-rich food group provides approximately 10% of adult daily requirements. Choose 8 or more servings per day. These also count towards servings from the other food groups in the guide. For example, 1/2 cup (125 mL) of fortified fruit juice counts as a calcium-rich food and also counts towards servings from the fruit group.
4. Include 2 servings every day of foods that supply n-3 fats. Foods rich in n-3 fat are found in the legumes/nuts group and in the fats group. A serving is 1 teaspoon (5 mL) of flaxseed oil, 3 teaspoons (15 mL) of canola or soybean oil, 1 tablespoon (15 mL) of ground flaxseed, or 1/4 cup (60 mL) walnuts. For the best balance of fats in your diet, olive and canola oils are the best choices for cooking.
5. Servings of nuts and seeds may be used in place of servings from the fats group.
6. Be sure to get adequate vitamin D from daily sun exposure or through fortified foods or supplements. Cow's milk and some brands of soymilk and breakfast cereals are fortified with vitamin D.
7. Include at least 3 good food sources of vitamin B-12 in your diet every day. These include 1 Tbsp (15 mL) of *Red Star* Vegetarian Support Formula nutritional yeast, 1 cup (250 mL) fortified soymilk, 1/2 cup (125 mL) cow's milk, 3/4 cup (185 mL) yogurt, 1 large egg, 1 ounce (28 g) of fortified breakfast cereal, 1-1/2 oz (42g) of fortified meat analog. If you don't eat these foods regularly (at least 3 servings per day), take a daily vitamin B-12 supplement of 5 to 10 µg or a weekly B-12 supplement of 2000 µg.
8. If you include sweets or alcohol in your diet, consume these foods in moderation. Get most of your daily calories from the foods in the Vegetarian Food Guide.

- To include guidelines that focus on specific nutrients of particular interest in vegetarian diets, as discussed in the American Dietetic Association (ADA) and Dietitians of Canada's joint

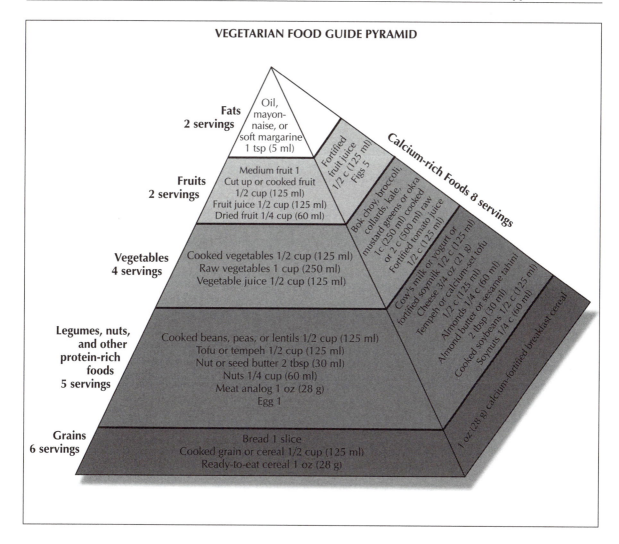

VEGETARIAN FOOD GUIDE PYRAMID

Fats 2 servings — Oil, mayonnaise, or soft margarine 1 tsp (5 ml)

Fruits 2 servings — Medium fruit 1 / Cut up or cooked fruit 1/2 cup (125 ml) / Fruit juice 1/2 cup (125 ml) / Dried fruit 1/4 cup (60 ml)

Vegetables 4 servings — Cooked vegetables 1/2 cup (125 ml) / Raw vegetables 1 cup (250 ml) / Vegetable juice 1/2 cup (125 ml)

Legumes, nuts, and other protein-rich foods 5 servings — Cooked beans, peas, or lentils 1/2 cup (125 ml) / Tofu or tempeh 1/2 cup (125 ml) / Nut or seed butter 2 tbsp (30 ml) / Nuts 1/4 cup (60 ml) / Meat analog 1 oz (28 g) / Egg 1

Grains 6 servings — Bread 1 slice / Cooked grain or cereal 1/2 cup (125 ml) / Ready-to-eat cereal 1 oz (28 g)

Calcium-rich Foods 8 servings — Fortified fruit juice 1/2 c (125 ml) / Figs 5 / Bok choy, broccoli, collards, kale, mustard greens or okra 1c (250 ml) cooked or 2 c (500 ml) raw / Fortified tomato juice 1/2 c (125 ml) / Cow's milk or yogurt or fortified soymilk 1/2 c (125 ml) / Cheese 3/4 oz (21 g) / Tempeh or calcium-set tofu 1/2 c (125 ml) / Almonds 1/4 c (60 ml) / Almond butter or sesame tahini 2 tbsp (30 ml) / Cooked soybeans 1/2 c (125 ml) / Soynuts 1/4 c (60 ml) / 1 oz (28 g) calcium-fortified breakfast cereal

position on vegetarian diets in this issue of the *Journal of the American Dietetic Association* (7,8);

- To include a wide variety of foods that are consumed by vegetarians; and
- To increase awareness about the availability of calcium from nondairy foods.

In addition, we strived to meet the challenge spelled out in the 1981 issue of the *Journal of Nutrition Education* by then US Food and Drug Administration (FDA) nutritionist Jean Pennington for an "instrument which converts the professional's scien-tific knowledge of food composition and nutrient requirements for health into a practical plan for food selection by those without training in nutrition" (9).

Challenges in designing such a guide exist regardless of dietary pattern. Individual food preferences, habits, and choices within food groups will all impact diet quality. Although no food guide is completely reliable, a food guide can maximize the chances that consumers will choose healthful diets. The inclusion of "Eight Tips for Meal Planning" [previous page] provides additional help to vegetarians in planning healthful diets.

Food Groups

The food guide principle that has been in use in North America since 1916 is based on an approach that classifies foods into groups based on similar nutrient content. We have adhered to this principle, with some modification. In the vegetarian food guide, calcium needs are met through choices from several food groups.

In keeping with familiar and widely used approaches to food guide presentation in North America, we have designed our guide in the forms of both a pyramid and a rainbow; the latter is the graphic used in Canada. Both guides use the same food groupings, specify the same number of servings, and can be used interchangeably.

Foods are grouped as follows:

Grains At the base of the pyramid and in the widest arc of the rainbow, these foods form the foundation of the diet. Grains provide energy, complex carbohydrates, fiber, iron, and B-vitamins. Whole grains are an important source of zinc and other minerals. Vegetarians should choose whole grains often, but enriched refined grains can play a role in vegetarian diets and may be especially valuable for children.

Vegetables and fruits Vegetables have been grouped separately from fruits to encourage vege-

tarians to choose a variety of both types of food rather than to focus on one or the other for most choices. A higher number of servings of vegetables is specified because of the greater nutrient density and phytochemical content of vegetables compared with fruits.

Legumes, nuts, and other protein-rich foods This group includes foods that are good sources of protein, B-vitamins, and many trace minerals. It includes all legumes, including soy products such as soy milk and tofu, as well as nuts, seeds, nut and seed butters, eggs, and meat analogs. In a departure from most existing food guides, we have placed dairy foods in this group as well. This groups dairy products with other foods that offer similar amounts of protein per serving. It makes dairy an available but optional choice for vegetarians, while ensuring that protein needs will be met whether or not dairy foods are included in the diet. Categorizing dairy foods with other protein sources also meets the goal of emphasizing the availability of calcium from all of the food groups. Most of the foods in this group provide iron, which is well absorbed when a source of vitamin C is consumed with the meal (10). Dairy foods are the exception here, and those vegetarians who consume frequent servings of dairy foods should be advised to ensure that they are including adequate sources of iron in their meals.

Fats Vegetarians and others who do not eat fish require small amounts of plant sources of n-3 fats. In addition, research suggests that moderate intake of certain healthful plant fats may reduce risk for cardiovascular disease (11), may improve nutrient intake (12), and may even aid in weight control (12). Ideally, most of the fat in vegetarian diets should come from fat-rich whole plant foods such as nuts, seeds, and avocado. To ensure an optimal fat intake and to support a practical approach to meal planning, we have specified a minimum of two servings of fats per day. Figure 1 indicates that nuts or seeds may be used in place of these fats and also directs vegetarians toward choosing the most healthful fats.

Calcium-rich foods Adults should choose a minimum of eight servings of calcium-rich foods daily. Each serving also counts toward choices from one of the other food groups in the guide. For example, 1 cup of certain cooked leafy green vegetables counts as a serving from the calcium-rich foods group and as 2 servings from the vegetable group.

MODIFICATIONS TO THE VEGETARIAN FOOD GUIDE FOR CHILDREN, ADOLESCENTS, AND PREGNANT AND LACTATING WOMEN

| Life cycle | Food group[a] | | |
	B-12-rich foods (servings)	Beans/nuts/ seeds/egg (servings)	Calcium-rich foods (servings)
Child[b]	2	5	6
Adolescent[c]	2	6	10
Adolescent[d]	3	6	10
Pregnancy	4	7	8
Lactation	4	8	8

[a]The number of servings in each group is the minimum amount needed. The minimum number of servings from other groups is not different from the vegetarian food guide. Additional foods can be chosen from any of the groups in the vegetarian food guide to meet energy needs.
[b]4 to 8 years.
[c]9 to 13 years.
[d]14 to 18 years.

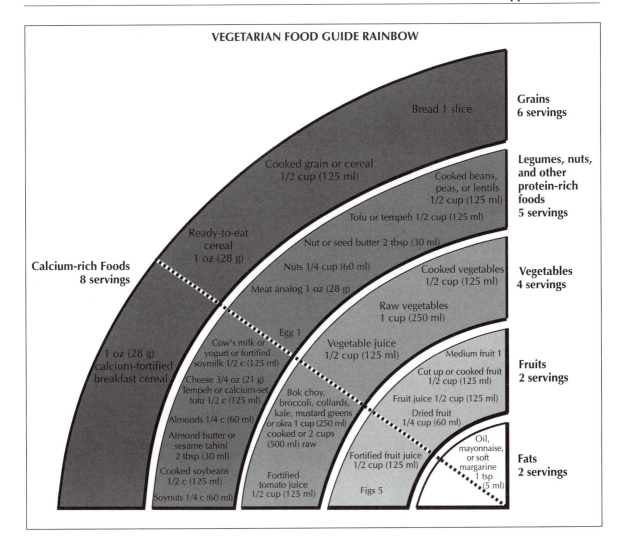

VEGETARIAN FOOD GUIDE RAINBOW

**Grains
6 servings**

Bread 1 slice

Cooked grain or cereal
1/2 cup (125 ml)

Ready-to-eat
cereal
1 oz (28 g)

**Legumes, nuts,
and other
protein-rich
foods
5 servings**

Cooked beans,
peas, or lentils
1/2 cup (125 ml)

Tofu or tempeh 1/2 cup (125 ml)

Nut or seed butter 2 tbsp (30 ml)

Nuts 1/4 cup (60 ml)

Meat analog 1 oz (28 g)

**Calcium-rich Foods
8 servings**

Cooked vegetables
1/2 cup (125 ml)

**Vegetables
4 servings**

Raw vegetables
1 cup (250 ml)

Egg 1

1 oz (28 g)
calcium-fortified
breakfast cereal

Cow's milk or
yogurt or fortified
soymilk 1/2 c (125 ml)

Cheese 3/4 oz (21 g)
Tempeh or calcium-set
tofu 1/2 c (125 ml)

Almonds 1/4 c (60 ml)

Almond butter or
sesame tahini
2 tbsp (30 ml)

Cooked soybeans
1/2 c (125 ml)

Soynuts 1/4 c (60 ml)

Bok choy,
broccoli, collards,
kale, mustard greens
or okra 1 cup (250 ml)
cooked or 2 cups
(500 ml) raw

Fortified
tomato juice
1/2 cup (125 ml)

Vegetable juice
1/2 cup (125 ml)

Fortified fruit juice
1/2 cup (125 ml)

Figs 5

Medium fruit 1

Cut up or cooked fruit
1/2 cup (125 ml)

Fruit juice 1/2 cup (125 ml)

Dried fruit
1/4 cup (60 ml)

**Fruits
2 servings**

Oil,
mayonnaise,
or soft
margarine
1 tsp
(5 ml)

**Fats
2 servings**

Placement of the calcium food group adjacent to each of the other food groups allows this concept to be presented in a clear visual way. It also emphasizes the fact that calcium needs are met by choosing a variety of foods from across the food groups.

Diets based on the minimum specified servings from each of the food groups provide approximately 1,400 to 1,500 calories per day, which may be an inadequate energy intake for many vegetarians. Because the numbers of servings in the food guide are minimum recommendations, consumers can meet higher energy needs by choosing more servings from any of the food groups. Regardless of energy needs, most food choices should come from

these groups, with only moderate servings of sweets and alcohol at most.

Expanded Choices for Meeting Calcium Needs

Survey data suggest that vegans account for as much as 40% of the actual vegetarian population (13). Actual vegetarians are those who never eat meat, in contrast to self-described vegetarians, many of whom actually eat some type of animal flesh regularly. Therefore, any guide aimed at vegetarians must consider the needs of vegans. Studies also indicate that a substantial percentage of vegan women as well as some lacto-ovo-vegetarian women (lacto-ovo-vegetarians are those vegetarians who use dairy products and eggs) have calcium intakes that are too low, which suggests that calcium deserves special attention in vegetarian food guides (14). With few exceptions, vegetarian food guides have not provided appropriate guidelines for vegans. A number of guides have included an optional dairy group, which presents the risk that consumers will choose diets that are deficient in both calcium and protein. Other guides have included a dairy group that also includes fortified soy milk. However, not all vegans choose to consume soy milk daily. Those who do may not wish to consume the two to three recommended servings. For many families, the expense of soy milk compared with cow's milk makes it an unrealistic choice as the primary source of calcium in the diet.

This food guide illustrates acceptable choices in addition to dairy foods and fortified soy milk for meeting calcium needs. It incorporates the principles of variety and moderation and encourages consumers to consider more plant foods as sources of nutrients. This is in keeping with government recommendations. Although this food guide does not emphasize the value of one calcium source over another, there may be an advantage to including more plant sources of calcium in diets because research suggests that other compounds in plant foods, such as isoflavones in soy foods (15) and potassium (16) and vitamin K (17) in fruits and vegetables, may favorably impact bone health.

By including foods that provide approximately 10% to 15% (100 to 150 mg) per serving of the adult adequate intake for calcium, we have allowed consumers to meet calcium needs using a variety of foods in realistic serving sizes. Although the serving size of one-half cup for milk differs from many other food guides, it is consistent with common serving sizes on many food labels, such as on puddings or for use with breakfast cereals.

It should be noted that this approach of emphasizing the variety of calcium-rich foods in different food groups is not specific to the needs of vegetarians but could be adopted for those who consume nonvegetarian diets as well. The advantages of this approach are relevant for all consumers regardless of diet choices.

Special Considerations for Vegetarians

Unsupplemented vegan diets do not provide vitamin B-12. Dairy products and eggs supply vitamin B-12; however, depending on food choices, some lacto-ovo-vegetarians may have inadequate intakes as well. The Institute of Medicine has recommended that all people over the age of 50, regardless of type of diet, take vitamin B-12 in the form found in supplements and fortified foods for optimal absorption (18). Vitamin B-12 is well absorbed from fortified nondairy milks and from breakfast cereals, as well as from supplements. Because vitamin B-12 absorption is inversely related to dosage, we have recommended a daily supplement of at least 5 μg or a weekly supplement of 2,000 μg.

In addition to regular supplementation with vitamin B-12, vegans require a dietary source of vitamin D when sun exposure is insufficient. This occurs at northern latitudes and in certain other situations. Many fortified nondairy milks and breakfast cereals provide vitamin D, although the form used to fortify cereals is often not vegan. Vegetarians may also choose vitamin D supplements.

The vegetarian food guide is based on the nutrient needs of adults. It can be modified to meet the needs of people at different stages of the life cycle. The Table shows modifications in food group servings for different age groups.

Summary

In summary, this vegetarian food guide has a number of advantages over previous guides designed for this population:

- It is based on current nutritional science. This guide aims to provide sufficient nutrient intake based on the most recent dietary reference intakes and addresses concerns such as balance of fats in diets.

- It provides information about how to meet calcium needs that is appropriate to a wide range of individuals, including those who follow lacto-ovo-vegetarian diets and vegan diets.

- It promotes the concepts of variety and moderation. Many other guides for both vegetarians and nonvegetarians direct consumers only to dairy foods to meet calcium needs, whereas this guide emphasizes the wide variety of foods that can meet calcium requirements.

- It focuses on foods that are commonly consumed by vegetarians.

REFERENCES

1. Hertzler AA, Anderson HL. Food guides in the United States. *J Am Diet Assoc.* 1974;64:19–28.

2. Health Canada, Office of Nutrition Policy and Promotion. Canada's Food Guides From 1942 to 1992. Available at: http://www.hc-sc.gc.ca/hpfb-dgpsa/onpp-bppn/food_guide_history_int_e.html. Accessed April 3, 2003.

3. *Food Guide Pyramid: A Guide to Daily Food Choices.* Washington, DC: US Dept of Agriculture, Human Nutrition Information Service; 1992. Home and Garden Bulletin No. 252.

4. Welsh SO, Davis C, Shaw A. *USDA's Food Guide: Background and Development.* Hyattsville, MD: United States Department of Agriculture, Human Nutrition Information Service; 1993. Publication Number 1514.

5. Mutch PB. Food guides for the vegetarian. *Am J Clin Nutr.* 1988;48:913–919.

6. Messina MJ, Messina VL. *The Dietitian's Guide to Vegetarian Diets: Issues and Applications.* Gaithersburg, MD: Aspen Publishers; 1996.

7. Position of the American Dietetic Association and Dietitians of Canada: Vegetarian Diets. *J Am Diet Assoc.* 2003;103:748–765.

8. Position of the American Dietetic Association and Dietitians of Canada: Vegetarian Diets. *Can J Diet Pract Res.* 2003;64(2).

9. Pennington JT. Considerations for a new food guide. *J Nutr Educ.* 1981;13:53–55.

10. Sandstrom B. Micronutrient interactions: effects on absorption and bio-availability. *Br J Nutr.* 2001;85 (suppl 2):S181–185.

11. Kris-Etherton PM. AHA Science Advisory. Monounsaturated fatty acids and risk of cardiovascular disease. American Heart Association. Nutrition Committee. *Circulation.* 1999;100:1253–1258.

12. McManus K, Antinoro L, Sacks F. A randomized controlled trial of a moderate-fat, low-energy diet compared with a low-fat, low-energy diet for weight loss in overweight adults. *Int J Obes Relat Metab Disord.* 2001;25:1503–1511.

13. Vegetarian Resource Group. How many vegetarians are there? Available at http://www.vrg.org/nutshell/poll2000.htm. Accessed April 3, 2002.

14. Janelle KC, Barr SI. Nutrient intakes and eating behavior scores of vegetarian and nonvegetarian women. *J Am Diet Assoc.* 1995;95:180–189.

15. Arjmandi BH, Smith BJ. Soy isoflavones' osteoprotective role in post-menopausal women: Mechanism of action. *J Nutr Biochem.* 2002;13:130–137.

16. Lemann J Jr, Pleuss JA, Gray RW. Potassium causes calcium retention in healthy adults. *J Nutr.* 1993;123:1623–1636.

17. Booth SL, Broe KE, Gagnon DR, Tucker KL, Hannan MT, McLean RR, Dawson-Hughes B, Wilson PWF, Cupples LA, Kiel DP. Vitamin K intake and bone mineral density in women and men. *Am J Clin Nutr.* 2003;77:512–516.

18. Food and Nutrition Board, Institute of Medicine. *Dietary Reference Intakes for Thiamin, Riboflavin, Niacin, Vitamin B$_6$, Folate, Vitamin B$_{12}$, Pantothenic Acid, Biotin, and Choline.* Washington, DC: National Academy Press; 1998.

*Messina is a nutrition consultant with Nutrition Matters, Inc., Port Townsend, WA. V. Melina is a nutrition consultant with Nutrispeak.com, Langley, BC, Canada. A. R. Mangels is a nutrition advisor to The Vegetarian Resource Group, Baltimore, MD.

Address correspondence to: Virginia Messina, MPH, RD, 439 Calhoun St, Port Townsend, WA 98368. E-mail: messina@olympus.net

APPENDIX VI
DIETARY SUPPLEMENT HEALTH AND EDUCATION ACT OF 1994

For Legislative History of Act, see Report for P.L. 103–417 in U.S.C.C. & A.N. Legislative History Section.

An Act to amend the Federal Food, Drug, and Cosmetic Act to establish standards with respect to dietary supplements, and for other purposes.

Be it enacted by the Senate and House of Representatives of the United States of America in Congress assembled.

SEC. 1. SHORT TITLE: REFERENCE; TABLE OF CONTENTS.

(a) SHORT TITLE.—This Act may be cited as the "Dietary Supplement Health and Education Act of 1994."

(b) REFERENCE.—Whenever in this Act an amendment or repeal is expressed in terms of an amendment to, or repeal of, a section or other provision, the reference shall be considered to be made to a section or other provision of the Federal Food, Drug, and Cosmetic Act.

(c) TABLE OF CONTENTS.—The table of contents of this Act is as follows:

SEC. 2. FINDINGS.

Congress finds that—

(1) improving the health status of United States citizens ranks at the top of the national priorities of the Federal Government;

(2) the importance of nutrition and the benefits of dietary supplements to health promotion and disease prevention have been documented increasingly in scientific studies;

(3)(A) there is a link between the ingestion of certain nutrients or dietary supplements and the prevention of chronic diseases such as cancer, heart disease, and osteoporosis; and

(B) clinical research has shown that several chronic diseases can be prevented simply with a healthful diet, such as a diet that is low in fat, saturated fat, cholesterol, and sodium, with a high proportion of plant-based foods;

(4) healthful diets may mitigate the need for expensive medical procedures, such as coronary bypass surgery or angioplasty;

(5) preventive health measures, including education, good nutrition, and appropriate use of safe nutritional supplements will limit the

incidence of chronic diseases, and reduce long-term health care expenditures;

(6)(A) promotion of good health and healthy lifestyles improves and extends lives while reducing health care expenditures; and

(B) reduction in health care expenditures is of paramount importance to the future of the country and the economic well-being of the country;

(7) there is a growing need for emphasis on the dissemination of information linking nutrition and long-term good health;

(8) consumers should be empowered to make choices about preventive health care programs based on data from scientific studies of health benefits related to particular dietary supplements;

(9) national surveys have revealed that almost 50 percent of the 260,000,000 Americans regularly consume dietary supplements of vitamins, minerals, or herbs as a means of improving their nutrition;

(10) studies indicate that consumers are placing increased reliance on the use of nontraditional health care providers to avoid the excessive costs of traditional medical services and to obtain more holistic consideration of their needs;

(11) the United States will spend over $1,000,000,000,000 on health care in 1994, which is about 12 percent of the Gross National Product of the United States, and this amount and percentage will continue to increase unless significant efforts are undertaken to reverse the increase;

(12)(A) the nutritional supplement industry is an integral part of the economy of the United States;

(B) the industry consistently projects a positive trade balance; and

(C) the estimated 600 dietary supplement manufacturers in the United States produce approximately 4,000 products, with total annual sales of such products alone reaching at least $4,000,000,000;

(13) although the Federal Government should take swift action against products that are unsafe or adulterated, the Federal Government should not take any actions to impose unreasonable regulatory barriers limiting or slowing the flow of safe products and accurate information to consumers;

(14) dietary supplements are safe within a broad range of intake, and safety problems with the supplements are relatively rare; and

(15)(A) legislative action that protects the right of access of consumers to safe dietary supplements is necessary in order to promote wellness; and

(B) a rational Federal framework must be established to supersede the current ad hoc, patchwork regulatory policy on dietary supplements.

SEC. 3. DEFINITIONS.

(a) DEFINITION OF CERTAIN FOODS AS DIETARY SUPPLEMENTS.—Section 201 (21 U.S.C. 321) is amended by adding at the end the following:

"(ff) The term 'dietary supplement'—

"(1) means a product (other than tobacco) intended to supplement the diet that bears or contains one or more of the following dietary ingredients:

"(A) a vitamin;

"(B) a mineral;

"(C) an herb or other botanical;

"(D) an amino acid;

"(E) a dietary substance for use by man to supplement the diet by increasing the total dietary intake; or

"(F) a concentrate, metabolite, constituent, extract, or combination of any ingredient described in clause (A), (B), (C), (D), or (E);

"(2) means a product that—

"(A)(i) is intended for ingestion in a form described in section 411(c)(1)(B)(i); or

"(ii) complies with section 411(C)(1)(B)(ii);

"(B) is not represented for use as a conventional food or as a sole item of a meal or the diet; and

"(C) is labeled as a dietary supplement; and

"(3) does—

"(A) include an article that is approved as a new drug under section 505, certified as an antibiotic under section 507, or licensed as a biologic under section 351 of the Public Health Service Act (42 U.S.C. 262) and was, prior to such approval, certification, or license, marketed as a dietary supplement or as a food unless the Secretary has issued a regulation, after notice and comment, finding that the article, when used as or in a dietary supplement under the conditions of use and dosages set forth in the labeling for such dietary supplement, is unlawful under section 402(f); and

"(B) not include—

"(i) an article that is approved as a new drug under section 505, certified as an antibiotic under section 507, or licensed as a biologic under section 351 of the Public Health Service Act (42 U.S.C. 262), or

"(ii) an article authorized for investigation as a new drug, antibiotic, or biological for which substantial clinical investigations have been instituted and for which the existence of such investigations has been made public,

which was not before such approval, certification, licensing, or authorization marketed as a dietary supplement or as a food unless the Secretary, in the Secretary's discretion, has issued a regulation, after notice and comment, finding that the article would be lawful under this Act.

Except for purposes of section 201(g), a dietary supplement shall be deemed to be a food within the meaning of this Act."

(b) EXCLUSION FROM DEFINITION OF FOOD ADDITIVE.—Section 201(s) (21 U.S.C. 321(s)) is amended—

(1) by striking "or" at the end of subparagraph (4);

(2) by striking the period at the end of subparagraph (5) and inserting "or"; and

(3) by adding at the end the following new subparagraph

"(6) an ingredient described in paragraph (ff) in, or intended for us in, a dietary supplement.".

(c) FORM OF INGESTION.—Section 411(c)(1)(B) (21 U.S.C. 350(c)(B)) is amended—

(1) in clause (i), by inserting "powder, softgel, gelcap," after "capsule,"; and

(2) in clause (ii), by striking "does not simulate and."

SEC. 4. SAFETY OF DIETARY SUPPLEMENTS AND BURDEN OF PROOF ON FDA.

Section 402 (21 U.S.C. 342) is amended by adding at the end the following:

"(f)(1) If it is a dietary supplement or contains a dietary ingredient that—

"(A) presents a significant or unreasonable risk of illness or injury under—

"(i) conditions of use recommended or suggested in labeling, or

"(ii) if no condition of use are suggested or recommended in the labeling, under ordinary conditions of use;

"(B) is a new dietary ingredient for which there is inadequate information to provide reasonable assurance that such ingredient does not present a significant or unreasonable risk of illness or injury;

"(C) the Secretary declares to pose an imminent hazard to public health or safety, except that the authority to make such declaration shall not be delegated and the Secretary shall promptly after such a declaration initiate a proceeding in accordance with sections 554 and 556 of title 5, United States Code, to affirm or withdraw the declaration; or

"(D) is or contains a dietary ingredient that renders it adulterated under paragraph (a)(1) under the conditions of use recommended or suggested in the labeling of such dietary supplement.

In any proceeding under this subparagraph, the United States shall bear the burden of proof on each element to show that a dietary supplement is adulterated. The court shall decide any issue under this paragraph on a de novo basis.

"(2) Before the Secretary may report to a United States attorney a violation of paragraph (1)(A) for a civil proceeding, the person against whom such proceeding would be initiated shall be given appropriate notice and the opportunity to present views, orally and in writing, at least 10 days before such notice, with regard to such proceeding."

SEC. 5. DIETARY SUPPLEMENT CLAIMS.

Chapter IV (21 U.S.C. 341 et seq.) is amended by inserting after section 403A the following new section:

"DIETARY SUPPLEMENT LABELING EXEMPTIONS

"SEC. 403B. (a) IN GENERAL.—A publication, including an article, a chapter in a book, or an official abstract of a peer-reviewed scientific publication that appears in an article and was prepared by the author or the editors of the publication, which is reprinted in its entirety, shall not be defined as labeling when used in connection with the sale of a dietary supplement to consumers when it—

"(1) is not false or misleading;

"(2) does not promote a particular manufacturer or brand of a dietary supplement;

"(3) is displayed or presented, or is displayed or presented with other such items on the same subject matter, so as to present a balanced view of the available scientific information on a dietary supplement;

"(4) if displayed in an establishment, is physically separate from the dietary supplements; and

"(5) does not have appended to it any information by sticker or any other method.

"(b) APPLICATION.—Subsection (a) shall not apply to or restrict a retailer or wholesaler of dietary supplements in any way whatsoever in the sale of books or other publications as a part of the business of such retailer or wholesaler.

"(c) BURDEN OF PROOF.—In any proceeding brought under subsection (a), the burden of proof shall be on the United States to establish that an article or other such matter is false or misleading."

SEC. 6. STATEMENTS OF NUTRITIONAL SUPPORT.

Section 403(r) (21 U.S.C. 343(r)) is amended by adding at the end the following:

"(6) For purposes of paragraph (r)(1)(B), a statement for a dietary supplement may be made if—

"(A) the statement claims a benefit related to a classical nutrient deficiency disease and discloses the prevalence of such disease in the United States, describes the role of a nutrient or dietary ingredient intended to affect the structure or function in humans, characterizes the documented mechanism by which a nutrient or dietary ingredient acts to maintain such structure or function, or describes general well-being from consumption of a nutrient or dietary ingredient,

"(B) the manufacturer of the dietary supplement has substantiation that such statement is truthful and not misleading, and

"(C) the statement contains prominently displayed and in boldface type, the following: 'This statement has not been evaluated by the Food and Drug Administration. This product is not intended to diagnose, treat, cure, or prevent any disease.'. A statement under this subparagraph may not claim to diagnose, mitigate, treat, cure, or prevent a specific disease or class of diseases. If the manufacturer of a dietary supplement proposes to make a statement described in the first sentence of this subparagraph in the labeling of the dietary supplement, the manufacturer shall notify the Secretary no later than 30 days after the first marketing of the dietary supplement with such statement that such a statement is being made."

SEC. 7. DIETARY SUPPLEMENT INGREDIENT LABELING AND NUTRITION INFORMATION LABELING.

(a) MISBRANDED SUPPLEMENTS.—Section 403 (21 U.S.C. 343) is amended by adding at the end the following:

"(s) If—

"(1) it is a dietary supplement; and

"(2)(A) the label or labeling of the supplement fails to list—

"(i) the name of each ingredient of the supplement that is described in section 201(ff); and

"(ii)(I) the quantity of each such ingredient; or

"(II) with respect to a proprietary blend of such ingredients, the total quantity of all ingredients in the blend;

"(B) the label or labeling of the dietary supplement fails to identify the product by using the term 'dietary supplement', which term may be modified with the name of such an ingredient;

"(C) the supplement contains an ingredient described in section 201(ff)(1)(C), and the label or labeling of the supplement fails to identify any part of the plant from which the ingredient is derived;

"(D) the supplement—

"(i) is covered by the specifications of an official compendium;

"(ii) is represented as conforming to the specifications of an official compendium; and "(iii) fails to so conform; or

"(E) the supplement—

"(i) is not covered by the specifications of an official compendium; and

"(ii)(I) fails to have the identity and strength that the supplement is represented to have; or

"(II) fails to meet the quality (including tablet or capsule disintegration), purity, or compositional specifications, based on validated assay or other appropriate methods, that the supplement is represented to meet."

(b) SUPPLEMENT LISTING ON NUTRITION LABELING.— Section 403(q)(5)(F) (21 U.S.C. 343(q)(5)(F)) is amended to read as follows:

"(F) A dietary supplement product (including a food to which section 411 applies) shall comply with the requirements of subparagraphs (1) and (2) in a manner which is appropriate for the product and which is specified in regulations of the Secretary which shall provide that—

"(i) nutrition information shall first list those dietary ingredients that are present in the product in a significant amount and for which a recommendation for daily consumption has been established by the Secretary, except that a dietary ingredient shall not be required to be listed if it is not present in a significant amount, and shall list any other dietary ingredient present and identified as having so such recommendation;

"(ii) the listing of dietary ingredients shall include the quantity of each such ingredient (or of a proprietary blend of such ingredients) per serving;

"(iii) the listing of dietary ingredients may include the source of a dietary ingredient; and

"(iv) the nutrition information shall immediately precede the ingredient information required under subclause (i), except that no ingredient identified pursuant to subclause (i) shall be required to be identified a second time."

(c) PERCENTAGE LEVEL CLAIMS.—Section 403(r)(2) (21 U.S.C. 343(r)(2)) is amended by adding after clause (E) the following:

"(F) Subclause (i) clause (A) does not apply to a statement in the labeling of a dietary supplement that characterizes the percentage level of a dietary ingredient for which the Secretary has not established a reference daily intake, daily recommended

value, or other recommendation for daily consumption."

(d) VITAMINS AND MINERALS.—Section 411(b)(2) (21 U.S.C. 350(b)(2)) is amended—

(1) by striking "vitamins or minerals" and inserting "dietary supplement ingredients described in section 201(ff)";

(2) by striking "(2)(A)" and inserting "(2)"; and

(3) by striking subparagraph (B).

(e) EFFECTIVE DATE.—Dietary supplements—

(1) may be labeled after the date of the enactment of this Act in accordance with the amendments made by this section, and

(2) shall be labeled after December 31, 1996, in accordance with such amendments.

SEC. 8. NEW DIETARY INGREDIENTS.

Chapter IV of the Federal Food, Drug, and Cosmetic Act is amended by adding at the end the following:

"NEW DIETARY INGREDIENTS

"SEC. 413. (a) IN GENERAL.—A dietary supplement which contains a new dietary ingredient shall be deemed adulterated under section 402(f) unless it meets one of the following requirements:

"(1) The dietary supplement contains only dietary ingredients which have been present in the food supply as an article used for food in a form in which the food has not been chemically altered.

"(2) There is a history of use or other evidence of safety establishing that the dietary ingredient when used under the conditions recommended or suggested in the labeling of the dietary supplement will reasonably be expected to be safe and at least 75 days before being introduced or delivered for introduction into interstate commerce, the manufacturer or distributor of the dietary ingredient or dietary supplement provides the Secretary with information, including any citation to published articles, which is the basis on which the manufacturer or distributor has concluded that a dietary supplement containing such dietary ingredient will reasonably be expected to be safe.

The Secretary shall keep confidential any information provided under paragraph (2) for 90 days following its receipt. After the expiration of such 90 days, the Secretary shall place such information on public display, except matters in the information which are trade secrets or otherwise confidential, commercial information.

"(b) PETITION.—Any person may file with the Secretary a petition proposing the issuance of an order prescribing the conditions under which a new dietary ingredient under its intended conditions of use will reasonably be expected to be safe. The Secretary shall make a decision on such petition within 180 days of the date the petition is filed with the Secretary. For purposes of chapter 7 of title 5, United States Code, the decision of the Secretary shall be considered final agency action.

"(c) DEFINITION.—For purposes of this section, the term 'new dietary ingredient' means a dietary ingredient that was not marketed in the United States before October 15, 1994 and does not include and dietary ingredient which was marketed in the United States before October 15, 1994."

SEC. 9. GOOD MANUFACTURING PRACTICES.

Section 402 (21 U.S.C. 342), as amended by section 4, is amended by adding at the end the following:

"(g)(1) If it is a dietary supplement and it has been prepared, packed, or held under conditions that do not meet current good manufacturing practice regulations, including regulations requiring, when necessary, expiration date labeling, issued by the Secretary under subparagraph (2).

"(2) The Secretary may by regulation prescribe good manufacturing practices for dietary supplements. Such regulations shall be modeled after current good manufacturing practice regulations for food and may not impose standards for which there is no current and generally available analytical methodology. No standard of current good manufacturing practice may be imposed unless such standard is included in a regulation promulgated after notice and opportunity for comment in accordance with chapter 5 of title 5, United States Code."

SEC. 10. CONFORMING AMENDMENTS.

(a) SECTION 201.—The last sentence of section 201(g)(1) (21 U.S.C. 321(g)(1)) is amended to read as follows: "A food or dietary supplement for which a claim, subject to sections 403(r)(1)(B) and 403(r)(3) or sections 403(r)(1)(B) and 403(r)(5)(D), is made in accordance with the requirements of section 403(r) is not a drug solely because the label or the labeling contains such a claim. A food, dietary ingredient, or dietary supplement for which a truthful and not misleading statement is made in accordance with section 403(r)(6) is not a drug under clause (C) solely because the label or the labeling contains such a statement."

(b) SECTION 301.—Section 301 (21 U.S.C. 331) is amended by adding at the end the following:
"(u) The introduction or delivery for introduction into interstate commerce of a dietary supplement that is unsafe under section 413."

(c) SECTION 403.—Section 403 (21 U.S.C. 343), as amended by section 7, is amended by adding after paragraph (s) the following "A dietary supplement shall not be deemed misbranded solely because its label or labeling contains directions or conditions of use or warnings."

SEC. 11. WITHDRAWAL OF THE REGULATIONS AND NOTICE.

The advance notice of proposed rulemaking concerning dietary supplements published in the Federal Register of June 18, 1993 (58 FR 33690–33700) is null and void and of no force or effect insofar as it applies to dietary supplements. The Secretary of Health and Human Services shall publish a notice in the Federal Register to revoke the item declared to be null and void and of no force or effect under subsection (a).

SEC. 12. COMMISSION ON DIETARY SUPPLEMENT LABELS.

(a) ESTABLISHMENT.—There shall be established as an independent agency within the executive branch a commission to be known as the Commission on Dietary Supplement Labels (hereafter in this section referred to as the "Commission").

(b) MEMBERSHIP.—

(1) COMPOSITION.—The Commission shall be composed of 7 members who shall be appointed by the President.

(2) EXPERTISE REQUIREMENT.—The members of the Commission shall consist of individuals with expertise and experience in dietary supplements

and in the manufacture, regulation, distribution, and use of such supplements. At least three of the members of the Commission shall be qualified by scientific training and experience to evaluate the benefits to health of the use of dietary supplements and one of such three members shall have experience in pharmacognosy, medical botany, traditional herbal medicine, or other related sciences. Members and staff of the Commission shall be without bias on the issue of dietary supplements.

(c) FUNCTIONS OF THE COMMISSION.—The Commission shall conduct a study on, and provide recommendation for, the regulation of label claims and statements for dietary supplements, including the use of literature in connection with the sale of dietary supplements and procedures for the evaluation of such claims. In making such recommendations, the Commission shall evaluate how best to provide truthful, scientifically valid, and not misleading information to consumers so that such consumers may make informed and appropriate health care choices for themselves and their families.

(d) ADMINISTRATIVE POWERS OF THE COMMISSION.—

(1) HEARINGS.—The Commission may hold hearings, sit and act at such times and places, take such testimony, and receive such evidence as the Commission considers advisable to carry out the purposes of this section.

(2) INFORMATION FROM FEDERAL AGENCIES.—The Commission may secure directly from any Federal department or agency such information as the Commission considers necessary to carry out the provisions of this section.

(3) AUTHORIZATION OF APPROPRIATIONS.—There are authorized to be appropriated such sums as may be necessary to carry out this section.

(e) REPORTS AND RECOMMENDATIONS.—

(1) FINAL REPORT REQUIRED.—Not later than 24 months after the date of enactment of this Act, the Commission shall prepare and submit to the President and to the Congress a final report on the study required by this section.

(2) RECOMMENDATIONS.—The report described in paragraph (1) shall contain such recommendations, including recommendations for legislation, as the Commission deems appropriate.

(3) ACTION ON RECOMMENDATIONS.—Within 90 days of the issuance of the report under paragraph (1), the Secretary of Health and Human Services shall publish in the Federal Register a notice of any recommendation of Commission for changes in regulations of the Secretary for the regulation of dietary supplements and shall include in such notice a notice of proposed rulemaking on such changes together with an opportunity to present views on such changes. Such rulemaking shall be completed not later than 2 years after the date of the issuance of such report. If such rulemaking is not completed on or before the expiration of such 2 years, regulations of the Secretary published in 59 FR 395–426 on January 4, 1994, shall not be in effect.

SEC. 13. OFFICE OF DIETARY SUPPLEMENTS.

(a) IN GENERAL.—Title IV of the Public Health Service Act is amended by inserting after section 485B (42 U.S.C. 287c-3) the following:

"Subpart 4—Office of Dietary Supplements

"SEC. 485C. DIETARY SUPPLEMENTS.

"(a) ESTABLISHMENT.—The Secretary shall establish an Office of Dietary Supplements within the National Institutes of Health.

"(b) PURPOSE.—The purposes of the Office are—

"(1) to explore more fully the potential role of dietary supplements as a significant part of the efforts of the United States to improve health care; and

"(2) to promote scientific study of the benefits of dietary supplements in maintaining health and preventing chronic disease and other health-related conditions.

"(c) DUTIES.—The Director of the Office of Dietary Supplements shall—

"(1) conduct and coordinate scientific research within the National Institutes of Health relating to dietary supplements and the extent to which the use of dietary supplements can limit or reduce the risk of diseases such as heart disease, cancer, birth defects, osteoporosis, cataracts, or prostatism;

"(2) collect and compile the results of scientific research relating to dietary supplements, including scientific data from foreign sources or the Office of Alternative Medicine;

"(3) serve as the principal advisor to the Secretary and to the Assistant Secretary for Health and provide advice to the Director of the National Institutes of Health, the Director of the Centers for Disease Control and Prevention, and the Commissioner of Food and Drugs on issues relating to dietary supplements including—

"(A) dietary intake regulations;

"(B) the safety of dietary supplements;

"(C) claims characterizing the relationship between—

"(i) dietary supplements; and

"(ii)(I) prevention of disease or other health-related conditions; and

"(II) maintenance of health; and

"(D) scientific issues arising in connection with the labeling and composition of dietary supplements;

"(4) compile a database of scientific research on dietary supplements and individual nutrients; and

"(5) coordinate funding relating to dietary supplements for the National Institutes of Health.

"(d) Definition.—As used in this section, the term 'dietary supplement' has the meaning given the term in section 201(ff) of the Federal Food, Drug, and Cosmetic Act.

"(e) Authorization of Appropriations.—There are authorized to be appropriated to carry out this section $5,000,000 for fiscal year 1994 and such sums as may be necessary for each subsequent fiscal year."

(b) Conforming Amendment.—Section 401(b)(2) of the Public Health Service Act (42 U.S.C. 281(b)(2)) is amended by adding at the end the following:

"(E) The Office of Dietary Supplements."

Approved October 25, 1994.

APPENDIX VII
THE NEW FOOD LABEL

FDA regulates dietary supplements under a different set of regulations than those covering "conventional" foods and drug products (prescription and Over-the-Counter). Under the Dietary Supplement Health and Education Act of 1994 (DSHEA), the dietary supplement manufacturer is responsible for ensuring that a dietary supplement is safe before it is marketed. FDA is responsible for taking action against any unsafe dietary supplement product after it reaches the market. Generally, manufacturers do not need to register with FDA nor get FDA approval before producing or selling dietary supplements. Manufacturers must make sure that product label information is truthful and not misleading.

FDA's post-marketing responsibilities include monitoring safety, e.g. voluntary dietary supplement adverse event reporting, and product information, such as labeling, claims, package inserts, and accompanying literature. The Federal Trade Commission regulates dietary supplement advertising.

THE FOOD LABEL

Grocery store aisles are avenues to greater nutritional knowledge. Under regulations from the Food and Drug Administration of the Department of Health and Human Services and the Food Safety and Inspection Service of the U.S. Department of Agriculture, the food label offers more complete, useful and accurate nutrition information than ever before.

With today's food labels, consumers get:

- nutrition information about almost every food in the grocery store
- distinctive, easy-to-read formats that enable consumers to more quickly find the information they need to make healthful food choices
- information on the amount per serving of saturated fat, cholesterol, dietary fiber, and other nutrients of major health concern
- nutrient reference values, expressed as % Daily Values, that help consumers see how a food fits into an overall daily diet
- uniform definitions for terms that describe a food's nutrient content—such as "light," "low-fat," and "high-fiber"—to ensure that such terms mean the same for any product on which they appear
- claims about the relationship between a nutrient or food and a disease or health-related condition, such as calcium and osteoporosis, and fat and cancer. These are helpful for people who are concerned about eating foods that may help keep them healthier longer.
- standardized serving sizes that make nutritional comparisons of similar products easier
- declaration of total percentage of juice in juice drinks. This enables consumers to know exactly how much juice is in a product.

NLEA

These and other changes are part of final rules published in the *Federal Register* in 1992 and 1993. FDA's rules implement the provisions of the Nutrition Labeling and Education Act of 1990 (NLEA), which, among other things, requires nutrition labeling for most foods (except meat and poultry) and authorizes the use of nutrient content claims and appropriate FDA-approved health claims. Meat and poultry products regulated by USDA are not covered by NLEA. However, USDA's regulations closely parallel FDA's rules, summarized here.

NUTRITION LABELING—APPLICABLE FOODS

Under these rules, nutrition labeling is required for most foods. In addition, voluntary nutrition information is available for many raw foods: the 20 most frequently eaten raw fruits, vegetables and fish each, under FDA's voluntary point-of-purchase nutrition information program, and the 45 best-selling cuts of meat, under USDA's program.

Although voluntary, FDA's program for raw produce and fish carries a strong incentive for retailers to participate. The program will remain voluntary only if at least 60 percent of a nationwide sample of retailers continue to provide the necessary information. (In a 1996 survey, FDA found that more than 70 percent of U.S. food stores were complying.)

Also nutrition information is required for some restaurant foods. FDA requires nutrition information for foods about which health or nutrient-content claims are made on restaurant menus, signs or placards. Restaurants have to provide a "reasonable basis" for making claims, although they are given some flexibility in demonstrating that reasonable basis. For example, they could rely on recipes endorsed by medical or dietary groups.

NUTRITION LABELING—EXEMPTIONS

Under NLEA, some foods are exempt from nutrition labeling. These include:

- food served for immediate consumption, such as that served in hospital cafeterias and airplanes, and that sold by food service vendors—for example, mall cookie counters, sidewalk vendors, and vending machines
- ready-to-eat food that is not for immediate consumption but is prepared primarily on site—for example, bakery, deli, and candy store items
- food shipped in bulk, as long as it is not for sale in that form to consumers
- medical foods, such as those used to address the nutritional needs of patients with certain diseases
- plain coffee and tea, some spices, and other foods that contain no significant amounts of any nutrients.

Food produced by small businesses also may be exempt, under 1993 amendments to the NLEA.

Businesses with fewer than 100 full-time equivalent employees may claim an exemption for food products that have U.S. sales of fewer than 100,000 units annually. Companies claiming this exemption must notify FDA that they meet the criteria before they begin marketing their products. U.S. companies, other than importers, with fewer than 10 full-time equivalent employees and selling fewer than 10,000 units of a food in a year also are exempt but do not need to notify FDA. Also exempt are retailers with annual gross sales in the United States of less than $500,000 or with annual gross sales of food to consumers in the United States of less than $50,000.

Although certain foods may be exempt, they are free to carry nutrition information, when appropriate—as long as it complies with regulations. Also, these foods will lose their exemption if their labels carry a nutrient content or health claim or any other nutrition information.

Nutrition information about game meats—such as deer, bison, rabbit, quail, wild turkey, and ostrich—is not required on individual packages. Instead, it can be given on counter cards, signs, or other point-of-purchase materials. Because few nutrient data exist for these foods, FDA believes that allowing this option will enable game meat producers to give first priority to collecting appropriate data and make it easier for them to update the information as it becomes available.

NUTRITION INFORMATION PANEL

Under the label's "Nutrition Facts" panel, manufacturers are required to provide information on certain nutrients. The mandatory (underlined) and voluntary components and the order in which they must appear are:

- total calories
- calories from fat
- calories from saturated fat
- total fat
- saturated fat
- polyunsaturated fat
- monounsaturated fat
- cholesterol

- sodium
- potassium
- total carbohydrate
- dietary fiber
- soluble fiber
- insoluble fiber
- sugars
- sugar alcohol (for example, the sugar substitutes xylitol, mannitol, and sorbitol)
- other carbohydrate (the difference between total carbohydrate and the sum of dietary fiber, sugars, and sugar alcohol if declared)
- protein
- vitamin A
- percent of vitamin A present as beta-carotene
- vitamin C
- calcium
- iron
- other essential vitamins and minerals

If a claim is made about any of the optional components, or if a food is fortified or enriched with any of them, nutrition information for these components becomes mandatory.

These mandatory and voluntary components are the only ones allowed on the Nutrition Facts panel. The listing of single amino acids, maltodextrin, calories from polyunsaturated fat, and calories from carbohydrates, for example, may not appear as part of the Nutrition Facts on the label.

The required nutrients were selected because they address today's health concerns. The order in which they must appear reflects the priority of current dietary recommendations.

NUTRITION PANEL FORMAT

All nutrients must be declared as percentages of the Daily Values which are label reference values. The amount, in grams or milligrams, of macronutrients (such as fat, cholesterol, sodium, carbohydrates, and protein) are still listed to the immediate right of these nutrients. But, for the first time, a column headed "% Daily Value" appears on the far right side.

Declaring nutrients as a percentage of the Daily Values is intended to prevent misinterpretations that arise with quantitative values. For example, a food with 140 milligrams (mg) of sodium could be mistaken for a high-sodium food because 140 is a relatively large number. In actuality, however, that amount represents less than 6 percent of the Daily Value for sodium, which is 2,400 mg.

On the other hand, a food with 5 g of saturated fat could be construed as being low in that nutrient. In fact, that food would provide one-fourth the total Daily Value because 20 g is the Daily Value for saturated fat.

NUTRITION PANEL FOOTNOTE

The % Daily Value listing carries a footnote saying that the percentages are based on a 2,000-calorie diet. Some nutrition labels—at least those on larger packages—have these additional footnotes:

- a sentence noting that a person's individual nutrient goals are based on his or her calorie needs
- lists of the daily values for selected nutrients for a 2,000- and a 2,500-calorie diet.

An optional footnote for packages of any size is the number of calories per gram of fat (9), and carbohydrate and protein (4).

FORMAT MODIFICATIONS

In some circumstances, variations in the format of the nutrition panel are allowed. Some are mandatory. For example, the labels of foods for children under 2 (except infant formula, which has special labeling rules under the Infant Formula Act of 1980) may not carry information about saturated fat, polyunsaturated fat, monounsaturated fat, cholesterol, calories from fat, or calories from saturated fat.

The reason is to prevent parents from wrongly assuming that infants and toddlers should restrict their fat intake, when, in fact, they should not. Fat is important during these years to ensure adequate growth and development.

The labels of foods for children under 4 may not include the % Daily Values for total fat, saturated fat, cholesterol, sodium, potassium, total carbohydrate, and dietary fiber. They may carry % Daily

Values for protein, vitamins and minerals, however. These nutrients are the only ones for which FDA has set Daily Values for this age group.

Thus, the top portion of the "Nutrition Facts" panels of foods for children under 4 will consist of two columns. The nutrients' names will be listed on the left and their quantitative amounts will be on the right. The bottom portion will provide the % Daily Values for protein, vitamins and minerals. Only the calorie conversion information may be given as a footnote.

Some foods qualify for a simplified label format. This format is allowed when the food contains insignificant amounts of seven or more of the mandatory nutrients and total calories. "Insignificant" means that a declaration of zero could be made in nutrition labeling, or, for total carbohydrate, dietary fiber, and protein, the declaration states "less than 1 g."

For foods for children under 2, the simplified format may be used if the product contains insignificant amounts of six or more of the following: calories, total fat, sodium, total carbohydrate, dietary fiber, sugars, protein, vitamins A and C, calcium, and iron.

If the simplified format is used, information on total calories, total fat, total carbohydrate, protein, and sodium—even if they are present in insignificant amounts—must be listed. Other nutrients, along with calories from fat, must be shown if they are present in more than insignificant amounts. Nutrients added to the food must be listed, too.

Some format exceptions exist for small and medium-size packages. Packages with less than 12 square inches of available labeling space (about the size of a package of chewing gum) do not have to carry nutrition information unless a nutrient content or health claim is made for the product. However, they must provide an address or telephone number for consumers to obtain the required nutrition information.

If manufacturers wish to provide nutrition information on these packages voluntarily, they have several options: (1) present the information in a smaller type size than that required for larger packages, or (2) present the information in a tabular or linear (string) format.

The tabular and linear formats also may be used on packages that have less than 40 square inches available for labeling and insufficient space for the full vertical format. Other options for packages with less than 40 square inches of label space are:

- abbreviating names of dietary components
- omitting all footnotes, except for the statement that "Percent Daily Values are based on a 2,000-calorie diet"
- placing nutrition information on other panels readily seen by consumers.

A select group of packages with more than 40 square inches of labeling space is allowed a format exception, too. These are packages with insufficient vertical space (about 3 inches) to accommodate the required information. Some examples are bread bags, pie boxes, and bags of frozen vegetables. On these packages, the "Nutrition Facts" panel may appear, in tabular format, with the footnote information appearing to the far right.

For larger packages in which there is not sufficient space on the principal display panel or the information panel (the panel to the right of the principal display), FDA allows nutrition information to appear on any label panel that is readily seen by consumers. This lessens the chances of overcrowding of information and encourages manufacturers to provide the greatest amount of nutrition information possible.

For products that require additional preparation before eating, such as dry cake mixes and dry pasta dinners, or that are usually eaten with one or more additional foods, such as breakfast cereals with milk, FDA encourages manufacturers to provide voluntarily a second column of nutrition information. This is known as dual declaration.

With this variation, the first column, which is mandatory, contains nutrition information for the food as purchased. The second gives information about the food as prepared and eaten.

Still another variation is the aggregate display. This is allowed on labels of variety-pack food items, such as ready-to-eat cereals and assorted flavors of individual ice cream cups. With this display, the quantitative amount and % Daily Value for each nutrient are listed in separate columns under the name of each food.

SERVING SIZES

The serving size remains the basis for reporting each food's nutrient content. However, unlike in the past, when the serving size was up to the discretion of the food manufacturer, serving sizes now are more uniform and reflect the amounts people actually eat. They also must be expressed in both common household and metric measures.

FDA allows as common household measures: the cup, tablespoon, teaspoon, piece, slice, fraction (such as "1/4 pizza"), and common household containers used to package food products (such as a jar or tray). Ounces may be used, but only if a common household unit is not applicable and an appropriate visual unit is given—for example, 1 oz (28g/about 1/2 pickle).

Grams (g) and milliliters (mL) are the metric units that are used in serving size statements.

NLEA defines serving size as the amount of food customarily eaten at one time. The serving sizes that appear on food labels are based on FDA-established lists of "Reference Amounts Customarily Consumed Per Eating Occasion."

These reference amounts, which are part of the regulations, are broken down into 139 FDA-regulated food product categories, including 11 groups of foods specially formulated or processed for infants or children under 4. They list the amounts of food customarily consumed per eating occasion for each category, based primarily on national food consumption surveys. FDA's list also gives the suggested label statement for serving size declaration. For example, the category "breads (excluding sweet quick type), rolls" has a reference amount of 50 g, and the appropriate label statement for sliced bread or roll is "___ piece(s) (_ g)" or, for unsliced bread, "2 oz (56 g/_ inch slice)."

The serving size of products that come in discrete units, such as cookies, candy bars, and sliced products, is the number of whole units that most closely approximates the reference amount. Cookies are an example. Under the "bakery products" category, cookies have a reference amount of 30 g. The household measure closest to that amount is the number of cookies that comes closest to weighing 30 g. Thus, the serving size on the label of a package of cookies in which each cookie weighs 13 g would read "2 cookies (26 g)."

If one unit weighs more than 50 percent but less than 200 percent of the reference amount, the serving size is one unit. For example, the reference amount for bread is 50 g; therefore, the label of a loaf of bread in which each slice weighs more than 25 g would state a serving size of one slice.

Certain rules apply to food products that are packaged and sold individually. If such an individual package is less than 200 percent of the applicable reference amount, the item qualifies as one serving. Thus, a 360-mL (12-fluid-ounce) can of soda is one serving, since the reference amount for carbonated beverages is 240 mL (8 ounces).

However, if the product has a reference amount of 100 g or 100 mL or more and the package contains more than 150 percent but less than 200 percent of the reference amount, manufacturers have the option of deciding whether the product can be one or two servings.

An example is a 15-ounce (420 g) can of soup. The serving size reference amount for soup is 245 g. Therefore, the manufacturer has the option to declare the can of soup as one or two servings.

DAILY VALUES—DRVS

The new label reference value, Daily Value, comprises two sets of dietary standards: Daily Reference Values (DRVs) and Reference Daily Intakes (RDIs). Only the Daily Value term appears on the label, though, to make label reading less confusing.

DRVs have been established for macronutrients that are sources of energy: fat, saturated fat, total carbohydrate (including fiber), and protein; and for cholesterol, sodium and potassium, which do not contribute calories.

DRVs for the energy-producing nutrients are based on the number of calories consumed per day. A daily intake of 2,000 calories has been established as the reference. This level was chosen, in part, because it approximates the caloric requirements for postmenopausal women. This group has the highest risk for excessive intake of calories and fat.

DRVs for the energy-producing nutrients are calculated as follows:

- fat based on 30 percent of calories
- saturated fat based on 10 percent of calories
- carbohydrate based on 60 percent of calories
- protein based on 10 percent of calories. (The DRV for protein applies only to adults and chil-

dren over 4. RDIs for protein for special groups have been established.)

- fiber based on 11.5 g of fiber per 1,000 calories.

Because of current public health recommendations, DRVs for some nutrients represent the uppermost limit that is considered desirable. The DRVs for total fat, saturated fat, cholesterol, and sodium are:

- total fat: less than 65 g
- saturated fat: less than 20 g
- cholesterol: less than 300 mg
- sodium: less than 2,400 mg

DAILY VALUES—RDIS

"Reference Daily Intake" replaces the term "U.S. RDA," which was introduced in 1973 as a label reference value for vitamins, minerals and protein in voluntary nutrition labeling. The name change was sought because of confusion that existed over "U.S. RDAs," the values determined by FDA and used on food labels, and "RDAs" (Recommended Dietary Allowances), the values determined by the National Academy of Sciences for various population groups and used by FDA to figure the U.S. RDAs.

However, the values for the new RDIs remain the same as the old U.S. RDAs for the time being.

NUTRIENT CONTENT CLAIMS

The regulations also spell out what terms may be used to describe the level of a nutrient in a food and how they can be used. These are the core terms:

- **Free.** This term means that a product contains no amount of, or only trivial or "physiologically inconsequential" amounts of, one or more of these components: fat, saturated fat, cholesterol, sodium, sugars, and calories. For example, "calorie-free" means fewer than 5 calories per serving, and "sugar-free" and "fat-free" both mean less than 0.5 g per serving. Synonyms for "free" include "without," "no" and "zero." A synonym for fat-free milk is "skim".

- **Low.** This term can be used on foods that can be eaten frequently without exceeding dietary guidelines for one or more of these components:

fat, saturated fat, cholesterol, sodium, and calories. Thus, descriptors are defined as follows:

- **low-fat:** 3 g or less per serving
- **low-saturated fat:** 1 g or less per serving
- **low-sodium:** 140 mg or less per serving
- **very low sodium:** 35 mg or less per serving
- **low-cholesterol:** 20 mg or less and 2 g or less of saturated fat per serving
- **low-calorie:** 40 calories or less per serving.

Synonyms for low include "little," "few," "low source of," and "contains a small amount of."

- **Lean and extra lean.** These terms can be used to describe the fat content of meat, poultry, seafood, and game meats.

- **lean:** less than 10 g fat, 4.5 g or less saturated fat, and less than 95 mg cholesterol per serving and per 100 g.
- **extra lean:** less than 5 g fat, less than 2 g saturated fat, and less than 95 mg cholesterol per serving and per 100 g.

- **High.** This term can be used if the food contains 20 percent or more of the Daily Value for a particular nutrient in a serving.

- **Good source.** This term means that one serving of a food contains 10 to 19 percent of the Daily Value for a particular nutrient.

- **Reduced.** This term means that a nutritionally altered product contains at least 25 percent less of a nutrient or of calories than the regular, or reference, product. However, a reduced claim can't be made on a product if its reference food already meets the requirement for a "low" claim.

- **Less.** This term means that a food, whether altered or not, contains 25 percent less of a nutrient or of calories than the reference food. For example, pretzels that have 25 percent less fat than potato chips could carry a "less" claim. "Fewer" is an acceptable synonym.

- **Light.** This descriptor can mean two things:

- First, that a nutritionally altered product contains one-third fewer calories or half the fat of the reference food. If the food derives 50 percent or more of its calories from fat, the reduction must be 50 percent of the fat.

○ Second, that the sodium content of a low-calorie, low-fat food has been reduced by 50 percent. In addition, "light in sodium" may be used on food in which the sodium content has been reduced by at least 50 percent.

The term "light" still can be used to describe such properties as texture and color, as long as the label explains the intent—for example, "light brown sugar" and "light and fluffy."

- **More.** This term means that a serving of food, whether altered or not, contains a nutrient that is at least 10 percent of the Daily Value more than the reference food. The 10 percent of Daily Value also applies to "fortified," "enriched" and "added" "extra and plus" claims, but in those cases, the food must be altered. Alternative spelling of these descriptive terms and their synonyms is allowed—for example, "hi" and "lo"—as long as the alternatives are not misleading.

- **Healthy.** A "healthy" food must be low in fat and saturated fat and contain limited amounts of cholesterol and sodium. In addition, if it's a single-item food, it must provide at least 10 percent of one or more of vitamins A or C, iron, calcium, protein, or fiber. Exempt from this "10-percent" rule are certain raw, canned and frozen fruits and vegetables and certain cereal-grain products. These foods can be labeled "healthy," if they do not contain ingredients that change the nutritional profile, and, in the case of enriched grain products, conform to standards of identity, which call for certain required ingredients. If it's a meal-type product, such as frozen entrees and multi-course frozen dinners, it must provide 10 percent of two or three of these vitamins or minerals or of protein or fiber, in addition to meeting the other criteria. The sodium content cannot exceed 360 mg per serving for individual foods and 480 mg per serving for meal-type products.

OTHER DEFINITIONS

The regulations also address other claims. Among them:

- **Percent fat free:** A product bearing this claim must be a low-fat or a fat-free product. In addition, the claim must accurately reflect the amount of fat present in 100 g of the food. Thus,

if a food contains 2.5 g fat per 50 g, the claim must be "95 percent fat free."

- **Implied:** These types of claims are prohibited when they wrongfully imply that a food contains or does not contain a meaningful level of a nutrient. For example, a product claiming to be made with an ingredient known to be a source of fiber (such as "made with oat bran") is not allowed unless the product contains enough of that ingredient (for example, oat bran) to meet the definition for "good source" of fiber. As another example, a claim that a product contains "no tropical oils" is allowed—but only on foods that are "low" in saturated fat because consumers have come to equate tropical oils with high saturated fat.

- **Meals and main dishes:** Claims that a meal or main dish is "free" of a nutrient, such as sodium or cholesterol, must meet the same requirements as those for individual foods. Other claims can be used under special circumstances. For example, "low-calorie" means the meal or main dish contains 120 calories or less per 100 g. "Low-sodium" means the food has 140 mg or less per 100 g. "Low-cholesterol" means the food contains 20 mg cholesterol or less per 100 g and no more than 2 g saturated fat. "Light" means the meal or main dish is low-fat or low-calorie.

- **Standardized foods:** Any nutrient content claim, such as "reduced fat," "low calorie," and "light," may be used in conjunction with a standardized term if the new product has been specifically formulated to meet FDA's criteria for that claim, if the product is not nutritionally inferior to the traditional standardized food, and the new product complies with certain compositional requirements set by FDA. A new product bearing a claim also must have performance characteristics similar to the referenced traditional standardized food. If the product doesn't, and the differences materially limit the product's use, its label must state the differences (for example, not recommended for baking) to inform consumers.

"FRESH"

Although not mandated by NLEA, FDA has issued a regulation for the term "fresh." The agency took this step because of concern over the term's possible misuse on some food labels.

The regulation defines the term "fresh" when it is used to suggest that a food is raw or unprocessed. In this context, "fresh" can be used only on a food that is raw, has never been frozen or heated, and contains no preservatives. (Irradiation at low levels is allowed.) "Fresh frozen," "frozen fresh," and "freshly frozen" can be used for foods that are quickly frozen while still fresh. Blanching (brief scalding before freezing to prevent nutrient breakdown) is allowed.

Other uses of the term "fresh," such as in "fresh milk" or "freshly baked bread," are not affected.

BABY FOODS

FDA is not allowing broad use of nutrient claims on infant and toddler foods. However, the agency may propose claims specifically for these foods at a later date. The terms "unsweetened" and "unsalted" are allowed on these foods, however, because they relate to taste and not nutrient content.

HEALTH CLAIMS

Claims for 10 relationships between a nutrient or a food and the risk of a disease or health-related condition are now allowed. They can be made in several ways: through third-party references (such as the National Cancer Institute), statements, symbols (such as a heart), and vignettes or descriptions. Whatever the case, the claim must meet the requirements for authorized health claims—for example, they cannot state the degree of risk reduction and can only use "may" or "might" in discussing the nutrient or food-disease relationship. And they must state that other factors play a role in that disease.

The claims also must be phrased so that consumers can understand the relationship between the nutrient and the disease and the nutrient's importance in relationship to a daily diet.

An example of an appropriate claim is: "While many factors affect heart disease, diets low in saturated fat and cholesterol may reduce the risk of this disease." The allowed nutrient-disease relationship claims and rules for their use are:

- **Calcium and osteoporosis:** To carry this claim, a food must contain 20 percent or more of the Daily Value for calcium (200 mg) per serving, have a calcium content that equals or exceeds the food's content of phosphorus, and contain a form of calcium that can be readily absorbed and used by the body. The claim must name the target group most in need of adequate calcium intakes (that is, teens and young adult white and Asian women) and state the need for exercise and a healthy diet. A product that contains 40 percent or more of the Daily Value for calcium must state on the label that a total dietary intake greater than 200 percent of the Daily Value for calcium (that is, 2,000 mg or more) has no further known benefit.

- **Fat and cancer:** To carry this claim, a food must meet the nutrient content claim requirements for "low-fat" or, if fish and game meats, for "extra lean."

- **Saturated fat and cholesterol and coronary heart disease (CHD):** This claim may be used if the food meets the definitions for the nutrient content claim "low saturated fat," "low-cholesterol," and "low-fat," or, if fish and game meats, for "extra lean." It may mention the link between reduced risk of CHD and lower saturated fat and cholesterol intakes to lower blood cholesterol levels.

- **Fiber-containing grain products, fruits and vegetables and cancer:** To carry this claim, a food must be or must contain a grain product, fruit or vegetable and meet the nutrient content claim requirements for "low-fat," and, without fortification, be a "good source" of dietary fiber.

- **Fruits, vegetables and grain products that contain fiber and risk of CHD:** To carry this claim, a food must be or must contain fruits, vegetables and grain products. It also must meet the nutrient content claim requirements for "low saturated fat," "low-cholesterol," and "low-fat" and contain, without fortification, at least 0.6 g soluble fiber per serving.

- **Sodium and hypertension (high blood pressure):** To carry this claim, a food must meet the nutrient content claim requirements for "low-sodium."

- **Fruits and vegetables and cancer:** This claim may be made for fruits and vegetables that meet the nutrient content claim requirements for "low-fat" and that, without fortification, for "good source" of at least one of the following: dietary fiber or vitamins A or C. This claim relates diets low in fat and rich in fruits and vegetables (and thus vitamins A and C and dietary fiber) to reduced cancer risk. FDA authorized this claim in place of an antioxidant vitamin and cancer claim.

- **Folic acid and neural tube defects:** Folic acid and neural tube defects: This claim is allowed on dietary supplements that contain sufficient folate and on conventional foods that are naturally good sources of folate, as long as they do not provide more than 100 percent of the Daily Value for vitamin A as retinol or preformed vitamin A or vitamin D. A sample claim is "healthful diets with adequate folate may reduce a woman's risk of having a child with a brain or spinal cord defect."

- **Dietary sugar alcohols and dental caries (cavities):** This claim applies to food products, such as candy or gum, containing the sugar alcohols xylitol, sorbitol, mannitol, maltitol, isomalt, lactitol, hydrogenated starch hydrolysates, hydrogenated glucose syrups, or a combination of any of these. If the food also contains a fermentable carbohydrate, such as sugar, the food cannot lower the pH of plaque in the mouth below 5.7. Besides the food ingredient's relationship to dental caries, the claim also must state that frequent between-meal consumption of foods high in sugars and starches promotes tooth decay. A shortened claim is allowed on food packages with less than 15 square inches of labeling surface area.

- **Soluble fiber from certain foods, such as whole oats and psyllium seed husk, and heart disease:** This claim must state that the fiber also needs to be part of a diet low in saturated fat and cholesterol, and the food must provide sufficient soluble fiber. The amount of soluble fiber in a serving of the food must be listed on the Nutrition Facts panel.

INGREDIENT LABELING

Ingredient declaration is required on all foods that have more than one ingredient. Because people may be allergic to certain additives and to help them better avoid them, the ingredient list must include, when appropriate:

- FDA-certified color additives, such as FD&C Blue No. 1, by name

- sources of protein hydrolysates, which are used in many foods as flavors and flavor enhancers

- declaration of caseinate as a milk derivative in the ingredient list of foods that claim to be non-dairy, such as coffee whiteners.

As required by NLEA, beverages that claim to contain juice must declare the total percentage of juice on the information panel. In addition, FDA's regulation establishes criteria for naming juice beverages. For example, when the label of a multi-juice beverage states one or more—but not all—of the juices present, and the predominantly named juice is present in minor amounts, the product's name must state that the beverage is flavored with that juice or declare the amount of the juice in a 5 percent range—for example, "raspberry-flavored juice blend" or "juice blend, 2 to 7 percent raspberry juice."

MORE INFORMATION

For more information, contact:

FDA
General Inquiries: (888) INFO-FDA (or (888) 463-6332, toll free)
Food Safety Hotline: (800) 332-4010
FDA's food label information on the Web:
www.cfsan.fda.gov/label.html.

USDA
Food Safety Education and Communication Office
1400 Independence Ave., S.W., Room 1180
Washington, DC 20250
Meat and Poultry Hotline: (800) 535-4555.

APPENDIX VIII
ILLNESSES AND INJURIES ASSOCIATED WITH THE USE OF SELECTED DIETARY SUPPLEMENTS

Products marketed as "dietary supplements" include a diverse range of products, from traditional nutrients, such as vitamins or minerals, to such substances as high-potency free amino acids, botanicals, enzymes, animal extracts, and bioflavanoids that often have no scientifically recognized role in nutrition.

There is currently no systematic evaluation of the safety of products marketed as dietary supplements. Dietary supplements routinely enter the marketplace without undergoing a safety review by FDA. Published studies on the safety of these products are extremely sparse. There is no systematic collection and review of adverse reaction reports for dietary supplements, as there is for drugs, and physicians rarely seek information about their patients' use of dietary supplements. Despite the lack of any system for gaining information about the risks of dietary supplements, an increased number of reports of adverse reactions to dietary supplement products has recently been recognized. Because of concern about these products. FDA has, in the last year, initiated an effort to collect and evaluate existing studies and case reports on safety problems associated with dietary supplements. As a result of that effort, FDA has begun to identify dietary supplements for which serious adverse reactions have been documented. A list of selected dietary supplements associated with serious safety problems follows. This list is not intended to include all hazardous ingredients in dietary supplements.

I. HERBALS

Herbal and other botanical ingredients of dietary supplements include processed or unprocessed plant parts (bark, leaves, flowers, fruits, and stems), as well as extracts and essential oils. They are available in a variety of forms, including water infusions (teas), powders, tablets, capsules, and elixirs, and may be marketed as single substances or in combination with other materials, such as vitamins, minerals, amino acids, and non-nutrient ingredients. Although data on the availability, consumer use, and health effects of herbals are very limited, some herbal ingredients have been associated with serious adverse health effects.

A. Chaparral (Larrea tridentata)

Chaparral, commonly called the creosote bush, is a desert shrub with a long history of use as a traditional medicine by Native Americans. Chaparral is marketed as a tea, as well as in table, capsule, and concentrated extract form, and has been promoted as a natural antioxidant "blood purifier," cancer cure, and acne treatment. At least six cases (five in the United States and one in Canada) of acute non-viral hepatitis (rapidly developing liver damage) have been associated with the consumption of chaparral as a dietary supplement. Additional cases have been reported and are under investigation. In the majority of the cases reported thus far, the injury to the liver resolves over time, after discontinuation of the product. In at least two patients, however, there is evidence that chaparral consumption causes irreversible liver damage. One patient suffered terminal liver failure requiring liver transplant.

Most of these cases are associated with the consumption of single ingredient chaparral capsules or tablets; however, a few of the more recent cases appear to be associated with consumption of multi-ingredient products (capsules, tablets or teas) that contain chaparral as one ingredient. Chemical analyses have identified no contaminants in the products associated with the cases of hepatitis. Products from at least four different distributors and from at least two different sources have been implicated thus far.

After FDA's health warning, many distributors of chaparral products voluntarily removed the products from the market in December of 1992. Some chaparral products remain on the market, however, and other distributors who removed their products from the market are seeking to clarify the status of these products.

B. Comfrey (Symphytum officinale (common comfrey), S. asperum (prickly comfrey), or S. X uplandicum (Russian comfrey))

Preparations of comfrey, a fast-growing leafy plant, are widely sold in the United States as teas, tables, capsules, tinctures, medicinal poultices, and lotions. Since 1985, at least seven cases of hepatic veno-occlusive disease—obstruction of blood flow for the liver with potential scarring (cirrhosis)—including one death, have been associated with the use of commercially available oral comfrey products.

Comfrey, like a number of other plants (e.g., *Senecio* species), contains pyrrolizidine alkaloids. The toxicity of pyrrolizidine alkaloids to humans is well-documented. Hepatic veno-occlusive disease, following ingestion of pyrrolizidine alkaloid-containing products, has been documented repeatedly throughout the world. Hepatic veno-occlusive disease is usually acute and may result in fatal liver failure. In less severe cases, liver disease may progress to a subacute form. Even after apparent recovery, chronic liver disease, including cirrhosis, has been noted. Individuals who ingest small amounts of pyrrolizidine alkaloids for a prolonged period may also be at risk for development of hepatic cirrhosis. The diagnosis of pyrrolizidine alkaloid-induced hepatic veno-occlusive disease is complex, and the condition is probably underdiagnosed.

The degree of injury caused by pyrrolizidine alkaloid-containing plants, like comfrey, is probably influenced by such factors as the age of the user, body mass, gender, and hepatic function, as well the total cumulative dose ingested and the type of exposure (i.e., whether exposure was to leaves or roots, infusions or capsules). Infants in general appear to be particularly susceptible to adverse effects of exposure to pyrrolizidine alkaloids: there are reports of infants developing hepatic veno-occlusive disease following acute exposure of less than one week. Transplacental pyrrolizidine poisoning has been suggested by the occurrence of hepatic disease in the newborn infant of a woman who consumed herbal tea during pregnancy.

Although liver damage is the major documented form of injury to humans from pyrrolizidine alkaloid-containing herbals, animal studies suggest that their toxicity is much broader. Animals exposed to pyrrolizidine alkaloids have developed a wide range of pulmonary, kidney and gastrointestinal pathologies. Pyrrolizidine alkaloid-containing plants, including comfrey, have also been shown to cause cancer in laboratory animals.

Four countries (the United Kingdom, Australia, Canada, and Germany) have recently restricted the availability of products containing comfrey, and other countries permit use of comfrey only under a physician's prescription.

C. Yohimbe (Pausinystalia yohimbe)

Yohimbe is a tree bark containing a variety of pharmacologically active chemicals. It is marketed in a number of products for body building and "enhanced male performance." Serious adverse effects, including renal failure, seizures and death, have been reported to FDA with products containing yohimbe and are currently under investigation.

The major identified alkaloid in yohimbe is yohimbine, a chemical that causes vasodilation, thereby lowering blood pressure. Yohimbine is also a prescription drug in the United States. Side effects are well recognized and may include central nervous system stimulation that causes anxiety attacks. At high doses, yohimbine is a monoamine osidase (MAO) inhibitor. MAO inhibitors can cause serious adverse effects when taken concomitantly with tyramine-containing foods (e.g., liver, cheeses, red wine) or with over-the-counter (OTC) products containing phenylpropanolamme, such as nasal decongestants and diet aids. Individuals taking yohimbe should be warned to rigorously avoid these foods and OTC products because of the increased likelihood of adverse effects.

Yohimbe should also be avoided by individuals with hypotension (low blood pressure), diabetes, and heart, liver or kidney disease. Symptoms or overdosage include weakness and nervous stimulation followed by paralysis, fatigue, stomach disorders, and ultimately death.

D. Lobelia (Lobelia inflata)

Lobelia, also known as Indian tobacco, contains pyridine-derived alkaloids, primarily lobeline. These alkaloids have pharmacological actions similar to, although less potent than, nicotine. There have been several reported cases of adverse reactions associated with consumption of dietary supplements containing lobelia.

Depending on the dose, lobeline can cause either autonomic nervous system stimulation or depression. At low doses, it produces bronchial dilation and increased respiratory rate. Higher doses result in respiratory depression, as well as sweating, rapid heart rate, hypotension, and even coma and death. As little as 50 milligrams of dried herb or a single milliliter of lobelia tincture has caused these reactions.

Because of its similarity to nicotine, lobelia may be dangerous to susceptible populations, including children, pregnant women, and individuals with cardiac disease. Lobelia is nevertheless found in dietary supplement products that are marketed for use by children and infants, pregnant women, and smokers.

E. Germander (Teucrium genus)

Germander is the common name for a group of plants that are contained in medicinal teas, elixirs and capsules or tablets, either singly or in combination with other herbs, and marketed for the treatment of obesity and to facilitate weight loss.

Since 1986, at least 27 cases of acute nonviral hepatitis (liver disease), including one death, have been associated with the use of commercially available germander products in France. These cases show a clear temporal relationship between ingestion of germander and onset of hepatitis, as well as the resolution of symptoms when the use of ger-

mander was stopped. In 12 cases, re-administration of germander was followed by prompt recurrence of hepatitis. Recovery occurred gradually in most cases, approximately two to six months after withdrawal of germander. Analyses of these cases does not indicate a strong relationship between the dosage or duration of ingestion and the occurrence of hepatitis.

Although the constituent in germander responsible for its hepatic toxicity has not been identified, germander contains several chemicals, including polyphenols, tannins, diterpenoids, and flavonoids.

On the basis of the 27 French hepatitis cases, the French Ministry of Health has forbidden the use of germander in drugs. Its use has been restricted in other countries.

F. Willow Bark (Salix species)

Willow bark has long been used for its analgesic (pain-killing), antirheumatic, and antipyretic (fever-reducing) properties. Willow bark is widely promoted as an "aspirin-free" analgesic, including in dietary supplement products for children. Because it shares the same chemical properties and the same adverse effects as aspirin, this claim is highly misleading. The "aspirin-free" claim is particularly dangerous on products marketed, without warning labels, for use by children and other aspirin-sensitive individuals.

The pharmacologically active component in willow bark is "salicin," a compound that is converted to salicylic acid by the body after ingestion. Both willow bark and aspirin are salicylates, a class of compounds that work by virtue of their salicylic acid content. Aspirin (acetylsalicylic acid) is also converted to salicylic acid after ingestion.

All salicylates share substantially the same side effects. The major adverse effects include irritation of the gastric mucosa (a particular hazard to individuals with ulcer disease), adverse effects when used during pregnancy (including stillbirth, bleeding, prolonged gestation and labor, and low-birth-weight infants), stroke, and adverse effects in children with fever and dehydration. Children with influenza or chickenpox should avoid salicylates because their use, even in small doses, is associated with development of Reye syndrome, which is characterized by severe, sometimes fatal, liver injury. Salicylate intoxication (headache, dizziness, ringing in ears, difficulty hearing, dimness of vision, confusion, lassitude, drowsiness, sweating, hyperventilation, nausea, vomiting, and central nervous system disturbances in severe cases) may occur as the result of over-medication or kidney or liver insufficiency. Hypersensitivity, manifested by itching, bronchospasm and localized swelling (which may be life-threatening), can occur with very small doses of salicylates, and may occur even in those without a prior history of sensitivity to salicylates. Approximately 5 percent of the population is hypersensitive to salicylates.

G. Jin Bu Huan

Jin Bu Huan is a Chinese herbal product whose label claims that it is good for "insomnia due to pain," ulcer, "stomachic [sic] neuralgia, pain in shrunken womb after childbirth, nervous insomnia, spasmodic cough, and etc." Jin Bu Huan has been recently reported to be responsible for the poisoning of at least three young children (ages 13 months to 2 1/2 years), who accidentally ingested this product. The children were hospitalized with rapid-onset, life-threatening bradycardia (very low heart rate), and central nervous system and respiratory depression. One child required intubation (assisted breathing). All three ultimately recovered, following intensive medical care.

Although the product label identified the plant source for Jin Bu Huan as *Polygala chinensis,* this appears to be incorrect since preliminary analyses indicate the presence of tetrahydropalmatine (THP), a chemical not found in *Polygala.* THP is found, however, in high concentrations in plants of certain *Stephania* species. In animals, exposure to THP results in sedation, analgesia, and neuromuscular blockade (paralysis). The symptoms of the three children are consistent with these effects.

An additional case of THP toxicity, reported in the Netherlands, appears to be associated with the same product, and is being investigated.

H. Herbal Products Containing Stephania and Magnolia Species

A Chinese herbal preparation containing *Stephania* and *Magnolia* species that was sold as a weight-loss treatment in Belgium has been implicated recently

as a cause of severe kidney injury in at least 48 women. These cases were only discovered by diligent investigations by physicians treating two young women who presented with similar cases of rapidly progressing kidney disease that required renal dialysis. Once it was determined that both these women had used the herbal diet treatment, further investigation of kidney dialysis centers in Belgium found a total of 48 individuals with kidney injury who had used the herbal product.

At the time that a report of these adverse effects was published in February 1993, 18 of the 48 women had terminal kidney failure that will require either kidney transplantation or life-long renal dialysis.

I. Ma Huang

Ma huang is one of several names for herbal products containing members of the genus *Ephedra.* There are many common names for these evergreen plants, including squaw tea and Mormon tea. Serious adverse effects, including hypertension (elevated blood pressure), palpitations (rapid heart rate), neuropathy (nerve damage), myopathy (muscle injury), psychosis, stroke, and memory loss, have been reported to FDA with products containing Ma huang as ingredients and are currently under investigation.

The *Ephedras* have been shown to contain various chemical stimulants, including the alkaloids ephedrine, pseudoephedrine and norpseudoephedrine, as well as various tannins and related chemicals. The concentrations of these alkaloids depends upon the particular species of *Ephedra* used. Ephedrine and pseudoephedrine are amphetamine-like chemicals used in OTC and prescription drugs. Many of these stimulants have known serious side effects.

Ma huang is sold in products for weight control, as well as in products that boost energy levels. These products often contain other stimulants, such as caffeine, which may have synergistic effects and increase the potential for adverse effects.

II. AMINO ACIDS

Amino acids are the individual constituent parts of proteins. Consumption of foods containing intact proteins ordinarily provides sufficient amounts of the nine amino acids needed for growth and development in children and for maintenance of health of adults. The safety of amino acids in this form is generally not a concern. When marketed as dietary supplements, amino acids are sold as single compounds, in combinations of two or more amino acids, as components of protein powders, as chelated single compounds, or in chelated mixtures. Amino acids are promoted for a variety of uses, including body-building. Some are promoted for claimed pharmacologic effects.

The Federation of American Societies for Experimental Biology (FASEB) recently conducted an exhaustive search of available data on amino acids and concluded that there was insufficient information to establish a safe intake level for any amino acids in dietary supplements, and that their safety should not be assumed. FASEB warned that consuming amino acids in dietary supplement form posed potential risks for several subgroups of the general population, including women of childbearing age (especially if pregnant or nursing), infants, children, adolescents, the elderly, individuals with inherited disorders of amino acid metabolism, and individuals with certain diseases.

At least two of the amino acids consumed in dietary supplements have also been associated with serious injuries in healthy adults.

A. L-tryptophan

L-tryptophan is associated with the most serious recent outbreak of illness and death known to be due to consumption of dietary supplements. In 1989, public health officials realized that an epidemic of eosinophilia-myalgia syndrome (EMS) was associated with the ingestion of L-tryptophan in a dietary supplement. EMS is a systemic connective tissue disease characterized by severe muscle pain, an increase in white blood cells, and certain skin and neuromuscular manifestations.

More than 1,500 cases of L-tryptophan-related EMS have been reported to the national Centers for Disease Control and Prevention. At least 38 patients are known to have died. The true incidence of L-tryptophan-related EMS is thought to be much higher. Some of the individuals suffering from L-tryptophan-related EMS have recovered, while other individuals' illnesses have persisted or worsened over time.

Although initial epidemiologic studies suggested that the illnesses might be due to impurities in an L-tryptophan product from a single Japanese manufacturer, this hypothesis has not been verified, and additional evidence suggests that L-tryptophan itself may cause or contribute to development of EMS. Cases of EMS and related disorders have been found to be associated with ingestion of L-tryptophan from other batches or sources of L-tryptophan. These illnesses have also been associated with the use of L-5-hydroxytryptophan, a compound that is closely related to L-tryptophan, but is not produced using the manufacturing process that created the impurities in the particular Japanese product.

B. Phenylalanine

A number of illnesses, including those similar to the eosinophilia myalgia syndrome (EMS) associated with L-tryptophan consumption, have been reported to FDA in individuals using dietary supplements containing phenylalanine. There are also published reports of scleroderma/scleroderma-like illnesses, which have symptoms similar to EMS, occurring in children with poorly controlled blood phenylalanine levels, as well as in those with phenylketonuria (PKU), a genetic disorder characterized by the inability to metabolize phenylalanine.

III. VITAMINS AND MINERALS

Vitamin and mineral dietary supplements have a long history of use at levels consistent with the Recommended Dietary Allowances (RDA's) or at low multiplies of the RDA's, and are generally considered safe at these levels for the general population. Intakes above the RDA, however, vary widely in their potential for adverse effects. Certain vitamins and minerals that are safe when consumed at low levels are toxic at higher doses. The difference between a safe low dose and a toxic higher dose is quite large for some vitamins and minerals and quite small for others.

A. Vitamin A

Vitamin A is found in several forms in dietary supplements. Preformed vitamin A (vitamin A acetate and vitamin A palmitate) has well-recognized toxicity when consumed at levels of 25,000 International

Units (IU) per day, or higher. (Beta-carotene does not have the potential for adverse effects that the other forms of vitamin A do, because high intakes of beta-carotene are converted to vitamin A in the body at much lower levels.) The RDA for vitamin A is 1,000 retinol equivalents (RE) for men, which is equivalent to 3,300 IU of preformed vitamin A, and 80 percent of these amounts for women.

The adverse effects associated with consumption of vitamin A at 25,000+ IU include severe liver injury (including cirrhosis), bone and cartilage pathologies, elevated intracranial pressure, and birth defects in infants whose mothers consumed vitamin A during pregnancy. Groups especially vulnerable to vitamin A toxicity are children, pregnant women, and those with liver disease caused by a variety of factors, including alcohol, viral hepatitis, and severe protein-energy malnutrition.

There are some studies that suggest vitamin A toxicity has occurred at levels of ingestion below 25,000 IU. In addition, the severity of the injuries that occur at 25,000 IU suggests that substantial, but less severe and less readily recognized, injuries probably occur at somewhat lower intakes. Most experts recommend that vitamin A intake not exceed 10,000 IU for most adults or 8,000 IU for pregnant and nursing women.

B. Vitamin B_6

Neurologic toxicity, including ataxia (alteration in balance) and sensory neuropathy (changes in sensations due to nerve injury), is associated with intake of vitamin B_6 (pyridoxine) supplements at levels above 100 milligrams per day. As little as 50 milligrams per day has caused resumption of symptoms in an individual previously injured by higher intakes. The RDA for vitamin B_6 is 2 milligrams. Vitamin B_6 is marketed in capsules containing dosages in the 100-, 200- and 500- milligrams range.

C. Niacin (Nicotinic Acid and Nicotinamide)

Niacin taken in high doses is known to cause a wide range of adverse effects. The RDA for niacin is 20 milligrams. Niacin is marketed in dietary supplements at potencies of 250 mg, 400 mg, and 500 mg, in both immediate and slow-release formulations. Daily doses of 500 mg from slow-release formulations, and 750 mg of immediate-release

niacin, have been associated with severe adverse reactions, including gastrointestinal distress (burning pain, nausea, vomiting, bloating, cramping, and diarrhea) and mild to severe liver damage. Less common, but more serious (in some cases life-threatening), reactions include liver injury, myopathy (muscle disease), maculopathy of the eyes (injury to the eyes resulting in decreased vision), coagulopathy (increased bleeding problems), cytopenia (decreases in cell types in the blood), hypotensive myocardial ischemia (heart injury caused by too low blood pressure), and metabolic acidosis (increases in the acidity of the blood and urine).

Niacin (nicotinic acid) is approved as a prescription drug to lower cholesterol. Many of the observed adverse reactions have occurred when patients have switched to OTC formulations of niacin, and particularly when they have switched from immediate-release formulations to dietary supplements containing slow-release niacin formulations without the knowledge of their physicians.

D. Selenium

Selenium is a mineral found in dietary supplement products. At high doses (approximately 800 to 1,000 micrograms per day), selenium can cause tissue damage, especially in tissues or organs that concentrate the element. The toxicity of selenium depends upon the chemical form of selenium in the ingested supplement and upon the selenium levels in the foods consumed. Human injuries have occurred following ingestion of high doses over a few weeks.

IV. OTHER PRODUCTS MARKETED AS DIETARY SUPPLEMENTS

A. Germanium

Germanium is a nonessential element. Recently, germanium has been marketed in the form of inorganic germanium salts and novel organogermanium compounds, as a "dietary supplement." These products are promoted for their claimed immunomodulatory effects or as "health-promoting" elixirs. Germanium supplements, when used chronically, have caused nephrotoxicity (kidney injury) and death. Since 1982, there have been 20 reported cases of acute renal failure, including two deaths, attributed to oral intakes of germanium elixirs. In surviving patients, kidney function has improved after discontinuation of germanium, but none of the patients have recovered normal kidney function.

One particular organogermanium compound, an azaspiran organogermanium, has been studied for its potential use as an anticancer drug. Forty percent of the patients in this study experienced transient neurotoxicity (nerve damage), and two patients developed pulmonary toxicity. Because of these side effects, medically supervised administration of this drug with monitoring for toxicity has been recommended for those using germanium chronically.

APPENDIX IX

HEALTH AND HUMAN SERVICES ACTS TO REDUCE POTENTIAL RISKS OF DIETARY SUPPLEMENTS CONTAINING EPHEDRA

The following excerpt is taken from a press release issued by the Office of Public Affairs of the United States Food and Drug Administration, February 2003. Additional information on the topic may be found at the FDA website, http://www.fda.gov.

The Department of Health and Human Services (HHS) today announced a series of actions designed to protect Americans from potentially serious risks of dietary supplement products containing ephedra.

The results of a RAND Corporation study commissioned by the National Institutes of Health, as well as other recent studies, provide additional evidence that ephedra may be associated with important health risks. The RAND report also finds only limited evidence of health benefits resulting from ephedra use.

On the basis of new evidence in the medical literature and in adverse event reports, there are reasons for heightened concern that dietary supplements containing ephedra may present a significant and unreasonable risk of illness and injury.

To protect Americans from the potentially serious risks of these dietary supplements, HHS and FDA are going to:

- Seek rapid public comment on the new evidence on health risks associated with ephedra to establish an up-to-date record as quickly as possible to support new restrictions on ephedra-containing products.

- Seek rapid public comment on whether the currently available evidence and medical literature present a "significant or unreasonable risk of illness or injury" from dietary supplements containing ephedra.

- Seek rapid comment on a strong new warning label on any ephedra products that continue to be marketed.

- Immediately execute a series of actions against ephedra products making unsubstantiated claims about sports performance enhancement.

In addition, the nation's top public health officials issued strong statements cautioning about the use of ephedra-containing products, especially under conditions of strenuous exercise and in combination with other stimulants, including caffeine.

"We want to caution all Americans—particularly athletes and those who engage in strenuous activities—about using dietary supplements that contain ephedra," said Secretary of Health and Human Services Tommy G. Thompson. "There continue to be serious questions about the risks surrounding this particular dietary supplement."

"FDA will do all we can to protect Americans from potentially dangerous dietary supplements," said Commissioner of Food and Drugs Mark B. McClellan, M.D., Ph.D. "We are particularly concerned about the risks of using products containing ephedra during heavy workouts, with caffeine and other stimulants, in a diet program that stresses the cardiovascular system, or by people under the age of 18. We are also concerned about potential stresses to the body caused by the long-term use of ephedra. The standard for regulating the safety of dietary supplements is largely untested, but we are committed to finding the right public health solution."

Ephedra is a naturally occurring substance derived from the Chinese herbal Ma Huang. Its principal active ingredient is ephedrine, which when chemically synthesized is regulated as a drug. While products containing natural ephedrine alkaloids have long been used to treat certain respiratory symptoms in traditional Chinese medicine, in recent years they been extensively promoted and used with the goals of aiding weight loss, enhancing sports performance, and increasing energy.

Many of today's proposed actions involve a Federal Register notice, which went on display today, reopening for 30 days the comment period on a draft regulation FDA first proposed in 1997 and modified in 2000.

FDA's concerns about dietary supplements containing ephedra arise in part from ephedra's mechanism of action in the body. Ephedra is an adrenaline-like stimulant that can have potentially dangerous effects on the nervous system and heart.

In addition, evidence is accumulating about potentially serious safety problems following the use of ephedra-containing products. The RAND study has concluded that ephedra is associated with higher risks of mild to moderate side effects such as heart palpitations, psychiatric and upper gastrointestinal effects, and symptoms of autonomic hyperactivity such as tremor and insomnia, especially when it is taken with other stimulants.

Moreover, its review of some 16,000 adverse event reports revealed two deaths, four heart attacks, nine strokes, one seizure, and five psychiatric cases involving ephedra in which the records appeared thorough and no other contributing factors were identified. RAND called such cases "sentinel events," because they may indicate a safety problem but do not prove that ephedra caused the adverse event. The study recognized that such case studies are a weak form of scientific evidence. Other unmeasured factors may have contributed, and such serious adverse events are likely to happen (albeit at very low rates) among the millions of users of ephedra anyway. The study also identified other such events potentially associated with

ephedra, in which other factors may have contributed to the adverse events or in which records were inadequate.

Two recent studies of ephedra's safety were published too late to be included in the RAND Corporation's review, and each raises further concerns about ephedra. One, published this month in the *Annals of Internal Medicine*, found that although ephedra-products make up less than one percent of all dietary supplement sales, these products account for 64 percent of adverse events associated with dietary supplements.

Another "case-control" study, published in the journal *Neurology*, concluded that the rate of hemorrhagic (bleeding) strokes among ephedra users was statistically significantly higher than among non-users, for people who take doses above 32 milligrams a day. Many ephedra dietary supplement labels recommend that users take up to approximately 100 mg of ephedra daily.

Additional relevant evidence on whether the current system of regulating ephedra's safety is adequate comes from results under FDA's more extensive regulation of synthetic ephedrine, which is identical to the main active ingredient in ephedra. Ephedrine has long been available in some FDA-approved over-the-counter and prescription drugs. It appears that the more controlled availability of synthetic ephedrine products, which are available primarily for approved uses for respiratory symptoms and carry mandatory warning labels, has not been associated with the same kind of severe adverse events as have occurred with dietary supplements containing ephedra. This long experience with synthetic ephedrine (in over-the-counter drug products, not in dietary supplements) suggests that significant restrictions on labeling, marketing, and/or access to ephedrine might effectively address unreasonable risks associated with certain forms of ephedra today.

"Although the overall evidence suggests that serious adverse events from ephedra appear to be infrequent," said Dr. McClellan, "we know that such events can be very serious and possibly fatal. We believe that the current scientific evidence strongly suggests that at least some ephedra products present an unreasonable risk. We also believe that FDA's system for regulating synthetic versions of the chemicals in ephedra appears to have a much better track record of safety. To give us the strongest possible basis for further regulatory action, we are asking for quick comments on whether these dietary supplements present an unreasonable risk of harm, and whether it makes sense for FDA to seek new authority in this area."

Under the Dietary Supplement Health and Education Act of 1994, FDA does not review dietary supplements for safety and effectiveness before they are marketed. Rather, the law allows FDA to prohibit sale of a dietary supplement if it "presents a significant or unreasonable risk of injury." This legal standard of "significant or unreasonable risk" implies a risk-benefit calculation based on the best available scientific evidence. It strongly suggests that the agency must determine if a product's known or supposed risks outweigh any known or suspected benefits, based on the available scientific evidence, in light of the claims the product makes and in light of the product's being sold directly to consumers without medical supervision.

In seeking comment on these issues, FDA is reopening a proposed rule entitled "Dietary Supplements Containing Ephedrine Alkaloids." That proposal would have required a warning statement for these products, as well as restrictions on their potency and composition. FDA later withdrew parts of this proposed rule because of concerns about the specific scientific evidence in the proposal, expressed by the General Accounting Office.

In a broad action against potentially dangerous products, FDA today sent more than two dozen warning letters to firms marketing dietary supplements that contain ephedrine alkaloids. The letters, targeted particularly at products making claims for athletic performance, explain that any claims their products make about effects on the structure and function of the human body must be truthful and not misleading. They outline FDA's view in light of the RAND report that the claims being made are not adequately substantiated by scientific data, and they direct the companies to submit any data supporting the claims within 15 days.

The letters also warn firms that they must not make claims about their products' ability to treat or cure a disease or condition such as obesity. Under the Federal Food, Drug and Cosmetic Act, unapproved products making these "disease claims" are unapproved new drugs and therefore subject to other prompt regulatory actions, including injunctions against firms and seizures of their products.

FDA will also continue to work closely with the Federal Trade Commission to ensure that dietary supplement products containing ephedra do not make false and misleading claims. "If an ad says a product is 'safe,' the advertiser's must have competent and reliable evidence to prove the claim," said Timothy J. Muris, chairman of the Federal Trade Commission. "Consumers depend on advertising for factual information and deceptive ad claims can put a consumer's health at risk. That's why the FTC is currently investigating a number of weight loss products containing ephedra and we will continue to pursue aggressively marketers making unsubstantiated claims about product safety or effectiveness."

In addition, FDA today proposed a warning label for all ephedra-containing dietary supplements. The proposed label warns about the risks of serious adverse events, including heart attack, seizure, stroke, and death; cautions that the risk can increase with the dose, with strenuous exercise, and with other stimulants such as caffeine; specifies certain groups (such as women who are pregnant or breast feeding) who should never use these products; and lists other conditions, such as diseases and the use of certain medications, that rule out the use of ephedrine alkaloids.

"The steps being announced today demonstrate FDA's commitment to taking the most effective actions possible under current law, given the state of the scientific evidence," said Dr. McClellan. "It may be possible to use ephedra safely, in small doses, for some purposes. But in the face of continued serious adverse events following the use of ephedra, there is a problem. It is a problem we are determined to fix."

APPENDIX X
NCCAM CONSUMER ADVISORY ON EPHEDRA— REVISED FEBRUARY 28, 2003

Dietary supplements containing ephedra, which have been in the news recently because of the deaths of well-known athletes, may cause rare but serious health consequences. The U.S. Department of Health and Human Services (HHS) announced on Friday, February 28, 2003, a series of actions designed to protect the public from the risks of dietary supplements containing ephedra. HHS and its component agencies all caution the public that the use of ephedra poses health risks, especially when used for strenuous exercise and when used with other stimulants, such as caffeine.

WHAT IS EPHEDRA?

Herbal products containing ephedra (also known as herbal ephedrine alkaloids) are marketed in the United States as dietary supplements that claim to promote weight loss, increase energy, and enhance athletic performance. Ephedrine alkaloids, including the chemical known as ephedrine, are amphetamine-like compounds that potentially have powerful stimulant effects on the nervous system and heart. These alkaloids are found naturally in a number of plants, including the ephedra species of herbs (also known by its traditional Chinese medicine name—*ma huang* or Chinese Ephedra, or epitonin), but they can also be manufactured in the laboratory.

Like an amphetamine, ephedra stimulates the central nervous system, increasing blood pressure and heart rate, decreasing appetite, and making the user feel energetic. In synthetic form, ephedrine is regulated as a drug and is used as a decongestant for the short-term treatment of asthma, bronchitis, and allergic reactions by opening the air passages in the lungs.

WHAT ARE EPHEDRA'S SIDE EFFECTS AND RISKS?

Although dietary supplements containing ephedra are widely used, many adverse event (serious reactions and problems) reports have been received by the U.S. Food and Drug Administration (FDA). These reports have raised questions regarding ephedra's overall safety. Serious side effects reported in ephedra users include nausea and vomiting, psychiatric disturbances such as agitation and anxiety, high blood pressure, irregular heartbeat, and more rarely seizures, heart attack, stroke, and even death. The International Olympic Committee, the National Football League, the National Collegiate Athletic Association, minor league baseball, and the U.S. Armed Forces have all banned the use of ephedra.

SCIENTIFIC REVIEW OF EPHEDRA

NCCAM and the National Institutes of Health (NIH) Office of Dietary Supplements sponsored, through the Agency for Healthcare Research and Quality, a systematic review of the existing scientific literature on ephedra efficacy and safety in weight loss and athletic performance enhancement. The report, conducted by the RAND Corporation, is available at www.ahrq.gov/clinic/evrptfiles.htm#ephedra. The review was conducted to assist NIH in developing an appropriate research agenda, to identify gaps in knowledge, and to suggest study designs that would yield more definitive answers regarding its safety.

FDA SEEKING PUBLIC COMMENT

The FDA is reviewing whether ephedra-containing products should be on the market. Dietary supplements are not regulated the same way as drugs are. The Dietary Supplement Health and Education Act (DSHEA) requires proof of harm—a higher standard than used in prescription drug development—before a supplement like ephedra can be banned from the market. NIH-sponsored research like the recent RAND report provides the evidence on which decisions about the safety and effectiveness of products can be assessed. On February 28, 2003, the FDA announced that it is asking for public comment on whether, in light of the RAND report and other newly reported research findings, ephedra poses an unreasonable risk as currently marketed under DSHEA.

NCCAM EPHEDRA RESEARCH

In addition to supporting the RAND study with the NIH Office of Dietary Supplements and a recent study of reports to poison control centers of reactions to ephedra and other herbal products, NCCAM is funding two laboratory studies of ephedra to better understand the mechanism of action and chemical properties of this herb.

- Pharmacology of Combined Ephedrine/Caffeine Supplements, University of California, San Francisco
- Effects of Ephedra on Human Adrenoceptor Subtypes, University of Mississippi

The National Advisory Council on Complementary and Alternative Medicine will review the RAND report and additional research findings and discuss what further research studies concerning the safety or effectiveness of ephedra might be warranted. The Advisory Council will meet by conference call on March 17, 2003.

SUMMARY

At present, there is no evidence that ephedra products enhance athletic performance and only preliminary evidence that ephedra promotes small amounts of weight loss for a few months. There is evidence that ephedra is associated with an increased risk of side effects, possibly even fatal ones. NCCAM will be considering further research on ephedra, but in the meantime, people should be concerned about the significant risks it poses while offering limited benefits. While respecting the traditional uses of herbal medicines, their long history, and their potential health benefits, NCCAM believes that ephedra poses unique public health challenges that warrant the public's attention.

ADVICE TO CONSUMERS

Safety should be the primary concern for all users of ephedra. Consumers under the age of 18 or pregnant or nursing women should not use ephedra products.

Adults should consult a health care provider before using ephedra products if they have a history of high blood pressure, heart or thyroid disease, a seizure disorder, depression, diabetes, difficulty urinating, prostate enlargement, glaucoma, or are using any prescription drug.

Consumers should consult with a physician prior to using dietary supplements containing ephedra if they are also using a monoamine oxidase inhibitor (MAO inhibitors are drugs used in the treatment of selected atypical depressions) or any allergy, asthma, or cold medications containing ephedrine, pseudoephedrine, or phenylpropanolamine.

Consumers should discontinue use of ephedra and consult a physician if any of the following symptoms are experienced: rapid or irregular heartbeat, chest pain, severe headache, shortness of breath, dizziness, loss of consciousness, sleeplessness, or nausea.

APPENDIX XI
HEALTHY PEOPLE 2010

Healthy People 2010: Objectives for Improving Health is a set of goals and a plan for nationally increasing general health and health awareness. It discusses a wide range of health issues and preventive measures. The following excerpt, Chapter 19, covers nutrition. For more information on *Healthy People 2010,* go to http://www.healthypeople.gov.

NUTRITION AND OVERWEIGHT

Co-Lead Agencies: Food and Drug Administration and National Institutes of Health

Contents

GOAL

Promote health and reduce chronic disease associated with diet and weight.

OVERVIEW

Issues and Trends

Nutrition is essential for growth and development, health, and well-being. Behaviors to promote health should start early in life with breastfeeding[1] and continue through life with the development of healthful eating habits. Nutritional, or dietary, factors contribute substantially to the burden of preventable illnesses and prema-

ture deaths in the United States.[2] Indeed, dietary factors are associated with 4 of the 10 leading causes of death: coronary heart disease (CHD), some types of cancer, stroke, and type 2 diabetes.[3] These health conditions are estimated to cost society over $200 billion each year in medical expenses and lost productivity.[4] Dietary factors also are associated with osteoporosis, which affects more than 25 million persons in the United States and is the major underlying cause of bone fractures in postmenopausal women and elderly persons.[5]

Many dietary components are involved in the relationship between nutrition and health. A pri-

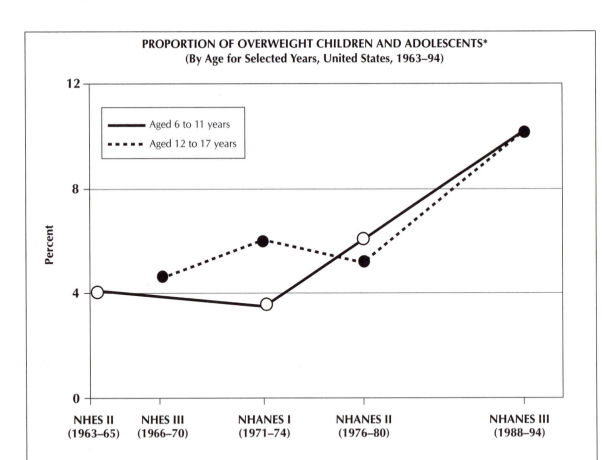

PROPORTION OF OVERWEIGHT CHILDREN AND ADOLESCENTS*
(By Age for Selected Years, United States, 1963–94)

*Overweight is defined as at or above the gender-and age-specific 95th percentile of body mass index (BMI) based on a preliminary analysis of data from the revised CDC Growth Charts for the United States.

Source: Adapted from Troiano, R.P., and Flegal K.M. Data as reported in: "Overweight children and adolescents: Description, epidemiology, and demographics." *Pediatrics* 101: 497–504, 1998.

mary concern is consuming too much saturated fat and too few vegetables, fruits, and grain products that are high in vitamins and minerals, carbohydrates (starch and dietary fiber), and other substances that are important to good health. The 2000 *Dietary Guidelines for Americans* recommend that, to stay healthy, persons aged 2 years and older should follow these ABCs for good health: **A**im for fitness, **B**uild a healthy base, and **C**hoose sensibly. To aim for fitness, aim for a healthy weight and be physically active each day. To build a healthy base, let the Pyramid guide food choices; choose a variety of grains daily, especially whole grains; choose a variety of fruits and vegetables daily; and keep food safe to eat. To choose sensibly, choose a diet that is low in saturated fat and cholesterol and moderate in total fat; choose beverages and foods to moderate intake of sugars; choose and prepare foods with less salt; and if consuming alcoholic beverages, do so in moderation.[6] The Food Guide Pyramid, introduced in 1992, is an educational tool that conveys recommendations about the number of servings from different food groups each day and other principles of the *Dietary Guidelines for Americans.*[7] [Note: In text that follows in this chapter, *Dietary Guidelines for Americans* will refer to the 2000 *Dietary Guidelines for Americans* unless otherwise noted.]

The *Dietary Guidelines for Americans* also emphasize the need for adequate consumption of iron-rich and calcium-rich foods.[6] Although some progress has been made since the 1970s in reducing the prevalence of iron deficiency among low-income children,[8] much more is needed to improve the health of children of all ages and of women who are pregnant or are of childbearing age. Since the start of this decade, consumption of calcium-rich foods, such as milk products, has generally decreased and is especially low among teenaged girls and young women.[9] Because important sources of calcium also can include other foods with calcium—occurring naturally or through fortification—as well as dietary supplements, the current emphasis is on tracking total calcium intake from all sources, as demonstrated by an objective in this focus area. In addition, in recent years there has been a concerted effort to increase the folic acid intake of females of child-bearing age through

fortication and other means to reduce the risk of neural tube defects.[10, 11] (See Focus Area 16. Maternal, Infant, and Child Health.)

In general, however, excesses and imbalances of some food components in the diet have replaced once commonplace nutrient deficiencies. Unfortunately, there has been an alarming increase in the number of overweight and obese persons.[12, 13] Overweight results when a person eats more calories from food (energy) than he or she expends, for example, through physical activity. This balance between energy intake and output is influenced by metabolic and genetic factors as well as behaviors affecting dietary intake and physical activity; environmental, cultural, and socioeconomic components also play a role.

When a body mass index (BMI) cut-point of 25 is used, nearly 55 percent of the U.S. adult population was defined as overweight or obese in 1988–94, compared to 46 percent in 1976–80.[12, 14, 15] In particular, the proportion of adults defined as obese by a BMI of 30 or greater has increased from 14.5 percent to 22.5 percent.[12] A similar increase in overweight and obesity also has been observed in children above age 6 years in both genders and in all population groups.[16]

Many diseases are associated with overweight and obesity. Persons who are overweight or obese are at increased risk for high blood pressure, type 2 diabetes, coronary heart disease, stroke, gallbladder disease, osteoarthritis, sleep apnea, respiratory problems, and some types of cancer. The health outcomes related to these diseases, however, often can be improved through weight loss or, at a minimum, no further weight gain. Total costs (medical costs and lost productivity) attributable to obesity alone amounted to an estimated $99 billion in 1995.[17]

Disparities

Disparities in health status indicators and risk factors for diet-related disease are evident in many segments of the population based on gender, age, race and ethnicity, and income. For example, overweight and obesity are observed in all population groups, but obesity is particularly common among Hispanic, African American, Native American, and Pacific Islander women. Furthermore, despite concerns about the increase in overweight and certain excesses in U.S. diets, segments of the population also suffer from undernutrition, including persons who are socially isolated and poor. Over the years, the recognition of the consequences of food insecurity (limited access to safe, nutritious food) has led to the development of national measures and surveys to evaluate food insecurity and hunger and to the ability to assess disparities among different population groups. With food security and other measures of undernutrition, such as growth retardation and iron deficiency, disparities are evident based not only on income but also on race and ethnicity.

In addition, there are concerns about the nutritional status of persons in hospitals, nursing homes, convalescent centers, and institutions; persons with disabilities, including physically, mentally, and developmentally disabled persons in community settings; children in child care facilities; persons living on reservations; persons in correctional facilities; and persons who are homeless. National data about these population groups are currently unavailable or limited. Data also are insufficient to target the fastest growing segment of the population, old and very old persons who live independently.

Opportunities

Establishing healthful dietary and physical activity behaviors needs to begin in childhood. Educating school-aged children about nutrition is important to help establish healthful eating habits early in life.[18, 19] Research suggests that parents who understand proper nutrition can help children in preschool choose healthful foods, but they have less influence on the choices of school-aged children.[20] Thus, the impact of nutrition education on health may be more effective if targeted directly at school-aged children. Unfortunately, a survey done in 1994 showed that only 69 percent of States and 80 percent of school districts required nutrition education for students in at least some grades from kindergarten through 12th grade.[21]

A well-designed curriculum that effectively addresses essential nutrition education topics can increase students' knowledge about nutrition, help shape appropriate attitudes, and help develop the behavioral skills students need to plan, prepare,

and select healthful meals and snacks.[18, 22, 23] Curricula that encourage specific, healthful eating behaviors and provide students with the skills needed to adopt and maintain those behaviors have led to favorable changes in student dietary behaviors and cardiovascular disease risk factors.[18, 22, 23] In order to enhance the effectiveness of these lessons, however, nutrition course work should be part of the core curriculum for the professional preparation of teachers of all grades and should be emphasized in continuing education activities for teachers.

Topics considered to be essential at the elementary, middle, junior high, and senior high school levels include using the Food Guide Pyramid; learning the benefits of healthful eating; making healthful food choices for meals and snacks; preparing healthy meals and snacks; using food labels; eating a variety of foods; eating more fruits, vegetables, and grains; eating foods low in saturated fat and total fat more often; eating more calcium-rich foods; balancing food intake and physical activity; accepting body size differences; and following food safety practices.[18, 24] In addition, the following topics are considered to be essential at the middle, junior high, and senior high school levels: the *Dietary Guidelines for Americans;* eating disorders; healthy weight maintenance; influences on food choices such as families, culture, and media; and goals for dietary improvement.[18]

Nutrition education should be taught as part of a comprehensive school health education program, and essential nutrition education topics should be integrated into science and other curricula to reinforce principles and messages learned in the health units. Nutrition education is addressed within a school health education objective. (See Focus Area 7. Educational and Community-Based Programs.) In addition, students must have access to healthful food choices to enhance further the likelihood of adopting healthful dietary practices. For these reasons, monitoring students' eating practices at school is important.

Although health promotion efforts should begin in childhood, they need to continue throughout adulthood. In particular, public education about the long-term health consequences and risks associated with overweight and how to achieve and maintain a healthy weight is necessary. While many persons attempt to lose weight, studies show that within 5 years a majority regain the weight.[25] To maintain weight loss, healthful dietary habits must be coupled with decreased sedentary behavior and increased physical activity and become permanent lifestyle changes. (See Focus Area 22. Physical Activity and Fitness.) Additionally, changes in the physical and social environment may help persons maintain the necessary long-term lifestyle changes for both diet and physical activity.

Policymakers and program planners at the national, State, and community levels can and should provide important leadership in fostering healthful diets and physical activity patterns among people in the United States. The family and others, such as health care practitioners, schools, worksites, institutional food services, and the media, can play a key role in this process. For example, registered dietitians and other qualified health care practitioners can improve health outcomes through efforts focused on nutrition screening, assessment, and primary and secondary prevention.

Food-related businesses also can help consumers achieve healthful diets by providing nutrition information for foods purchased in supermarkets, fast-food outlets, restaurants, and carryout operations. For example, the introduction of a new food label in 1993 has resulted in nutrition information on most processed packaged foods, along with credible health and nutrient content claims and standardized serving sizes.[26] While efforts were made in the 1990s to increase the availability of nutrition information, reduced-fat foods, and other healthful food choices in supermarkets, significant challenges remain on these fronts for away-from-home foods purchased at food service outlets. The importance of addressing these challenges is suggested by recent data indicating that nearly 40 percent of a family's food budget is spent on away-from-home food, including food from restaurants and fast-food outlets.[27] One analysis found that away-from-home foods are generally higher in saturated fat, total fat, cholesterol, and sodium and lower in dietary fiber, iron, and calcium than at-home foods.[27] Away-from-home sites include restaurants, fast-food outlets, school cafeterias, vending machines, and other food service outlets. This study also suggested that persons either eat larger amounts when they eat out, eat higher calorie foods, or both.

Many of the Healthy People 2010 objectives that address nutrition and overweight in the United States measure in some way the Nation's progress toward implementing the recommendations of the *Dietary Guidelines for Americans.* The recommendations for food and nutrient intake are not intended to be met every day but rather on average over a span of time. Although the Healthy People 2010 dietary intake objectives address the proportion of the population that consumes a specified level of certain foods or nutrients, it is also important to track and report the average amount eaten by different population groups to help interpret progress on these objectives. Other objectives target aspects of undernutrition, including iron deficiency, growth retardation, and food security.

In summary, several actions are recognized as fundamental in achieving this focus area's objectives:

- Improving accessibility of nutrition information, nutrition education, nutrition counseling and related services, and healthful foods in a variety of settings and for all population groups.

- Focusing on preventing chronic disease associated with diet and weight, beginning in youth.

- Strengthening the link between nutrition and physical activity in health promotion.

- Maintaining a strong national program for basic and applied nutrition research to provide a sound science base for dietary recommendations and effective interventions.

- Maintaining a strong national nutrition monitoring program to provide accurate, reliable, timely, and comparable data to assess status and progress and to be responsive to unmet data needs and emerging issues.

- Strengthening State and community data systems to be responsive to the data users at these levels.

- Building and sustaining broad-based initiatives and commitment to these objectives by public and private sector partners at the national State, and local levels.

INTERIM PROGRESS TOWARD YEAR 2000 OBJECTIVES

Of the 27 nutrition objectives, targets for 5 have been met, including 2 related to the availability of reduced-fat foods and prevalence of growth retardation.[28] The majority of the objectives have shown some progress, including those related to total fruit, vegetable, and grain product intake and total fat and saturated fat intake; availability of nutrition labeling on foods; breastfeeding; nutrition education in schools; and availability of worksite nutrition and weight management programs. For certain other objectives, such as consumer actions to reduce salt intake and home-delivered meals to elderly persons, there has been little or no progress. And for others, such as intake of calcium-rich food and overweight and obesity, movement has been away from the targets. In particular, the proportion of adults and children who are overweight or obese has increased substantially, and this represents one of the biggest challenges for Healthy People 2010.

Note: Unless otherwise noted, data are from the Centers for Disease Control and Prevention, National Center for Health Statistics, *Healthy People 2000 Review, 1998–99.*

HEALTHY PEOPLE 2010—SUMMARY OF OBJECTIVES

Nutrition and Overweight

Goal: Promote health and reduce chronic disease associated with diet and weight.

Number	Objective Short Title
Weight Status and Growth	
19-1	Healthy weight in adults
19-2	Obesity in adults
19-3	Overweight or obesity in children and adolescents
19-4	Growth retardation in children
Food and Nutrient Consumption	
19-5	Fruit intake
19-6	Vegetable intake
19-7	Grain product intake
19-8	Saturated fat intake
19-9	Total fat intake
19-10	Sodium intake
19-11	Calcium intake
Iron Deficiency and Anemia	
19-12	Iron deficiency in young children and in females of childbearing age
19-13	Anemia in low-income pregnant females
19-14	Iron deficiency in pregnant females
Schools, Worksites, and Nutrition Counseling	
19-15	Meals and snacks at school
19-16	Worksite promotion of nutrition education and weight management
19-17	Nutrition counseling for medical conditions
Food Security	
19-18	Food security

HEALTHY PEOPLE 2010 OBJECTIVES

Weight Status and Growth

19-1. Increase the proportion of adults who are at a healthy weight.

Target: 60 percent.

Baseline: 42 percent of adults aged 20 years and older were at a healthy weight (defined as a body mass index [BMI] equal to or greater than 18.5 and less than 25) in 1988–94 (age adjusted to the year 2000 standard population).

Target setting method: Better than the best.

Data source: National Health and Nutrition Examination Survey (NHANES), CDC, NCHS.

| | Healthy Weight | | |
	19-1. Both Genders	Females*	Males*
Adults Aged 20 Years and Older, 1988–94 (unless noted)	Percent		
TOTAL	42	45	38
Race and ethnicity			
American Indian or Alaska Native	DSU	DSU	DSU
Asian or Pacific Islander	DSU	DSU	DSU
Asian	DNC	DNC	DNC
Native Hawaiian and other Pacific Islander	DNC	DNC	DNC
Black or African American	34	29	40
White	42	47	37
Hispanic or Latino	DSU	DSU	DSU
Mexican American	30	31	30
Not Hispanic or Latino	43	47	39
Black or African American	34	29	40
White	43	49	38
Age			
20 to 39 years	51	55	48
40 to 59 years	36	40	31
60 years and older	36	37	33
Family income level†			
Lower income (≤130 percent of poverty threshold)	38	33	44
Higher income (>130 percent of poverty threshold)	43	48	37
Disability status			
Persons with disabilities	32 (1991–94)	35 (1991–94)	30 (1991–94)
Persons without disabilities	41 (1991–94)	45 (1991–94)	36 (1991–94)
Select populations			
Persons with arthritis	36 (1991–94)	37 (1991–94)	34 (1991–94)
Persons without arthritis	43 (1991–94)	47 (1991–94)	40 (1991–94)
Persons with diabetes	26	DNA	DNA
Persons without diabetes	43	DNA	DNA
Persons with high blood pressure	27	29	26
Persons without high blood pressure	46	50	42

DNA = Data have not been analyzed. DNC = Data are not collected. DSU = Data are statistically unreliable.

Note: Age adjusted to the year 2000 standard population.

*Data for females and males are displayed to further characterize the issue.

†A household income below 130 percent of poverty threshold is used by the Food Stamp Program.

19-2. Reduce the proportion of adults who are obese.

Target: 15 percent.

Baseline: 23 percent of adults aged 20 years and older were identified as obese (defined as a BMI of 30 or more) in 1988–94 (age adjusted to the year 2000 standard population).

Target setting method: Better than the best.

Data source: National Health and Nutrition Examination Survey (NHANES), CDC, NCHS.

| Adults Aged 20 Years and Older, 1988–94 (unless noted) | Obesity | | |
	19-2. Both Genders	Females*	Males*
	Percent		
TOTAL	23	25	20
Race and ethnicity			
American Indian or Alaska Native	DSU	DSU	DSU
Asian or Pacific Islander	DSU	DSU	DSU
Asian	DNC	DNC	DNC
Native Hawaiian and other Pacific Islander	DNC	DNC	DNC
Black or African American	30	38	21
White	22	24	21
Hispanic or Latino	DSU	DSU	DSU
Mexican American	29	35	24
Not Hispanic or Latino	22	25	20
Black or African American	30	38	21
White	22	23	20
Age (not age adjusted)			
20 to 39 years	18	21	15
40 to 59 years	28	30	25
60 years and older	24	26	21
Family income level†			
Lower income (≤130 percent of poverty threshold)	29	35	21
Higher income (>130 percent of poverty threshold)	22	23	20
Disability status			
Persons with disabilities	30 (1991–94)	38 (1991–94)	21 (1991–94)
Persons without disabilities	23 (1991–94)	25 (1991–94)	22 (1991–94)
Select populations			
Persons with arthritis	30	33	27
Persons without arthritis	21	23	19
Persons with diabetes	41	DNA	DNA
Persons without diabetes	22	DNA	DNA
Persons with high blood pressure	38	47	33
Persons without high blood pressure	18	20	16

DNA = Data have not been analyzed. DNC = Data are not collected. DSU = Data are statistically unreliable.

Note: Age adjusted to the year 2000 standard population.

*Data for females and males are displayed to further characterize the issue.

†A household income below 130 percent of poverty threshold is used by the Food Stamp Program.

19-3. Reduce the proportion of children and adolescents who are overweight or obese.

Target and baseline:

Objective	Reduction in Overweight or Obese Children and Adolescents*	1988–94 Baseline	2010 Target
		Percent	
19-3a.	Children aged 6 to 11 years	11	5
19-3b.	Adolescents aged 12 to 19 years	11	5
19-3c.	Children and adolescents aged 6 to 19 years	11	5

*Defined as at or above the gender- and age-specific 95th percentile of BMI based on the revised CDC Growth Charts for the United States.

Target setting method: Better than the best.

Data source: National Health and Nutrition Examination Survey (NHANES), CDC, NCHS.

	Overweight or Obese		
Children and Adolescents Aged 6 to 19 Years, 1988–94 (unless noted)	19-3a. Children Aged 6 to 11 Years	19-3b. Adolescents Aged 12 to 19 Years	19-3c. Children and Adolescents Aged 6 to 19 Years
	Percent		
TOTAL	11	11	11
Race and ethnicity			
American Indian or Alaska Native	DSU	DSU	DNA
Asian or Pacific Islander	DS7		
Asian	DNC	DNC	DNC
Native Hawaiian and other Pacific Islander	DNC	DNC	DNC
Black or African American	15	13	14
White	11	11	11
Hispanic or Latino	DSU	DSU	DSU
Mexican American	17	14	15
Not Hispanic or Latino	11	10	11
Black or African American	15	13	14
White	10	10	10
Gender			
Female	11	10	10
Male	12	11	12
Family income level*			
Lower income (≤130 percent of poverty threshold)	11	16	13
Higher income (>130 percent of poverty threshold)	11	8	10
Disability status			
Persons with disabilities	DSU (1991–94)	DSU (1991–94)	DSU (1991–94)
Persons without disabilities	13 (1991–94)	11 (1991–94)	12 (1991–94)

DNA = Data have not been analyzed. DNC = Data are not collected. DSU = Data are statistically unreliable.

*A household income below 130 percent of poverty threshold is used by the Food Stamp Program.

Maintenance of a healthy weight is a major goal in the effort to reduce the burden of illness and its consequent reduction in quality of life and life expectancy. The selection of a BMI cut-point to establish the upper limit of the healthy weight range is based on the relationship of overweight or obesity to risk factors for chronic disease or premature death. A BMI of less than 25 has been accepted by numerous groups as the upper limit of the healthy weight range, since chronic disease risk increases in most populations at or above this cut-point.[14, 15, 29] The lower cut-point for the healthy weight range (BMI of 18.5) was selected to be consistent with national and international recommendations.[14, 15] Problems associated with excessive thinness (BMI less than 18.5) include menstrual irregularity, infertility, and osteoporosis. There is some concern that the increased focus on overweight may result in more eating disorders, such as bulimia and anorexia nervosa. (See Focus Area 18. Mental Health and Mental Disorders.) However, no evidence currently exists that suggests the increased focus on overweight has resulted in additional cases of eating disorders.

Overweight and obesity are caused by many factors. These factors reflect the contributions of inherited, metabolic, behavioral, environmental, cultural, and socio-economic components. As weight increases, so does the prevalence of health risks. Simple, health-oriented definitions of overweight and obesity should be based on the amount of excess body fat at which health risks to individuals begin to increase. No such definitions currently exist. Most current clinical studies assessing the health effects of overweight rely on a measurement of body weight adjusted for height. BMI is the choice for many researchers and health professionals. While the relation of BMI to body fat differs by age and gender, it provides valid comparisons across racial and ethnic groups.[30] However, BMI does not provide information concerning body fat distribution, which has been identified as an independent predictor of health risk.[15, 29] Thus, until a better surrogate for body fat is developed, BMI often will be used to screen for overweight and obese individuals. Health risks also increase as waist measurement increases, and thus waist measurement also can be a useful indicator.[6]

Interpretations of data about overweight and obesity have differed because criteria for these terms have varied over time, from study to study, and from one part of the world to another. National and international organizations now support the use of a BMI of 30 or greater to identify obesity.[14, 15] These BMI cut-points are only a guide to the identification and treatment of overweight and obese individuals and allow for the comparison across populations and over time. However, the health risks associated with overweight and obesity are part of a continuum and do not conform to rigid cut-points.

Overweight and obesity affect a large proportion of the U.S. population—55 percent of adults. Between 1976 and 1994, the number of cases of obesity alone increased more than 50 percent—from 14.5 percent of the adult population to 22.5 percent. Approximately 25 percent of U.S. adult females and 20 percent of U.S. adult males are obese.[12] Because weight management is difficult for most persons, the Healthy People 2010 target of no more than 15 percent of adults aged 20 years and older having a BMI of 30 or more is ambitious. Nonetheless, the potential benefits from reduction in overweight and obesity are of considerable public health importance and deserve particular emphasis and attention. A concerted public effort will be needed to prevent further increases of overweight and obesity. Health care providers, health plans, and managed care organizations need to be alert to the development of overweight and obesity in their clients and should provide information concerning the associated risks. These groups need to provide guidance to help consumers address this health problem. To lose weight and keep it off, overweight persons will need long-term lifestyle changes in dietary and physical activity patterns that they can easily incorporate into their lives.

Patterns of healthful eating behavior need to begin in childhood and be maintained throughout adulthood. These patterns can be encouraged through nutrition education at schools and worksites that takes into account cultural and other factors influencing diet. Persons should be aware of the impact that away-from-home eating can have on weight management. In order to address physical activity needs, changes in the physical environment—such as access to walkways and bicycle paths—and the social environment—through social support and safe communities—will be needed to achieve long-term success.

There is much concern about the increasing prevalence of obesity in children and adolescents. Overweight and obesity acquired during childhood or adolescence may persist into adulthood and increase the risk for some chronic diseases later in life. Teenaged boys lose some fat accumulated before puberty during adolescence, but fat deposition continues in girls. Thus, without measures of sexual maturity, measures of body fat and body weight are difficult to interpret in children and adolescents. Therefore, the objective to reduce the prevalence of overweight and obesity among children and adolescents has a target set at no more than 5 percent and uses the gender- and age-specific 95th percentile of BMI from the revised Center for Disease Control and Prevention (CDC) Growth Charts for the United States. Interventions need to recognize that obese children also may experience psychological stress. The reduction of BMI in children and adolescents should be achieved by emphasizing physical activity and a properly balanced diet so that healthy growth is maintained. Additional research is needed to better define the prevalence and health consequences of overweight and obesity in children and adolescents and the implications of such findings for these persons as they become the next generation of adults.

19-4. Reduce growth retardation among low-income children under age 5 years.

Target: 5 percent.

Baseline: 8 percent of low-income children under age 5 years were growth retarded in 1997 (defined as height for age below the fifth percentile in the age-gender appropriate population using the 1977 NCHS/CDC growth charts;[31] preliminary data; not age adjusted).

Target setting method: Better than the best.

Data source: Pediatric Nutrition Surveillance System, CDC, NCCDPHP.

	Growth Retardation			
	19-4. Under Age 5 Years	Under Age 1 Year*	Aged 1 Year*	Aged 2 to 4 Years*
Low-Income Children Under Age 5 Years, 1997	Percent			
TOTAL	8	10	9	6
Race and ethnicity				
American Indian or Alaska Native	8	9	7	9
Asian or Pacific Islander	9	9	11	8
Asian	DNC	DNC	DNC	DNC
Native Hawaiian and other Pacific Islander	DNC	DNC	DNC	DNC
Black or African American	DNC	DNC	DNC	DNC
White	DNC	DNC	DNC	DNC
Hispanic or Latino	7	7	8	5
Not Hispanic or Latino	DNC	DNC	DNC	DNC
Black or African American	9	15	10	5
White	8	10	9	6
Gender				
Female	8	10	8	6
Male	8	10	10	6
Disability status				
Children with disabilities	DNC	DNC	DNC	DNC
Children without disabilities	DNC	DNC	DNC	DNC

DNA = Data have not been analyzed. DNC = Data are not collected. DSU = Data are statistically unreliable.

Note: Preliminary data; not age adjusted.

*Data for specific age groups under 5 years are displayed to further characterize the issue.

Retardation in linear growth in preschool children serves as an indicator of overall health and development and also may reflect the adequacy of a child's diet. Full growth potential may not be reached because of less than optimal nutrition, infectious diseases, chronic diseases, or poor health care. Inadequate maternal weight gain during pregnancy and other prenatal factors that influence birth weight also affect the prevalence of growth retardation among infants and young children.

Growth retardation is not a problem for the majority of young children in the United States. By definition, approximately 5 percent of healthy children are expected to be below the fifth percentile of height for age due to normal biologic variation. If more than 5 percent of a population group is below the fifth percentile, this suggests that full growth potential is not being reached by some children in that group. Among some age and ethnic groups of low-income children under age 5 years in the United States, up to 15 percent are below the fifth percentile. While progress has been made in reducing the prevalence of growth retardation among low-income Hispanic and Asian or Pacific Islander children, it remains especially high for African American children in the first year of life.

Interventions to improve children's linear growth potential include better nutrition; improvements in the prevention, diagnosis, and treatment of infectious and chronic diseases; and provision and use of adequate health services. Although the response of a population to interventions for growth retardation may not be as rapid as for iron deficiency or underweight, achievement of the objective by the year 2010 in all racial and ethnic, socioeconomic, and age groups should be possible. Special attention should be given to homeless children and those with special health care needs.

Food and Nutrient Consumption

19-5. Increase the proportion of persons aged 2 years and older who consume at least two daily servings of fruit.

Target: 75 percent.

Baseline: 28 percent of persons aged 2 years and older consumed at least two daily servings of fruit in 1994–96 (age adjusted to the year 2000 standard population).

Target setting method: Better than the best.

Data source: Continuing Survey of Food Intakes by Individuals (CSFII) (2-day average), USDA.

Persons Aged 2 Years and Older, 1994–96	Two or More Daily Servings of Fruit Percent
TOTAL	28
Race and ethnicity	
American Indian or Alaska Native	DSU
Asian or Pacific Islander	DSU
Asian	DNC
Native Hawaiian and other Pacific Islander	DNC
Black or African American	DNA
White	DNA
Hispanic or Latino	32
Mexican American	29
Other Hispanic	30
Not Hispanic or Latino	
Black or African American	24
White	27
Gender and age	
Female	
2 years and older	26
2 to 5 years (not age adjusted)	43
6 to 11 years (not age adjusted)	26
12 to 19 years (not age adjusted)	23
20 to 39 years (not age adjusted)	20
40 to 59 years (not age adjusted)	26
60 years and older (not age adjusted)	35
Male	
2 years and older	29
2 to 5 years (not age adjusted)	46
6 to 11 years (not age adjusted)	27
12 to 19 years (not age adjusted)	22
20 to 39 years (not age adjusted)	23
40 to 59 years (not age adjusted)	28
60 years and older (not age adjusted)	39
Household income level*	
Lower income (≤130 percent of poverty threshold)	23
Higher income (>130 percent of poverty threshold)	29
Disability status	
Persons with disabilities	DNC
Persons without disabilities	DNC

DNA = Data have not been analyzed. DNC = Data are not collected. DSU = Data are statistically unreliable.
Note: Age adjusted to the year 2000 standard population.
*A household income below 130 percent of poverty threshold is used by the Food Stamp Program.

19-6. Increase the proportion of persons aged 2 years and older who consume at least three daily servings of vegetables, with at least one-third being dark green or orange vegetables.

Target: 50 percent.

Baseline: 3 percent of persons aged 2 years and older consumed at least three daily servings of vegetables, with at least one-third of these servings being dark green or orange vegetables in 1994–96 (age adjusted to the year 2000 standard population).

Target setting method: Better than the best.

Data source: Continuing Survey of Food Intakes by Individuals (CSFII) (2-day average), USDA.

	Servings of Vegetables		
Persons Aged 2 Years and Older, 1994–96	19-6. Meet Both Recommendations	3 or More Daily Servings*	One-Third or More Servings From Dark Green or Orange Vegetables*
	Percent		
TOTAL	3	49	8
Race and ethnicity			
American Indian or Alaska Native	DSU	DSU	DSU
Asian or Pacific Islander	DSU	DSU	DSU
Asian	DNC	DNC	DNC
Native Hawaiian and other Pacific Islander	DNC	DNC	DNC
Black or African American	DNA	DNA	DNA
White	DNA	DNA	DNA
Hispanic or Latino	2	47	6
Mexican American	2	50	5
Other Hispanic	DSU	44	6
Not Hispanic or Latino	DNA	DNA	DNA
Black or African American	DNA	43	14
White	DNA	50	8
Gender and age			
Female			
2 years and older	4	41	10
2 to 5 years (not age adjusted)	DSU	23	9
6 to 11 years (not age adjusted)	DSU	24	7
12 to 19 years (not age adjusted)	2	38	7
20 to 39 years (not age adjusted)	4	43	10
40 to 59 years (not age adjusted)	4	49	11
60 years and older (not age adjusted)	6	43	13
Male			
2 years and older	3	57	7
2 to 5 years (not age adjusted)	DSU	23	8
6 to 11 years (not age adjusted)	DSU	27	6
12 to 19 years (not age adjusted)	DSU	55	4
20 to 39 years (not age adjusted)	3	68	4
40 to 59 years (not age adjusted)	4	64	9
60 years and older (not age adjusted)	6	57	11
Household income level†			
Lower income (≤130 percent of poverty threshold)	3	42	8
Higher income (>130 percent of poverty threshold)	4	50	8
Disability status			
Persons with disabilities	DNC	DNC	DNC
Persons without disabilities	DNC	DNC	DNC

DNA = Data have not been analyzed. DNC = Data are not collected. DSU = Data are statistically unreliable.

Note: Age adjusted to the year 2000 standard population.

*Data for number and type of daily servings are displayed to further characterize the issue.

†A household income below 130 percent of poverty threshold is used by the Food Stamp Program.

19-7. Increase the proportion of persons aged 2 years and older who consume at least six daily servings of grain products, with at least three being whole grains.

Target: 50 percent.

Baseline: 7 percent of persons aged 2 years and older consumed at least six daily servings of grain products, with at least three being whole grains in 1994–96 (age adjusted to the year 2000 standard population).

Target setting method: Better than the best.

Data source: Continuing Survey of Food Intakes by Individuals (CSFII)(2-day average), USDA.

	Servings of Grains		
	19-7. Meet Both Recommendations	**6 or More Daily Servings***	**3 or More Servings From Whole Grain***
Persons Aged 2 Years and Older, 1994–96	Percent		
TOTAL	7	51	7
Race and ethnicity			
American Indian or Alaska Native	DSU	DSU	DSU
Asian or Pacific Islander	DSU	DSU	DSU
Asian	DNC	DNC	DNC
Native Hawaiian and other Pacific Islander	DNC	DNC	DNC
Black or African American	DNA	DNA	DNA
White	DNA	DNA	DNA
Hispanic or Latino	4	46	4
Mexican American	3	46	4
Other Hispanic	4	46	4
Not Hispanic or Latino	DNA	DNA	DNA
Black or African American	3	40	4
White	7	54	8
Gender and age			
Female			
2 years and older	4	39	5
2 to 5 years (not age adjusted)	4	40	5
6 to 11 years (not age adjusted)	2	46	2
12 to 19 years (not age adjusted)	6	49	6
20 to 39 years (not age adjusted)	4	40	5
40 to 59 years (not age adjusted)	4	38	5
60 years and older (not age adjusted)	4	28	6
Male			
2 years and older	9	64	10
2 to 5 years (not age adjusted)	5	50	6
6 to 11 years (not age adjusted)	5	60	5
12 to 19 years (not age adjusted)	9	77	9
20 to 39 years (not age adjusted)	10	70	11
40 to 59 years (not age adjusted)	10	64	11
60 years and older (not age adjusted)	11	54	12
Household income level†			
Lower income (≤130 percent of poverty threshold)	4	44	5
Higher income (>130 percent of poverty threshold)	7	53	8
Disability status			
Persons with disabilities	DNC	DNC	DNC
Persons without disabilities	DNC	DNC	DNC

DNA = Data have not been analyzed. DNC = Data are not collected. DSU = Data are statistically unreliable.
Note: Age adjusted to the year 2000 standard population.
*Data for number and type of daily servings are displayed to further characterize the issue.
†A household income below 130 percent of poverty threshold is used by the Food Stamp Program.

The *Dietary Guidelines for Americans* recommend that Americans choose a variety of grains daily, especially whole grains, and a variety of fruits and vegetables daily.[6] In the United States, persons of all ages eat fewer than the recommended number of servings of grain products, vegetables, and fruits.[28] Vegetables (including legumes, such as beans and peas), fruits, and grains are good sources of vitamins and minerals, carbohydrates (starch and dietary fiber), and other substances that are important for good health. Some evidence from clinical studies suggests that water-soluble fibers from foods such as oat bran, beans, and certain fruits are associated with lower blood glucose and blood lipid levels.[32] Dietary patterns with higher intakes of vegetables (including legumes), fruits, and grains are associated with a variety of health benefits, including a decreased risk for some types of cancer.[32, 33, 34, 35, 36, 37]

The *Dietary Guidelines for Americans* recommend three to five servings from various vegetables and vegetable juices and two to four servings from various fruits and fruit juices, depending on calorie needs. Consumers can select from a plentiful supply of fresh, frozen, dried, and canned products throughout the year to obtain five or more servings of fruits and vegetables daily. The *Dietary Guidelines for Americans* recommend that persons choose dark green leafy vegetables, orange vegetables and fruits, and dry beans and peas often. In 1994–96, the average daily intake of fruits and vegetables was five servings, but only about 7 to 10 percent of vegetable servings were dark green or deep yellow (orange), and only about 5 to 6 percent were legumes.[38] In contrast, fried potatoes accounted for about one-third (32 percent) of vegetable servings consumed by youth aged 2 to 19 years. Consumption of fruits and vegetables also is tracked at the State level and is discussed in *Tracking Healthy People 2010.*

The *Dietary Guidelines for Americans* recommend 6 to 11 daily servings of grain products, depending on calorie needs, with several of these from whole-grain foods. Although grain product consumption increased during the 1990s, consumption of whole-grain products remains very low. In 1994–96, for the population aged 2 years and older, the average daily intake of grain products was nearly seven servings, but only about 14 to 15 percent of grain servings were whole grain.[38] The guidelines also recommend that grain products be prepared with little added saturated fat and moderate or low amounts of added sugars; however, considerable amounts of fats and sugars are contributed to U.S. diets by baked products such as cookies, cakes, and doughnuts.[39,40] No state-level data on grain intakes are available for adults, adolescents, and children.

Both the *Dietary Guidelines for Americans* and the National Cholesterol Education and Prevention Program recommend a diet that contains less than 10 percent of calories from saturated fat and no more than 30 percent of calories from total fat.[6, 33, 41] This can be achieved by obtaining most calories from plant foods (grains, fruits, vegetables) that have little added fat. Such a healthful diet also can include low-fat and lean foods from the milk group and the meat group. The increase of overweight and obesity in the United States indicates that more attention needs to be paid to serving size and total calorie content because a low-fat content does not, automatically, signify a lower calorie content.

The role of fat in the diet is complicated because different types of fatty acids have different effects on health. Evidence to date is complicated, but certain messages appear clear: persons in the United States consume too much dietary fat in general, and too much of the fat consumed is from saturated fatty acids—the type associated with an increased risk for heart disease. (See Focus Area 12, Heart Disease and Stroke.)

Strong evidence from human and animal studies shows that diets low in saturated fatty acids and cholesterol are associated with low risks and rates of coronary heart disease. Saturated fatty acids are the major dietary factors that raise blood low-density lipoprotein (LDL) cholesterol levels, increasing the risk for heart disease. Increasing evidence suggests that *trans*-fatty acids also can increase LDL-cholesterol levels.[42] Monounsaturated and polyunsaturated fatty acids do not raise blood cholesterol. Omega-3 polyunsaturated fatty acids, which are found in some fish such as salmon, tuna, and mackerel, are being studied to determine whether they offer protection against heart disease.[6]

19-8. Increase the proportion of persons aged 2 years and older who consume less than 10 percent of calories from saturated fat.

Target: 75 percent.

Baseline: 36 percent of persons aged 2 years and older consumed less than 10 percent of daily calories from saturated fat in 1994–96 (age adjusted to the year 2000 standard population).

Target setting method: Better than the best.

Data source: Continuing Survey of Food Intakes by Individuals (CSFII) (2-day average), USDA.

Persons Aged 2 Years and Older, 1994–96	Less than 10 Percent of Calories From Saturated Fat Percent
TOTAL	36
Race and ethnicity	
American Indian or Alaska Native	DSU
Asian or Pacific Islander	DSU
Asian	DNC
Native Hawaiian and other Pacific Islander	DNC
Black or African American	DNA
White	DNA
Hispanic or Latino	39
Mexican American	37
Other Hispanic	40
Not Hispanic or Latino	DNA
Black or African American	31
White	35
Gender and age	
Female	
2 years and older	39
2 to 5 years (not age adjusted)	23
6 to 11 years (not age adjusted)	23
12 to 19 years (not age adjusted)	34
20 to 39 years (not age adjusted)	41
40 to 59 years (not age adjusted)	42
60 years and older (not age adjusted)	47
Male	
2 years and older	32
2 to 5 years (not age adjusted)	23
6 to 11 years (not age adjusted)	25
12 to 19 years (not age adjusted)	27
20 to 39 years (not age adjusted)	32
40 to 59 years (not age adjusted)	33
60 years and older (not age adjusted)	42

Household income level*	
Lower income (≤130 percent of poverty threshold)	33
Higher income (>130 percent of poverty threshold)	36
Disability status	
Persons with disabilities	DNC
Persons without disabilities	DNC

DNA = Data have not been analyzed. DNC = Data are not collected. DSU = Data are statistically unreliable.
Note: Age adjusted to the year 2000 standard population.
*A household income below 130 percent of poverty threshold is used by the Food Stamp Program.

19-9. Increase the proportion of persons aged 2 years and older who consume no more than 30 percent of calories from total fat.

Target: 75 percent.

Baseline: 33 percent of persons aged 2 years and older consumed no more than 30 percent of daily calories from total fat in 1994–96 (age adjusted to the year 2000 standard population).

Target setting method: Better than the best.

Data source: Continuing Survey of Food Intakes by Individuals (CSFII) (2-day average), USDA.

Persons Aged 2 Years and Older, 1994–96	No More Than 30 Percent of Calories From Total Fat Percent
TOTAL	33
Race and ethnicity	
American Indian or Alaska Native	DSU
Asian or Pacific Islander	DSU
Asian	DNC
Native Hawaiian and other Pacific Islander	DNC
Black or African American	DNA
White	DNA
Hispanic or Latino	36
Mexican American	33
Other Hispanic	38
Not Hispanic or Latino	DNA
Black or African American	26
White	33

Gender and age

Female

2 years and older	36
2 to 5 years (not age adjusted)	35
6 to 11 years (not age adjusted)	34
12 to 19 years (not age adjusted)	36
20 to 39 years (not age adjusted)	38
40 to 59 years (not age adjusted)	33
60 years and older (not age adjusted)	40

Male

2 years and older	30
2 to 5 years (not age adjusted)	33
6 to 11 years (not age adjusted)	30
12 to 19 years (not age adjusted)	30
20 to 39 years (not age adjusted)	29
40 to 59 years (not age adjusted)	28
60 years and older (not age adjusted)	34

Household income level*

Lower income (≤130 percent of poverty threshold)	30
Higher income (>130 percent of poverty threshold)	34

Disability status

Persons with disabilities	DNC
Persons without disabilities	DNC

DNA = Data have not been analyzed. DNC = Data are not collected. DSU = Data are statistically unreliable.

Note: Age adjusted to the year 2000 standard population.

*A household income below 130 percent of poverty threshold is used by the Food Stamp Program.

A 1989 National Research Council report[33] indicated that diets high in total fat were associated with a higher risk of several cancers, especially cancer of the colon, prostate, and breast, but noted that findings were inconsistent. (See Focus Area 3. Cancer.) A 1996 review of the evidence showed that the relationship between the amount and type of fat and the risk of cancer continues to be uncertain.[43] To help clarify the relationship between total dietary fat and the risk of cancer, a randomized clinical trial called the Women's Health Initiative has been started. Set to conclude in 2003, it is a multicenter trial designed to test several risk factors for chronic disease in U.S. females.[44] A major emphasis is to reduce fat to 25 percent of dietary calories to determine whether a low-fat diet has any effect on breast cancer risk.

The proportion of calories in the U.S. diet provided by total fat is about 33 percent, saturated fat is about 11 percent, and *trans*-fat is about 2.6 percent.[45] The primary sources of saturated fat are meats and dairy products that contain fat. Thus, nonfat and low-fat dairy products and lean meats are choices that can help reduce saturated fat intake. *Trans*-fatty acids are formed when vegetable oil is hydrogenated to solidify the oils and increase the shelf life and flavor stability of the fats and the foods that contain them. Margarines that have been formulated to contain no *trans*-fats are available in most U.S. grocery stores. Other dietary sources of *trans*-fat are restaurant and fast-food fats (including frying fats), baked products, and some snack foods, such as chips.

The major vegetable sources of monounsaturated fatty acids include nuts, avocados, olive oil, canola oil, and high-oleic forms of safflower and sunflower seed oil. The major sources of polyunsaturated fatty acids are vegetable oils, including soybean oil, corn oil, and high-linoleic forms of safflower and sunflower seed oil and a few nuts, such as walnuts. Substituting monounsaturated and polyunsaturated fatty acids for saturated fatty acids can help lower health risks.

The proportion of all meals and snacks from away-from-home sources increased by more than two-thirds between 1977–78 and 1995, from 16 percent of all meals and snacks in 1977–78 to 27 percent of all meals and snacks in 1995.[27] Away-from-home food tends to have a higher saturated fat content, and persons tend to consume more calories when eating away from home than at home.[27] In 1995, the average total fat and saturated fat content of away-from-home foods, expressed as a percentage of calories, was 38 percent and 13 percent, respectively, compared with 32 percent and 11 percent for at-home foods.[27] Meals and snacks eaten by children at school had the highest saturated fat density of all food outlets. Thus, to help assess fat and saturated fat intake, as well as develop strategies to help children reduce the amount of fat they consume, additional tracking of saturated fat and total fat intake from foods eaten away from home as well as at home is important.

19-10. Increase the proportion of persons aged 2 years and older who consume 2,400 mg or less of sodium daily.

Target: 65 percent.

Baseline: 21 percent of persons aged 2 years and older consumed 2,400 mg or less of sodium daily (from foods, dietary supplements, tap water, and salt use at the table) in 1988–94 (age adjusted to the year 2000 standard population).

Target setting method: Better than the best.

Data source: National Health and Nutrition Examination Survey (NHANES), CDC, NCHS.

Persons Aged 2 Years and Older, 1988–94 (unless noted)	Consume 2,400 mg of Sodium or Less
	Percent
TOTAL	21
Race and ethnicity	
American Indian or Alaska Native	DSU
Asian or Pacific Islander	DSU
Asian	DNC
Native Hawaiian and other Pacific Islander	DNC
Black or African American	25
White	20
Hispanic or Latino	DSU
Mexican American	25
Not Hispanic or Latino	21
Black or African American	25
White	20
Gender and age	
Female	
2 years and older	32
2 to 5 years (not age adjusted)	64
6 to 11 years (not age adjusted)	26
12 to 19 years (not age adjusted)	29
20 years and older	30
Male	
2 years and older	9
2 to 5 years (not age adjusted)	50
6 to 11 years (not age adjusted)	16
12 to 19 years (not age adjusted)	4
20 years and older	6
Family income level*	
Lower income (≤130 percent of poverty threshold)	25
Higher income (>130 percent of poverty threshold)	20
Disability status (aged 20 years and older)	
Persons with disabilities	18 (1991–94)
Persons without disabilities	16 (1991–94)
Select populations	
Females with high blood pressure	32
Females without high blood pressure	29
Males with high blood pressure	7
Males without high blood pressure	5

DNA = Data have not been analyzed. DNC = Data are not collected. DSU = Data are statistically unreliable.

Note: Age adjusted to the year 2000 standard population.

*A household income below 130 percent of poverty threshold is used by the Food Stamp Program.

The *Dietary Guidelines for Americans* recommend choosing and preparing foods with less salt (salt consists of both sodium and chloride). Most studies in diverse populations have shown that salt intake is linked to increasing levels of blood pressure.[6, 46, 47, 48] (See Focus Area 12. Heart Disease and Stroke.) Persons who consume less salt or sodium have a lower risk of developing high blood pressure.[6] Data also show that high sodium intake may increase the amount of calcium excreted in the urine and therefore increase the body's need for calcium.[49] Eating less salt may decrease the loss of calcium from bone.[6]

Most persons in the United States consume more sodium than is needed, and reduction of sodium or salt or both to no more than 2,400 mg sodium or 6 g salt per day is recommended by some authorities.[33, 46] Data from the Continuing Survey of Food Intakes by Individuals show that, even without including salt added at the table, both home foods and away-from-home foods provide excessive amounts of sodium.[27] Higher sodium intakes also tend to be associated with higher calorie intakes; for example, males, who consume more calories than females, also consume more sodium.[27]

Sodium occurs naturally in foods. However, most dietary salt or sodium is added to foods during processing or preparation, with smaller amounts added at the discretion of the consumer in the form of table salt or use of condiments such as soy sauce.[50, 51] Thus, both the sodium content of foods and estimates of the amount of salt added have been used to assess dietary sodium consumption. Other contributing sources of sodium are water, dietary supplements, and medications such as antacids.

19-11. Increase the proportion of persons aged 2 years and older who meet dietary recommendations for calcium.

Target: 75 percent.

Baseline: 46 percent of persons aged 2 years and older were at or above approximated mean calcium requirements (based on consideration of calcium from foods, dietary supplements, and antacids) in 1988–94 (age adjusted to the year 2000 standard population).

Target setting method: Better than the best.

Data source: National Health and Nutrition Examination Survey (NHANES), CDC, NCHS.

Persons Aged 2 Years and Older, 1988–94 (unless noted)	Met Calcium Recommendations Percent
TOTAL	46
Race and ethnicity	
American Indian or Alaska Native	DSU
Asian or Pacific Islander	DSU
Asian	DNC
Native Hawaiian and other Pacific Islander	DNC
Black or African American	30
White	49
Hispanic or Latino	DSU
Mexican American	44
Not Hispanic or Latino	46
Black or African American	30
White	50
Gender and age	
Female	
2 years and older	36
2 to 8 years (not age adjusted)	79
9 to 19 years (not age adjusted)	19
20 to 49 years (not age adjusted)	40
50 years and older (not age adjusted)	27
Male	
2 years and older	56
2 to 8 years (not age adjusted)	89
9 to 19 years (not age adjusted)	52
20 to 49 years (not age adjusted)	64
50 years and older (not age adjusted)	35
Family income level*	
Lower income (≤130 percent of poverty threshold)	39
Higher income (>130 percent of poverty threshold)	48

Disability status (aged 20 years and older)	
Persons with disabilities	44 (1991–94)
Persons without disabilities	44 (1991–94)

DNA = Data have not been analyzed. DNC = Data are not collected. DSU = Data are statistically unreliable.
Note: Age adjusted to the year 2000 standard population.
*A household income below 130 percent of poverty threshold is used by the Food Stamp Program.

Calcium is essential for the formation and maintenance of bones and teeth.[32] The recommendations for adequate daily intakes of calcium are 500 mg for children aged 1 to 3 years, 800 mg for children aged 4 to 8 years, 1,300 mg for adolescents aged 9 to 18 years, 1,000 mg for adults aged 19 to 50 years, and 1,200 mg for adults aged 51 years and older.[52] Approximated mean calcium requirements are defined as 77 percent of the recommendations by the Institute of Medicine for adequate intakes of calcium.[52, 53] The bone mass achieved at full growth (peak bone mass) appears to be related to intake of calcium during childhood and adolescence.[33] Opinion is divided as to the age at which peak bone mass is achieved, although most of the accumulation of bone mineral occurs in humans by about age 20 years. After persons reach their adult height, a period of consolidation of bone density continues until approximately age 30 to 35 years. A high peak bone mass is thought to be protective against fractures in later life.

Osteoporosis is a complex disorder caused by many contributing factors. (See Focus Area 2. Arthritis, Osteoporosis, and Chronic Back Conditions.) Regular exercise and a diet with enough calcium help maintain good bone health and reduce the risk of osteoporosis later in life. However, the ideal level of calcium intake for development of peak bone mass is unknown. For the most part, young children appear to meet the approximate calcium requirements. In contrast, the majority of adolescent and adult females do not meet the average requirements. This is in part because of their lower food consumption, as well as the lower consumption of milk products relative to soft drinks in U.S. diets.[54] For example, in the period 1994–96, the amount of soft drinks consumed was about twice that consumed in the late 1970s and surpassed consumption of fluid milk. Thus, an increase in consumption of various sources of calcium is recommended for nearly all groups and especially for teenaged girls and women. In postmenopausal females—the group at highest risk for osteoporosis—estrogen replacement therapy under medical supervision is the most effective means to reduce the rate of bone loss and risk of fractures.[32]

The relationship between dietary calcium and blood pressure is uncertain. Results from studies that have used calcium supplements show a small reduction in systolic blood pressure in hypertensive individuals, with no significant reduction in diastolic blood pressure.[55] Among persons with normal blood pressure, there is no significant difference in blood pressure with calcium supplements.[56]

Dietary sources of calcium include milk and milk products such as cheese and yogurt, canned fish with soft bones such as sardines, dark green leafy vegetables such as kale and mustard or turnip greens, tofu made with calcium, tortillas made from lime-processed corn, calcium-enriched grain products, and other calcium-fortified foods and beverages.[6] In some locations, water is a source of calcium, but in amounts that cannot readily be determined. With current food selection practices, use of dairy products may constitute the difference between getting enough calcium in one's diet or not. Nonfat and low-fat dairy products are choices that help reduce the intake of saturated fat while still providing calcium, vitamin D, and other nutrients important for bone health. For those who have lactose intolerance, a range of lactose-reduced dairy products can provide calcium. Persons who do not (or cannot) consume and absorb adequate levels of calcium from dairy food sources may consider use of calcium-fortified foods, while persons with clinical evidence of inadequate intake should receive professional advice on the proper type and dosage of calcium supplements. Calcium supplements come in different forms, including calcium-containing antacids.

Fluid milk (but not yogurt or cheese) is an excellent source of vitamin D, which is essential for calcium utilization. Vitamin D also is synthesized in the skin upon exposure to sunlight.

Iron Deficiency and Anemia

19-12. Reduce iron deficiency among young children and females of childbearing age.

Target and Baseline:

Objective	Reduction in Iron Deficiency	1988–94 Baseline	2010 Target
		Percent	
19-12a.	Children aged 1 to 2 years	9	5
19-12b.	Children aged 3 to 4 years	4	1
19-12c.	Nonpregnant females aged 12 to 49 years	11	7

*Iron deficiency is defined as having abnormal results for two or more of the following tests: serum ferritin concentration, erythrocyte protoporphyrin, or transferrin saturation. Refer to *Tracking Healthy People 2010* for threshold values.

Target setting method: Better than the best.

Data source: National Health and Nutrition Examination Survey (NHANES), CDC, NCHS.

	Iron Deficiency		
	19-12a. Aged 1 to 2 Years	19-12b. Aged 3 to 4 Years	19-12c. Females of Childbearing Age
Select Populations, 1988–94 (unless noted)	Percent		
TOTAL	9	4	11
Race and ethnicity			
American Indian or Alaska Native	DSU	DSU	DSU
Asian or Pacific Islander	DSU	DSU	DSU
Asian	DNC	DNC	DNC
Native Hawaiian and other Pacific Islander	DNC	DNC	DNC
Black or African American	10	2	15
White	8	3	10
Hispanic or Latino	DSU	DSU	DSU
Mexican American	17	6	19
Not Hispanic or Latino	DNA	DNA	DNA
Black or African American	10	2	15
White	6	1	8
Family income level*			
Lower income (≤130 percent of poverty threshold)	12	5	16
Higher income (>130 percent of poverty threshold)	7	3	9
Disability status (aged 20 to 49 years)			
Persons with disabilities	DNC	DNC	4 (1991–94)
Persons without disabilities	DNC	DNC	12 (1991–94)

DNA = Data have not been analyzed. DNC = Data are not collected. DSU = Data are statistically unreliable.
*A household income below 130 percent of poverty threshold is used by the Food Stamp Program.

19-13. Reduce anemia among low-income pregnant females in their third trimester.

Target: 20 percent.

Baseline: 29 percent of low-income pregnant females in their third trimester were anemic (defined as hemoglobin <11.0 g/dL) in 1996.

Target setting method: Better than the best.

Data source: Pregnancy Nutrition Surveillance System, CDC, NCCDPHP.

Low-Income Pregnant Females, Third Trimester, 1996	Percent with Anemia
TOTAL	29
Race and ethnicity	
American Indian or Alaska Native	31
Asian or Pacific Islander	26
Asian	DNC
Native Hawaiian and other Pacific Islander	DNC
Black or African American	DNC
White	DNC
Hispanic or Latino	25
Not Hispanic or Latino	DNA
Black or African American	44
White	24
Disability status	
Females with disabilities	DNC
Females without disabilities	DNC

DNA = Data have not been analyzed. DNC = Data are not collected. DSU = Data are statistically unreliable.

19-14. (Developmental) Reduce iron deficiency among pregnant females.

Potential data source: National Health and Nutrition Examination Survey (NHANES), CDC, NCHS.

The terms anemia, iron deficiency, and iron deficiency anemia often are used interchangeably but are not equivalent. Iron deficiency ranges from depleted iron stores without functional or health impairment to iron deficiency with anemia, which affects the functioning of several organ systems. Iron deficiency anemia is more likely than iron deficiency without anemia to cause preterm births, low birth weight, and delays in infant and child development.[57, 58, 59] Iron deficiency (with and without anemia) in adolescent females has been associated with decreased verbal learning and memory.[60] The prevalence of iron deficiency anemia among children aged 1 to 2 years and 3 to 4 years and females aged 12 to 49 years in 1988 to 1994 was 3 percent, less than 1 percent, and 4 percent, respectively.

Anemia can be caused by many factors other than iron deficiency, including other nutrient deficiencies, infection, inflammation, and hereditary anemias. Anemia is used for monitoring risk of iron deficiency at the State and local levels because of the low cost and feasibility of measuring hemoglobin or hematocrit in the clinic setting.[61] Anemia is a good predictor of iron deficiency when the prevalence of iron deficiency is high, such as during the third trimester of pregnancy. It is not a good predictor of iron deficiency when the prevalence of iron deficiency is expected to be low, such as among white, non-Hispanic children aged 3 to 4 years in the United States. In that case, the majority of anemia is due to other causes.[8] However, changes in the prevalence of anemia over time at State and local levels can be used to evaluate the effectiveness of programs to decrease the prevalence of iron deficiency.

Iron deficiency and anemia among young children declined during the 1970s in association with increased iron intake.[8] Although the prevalence of iron deficiency among low-income children continued to decline from 1976–80 to 1988–94, the prevalence of iron deficiency among all young children remained the same, and the prevalence of iron deficiency among females of childbearing age actually increased.[9] From 1979 to 1996, the prevalence of third trimester anemia among low-income pregnant females did not change.[62, 63]

Iron deficiency is highest among toddlers and among certain racial, ethnic, and low-income children.[64] Iron deficiency can be prevented among young children by teaching families about child nutrition, including promoting breastfeeding of infants, with exclusive breastfeeding for 4 to 6 months; the use of iron-fortified formulas when formulas are used; delayed introduction of cow's milk until age 12 months; and age-appropriate introduction of iron-rich solid foods, such as iron-fortified infant cereals and pureed meats, and foods that enhance iron absorption such as vitamin C-rich fruits, vegetables, or juices.[61]

Nonpregnant females of childbearing age are at increased risk for iron deficiency because of iron loss during menstruation coupled with inadequate intake of iron.[61] Pregnant females are also at increased risk because of the increased iron requirements of pregnancy.[61, 63] Consequently, a Healthy People 2010 objective has been established to reduce the prevalence of anemia among low-income pregnant females in their third trimester. Although groups other than low-income females are considered at risk for iron deficiency during pregnancy, no nationally representative data exist on the prevalence of iron deficiency or iron deficiency anemia among pregnant females.

National data indicate that only one-fourth of all females of childbearing age (12 to 49 years) meet the U.S. recommended dietary allowance for iron (15 mg) through their diets.[65] Iron deficiency among females of childbearing age may be prevented by periodic anemia screening and appropriate treatment and by counseling them about better eating practices, such as selecting iron-rich foods, taking iron supplements during pregnancy, increasing consumption of foods that enhance iron absorption (for example, orange juice and other citrus products), and discouraging consumption of iron inhibitors (for example, coffee and tea) with iron-rich foods.[61] Some good sources of iron include ready-to-eat cereals with added iron; enriched and whole grain breads; lean meats; turkey dark meat; shellfish; spinach; and cooked dry beans, peas, and lentils.

Schools, Worksites, and Nutrition Counseling

19-15. (Developmental) Increase the proportion of children and adolescents aged 6 to 19 years whose intake of meals and snacks at school contributes to good overall dietary quality.

Potential data sources: Continuing Survey of Food Intakes by Individuals (CSFII), USDA; National Food and Nutrition Survey, USDA and CDC; National Health and Nutrition Examination Survey (NHANES), CDC, NCHS.

Students today have increased food options at school. Although students may understand that good nutrition and good health are connected, that understanding may not be reflected in their food choices and meal patterns. The U.S. Department of Agriculture (USDA) has established standards requiring schools to plan menus that meet the 1995 *Dietary Guidelines for Americans,* but these standards do not apply to à la carte foods; to foods sold in snack bars, school stores, and vending machines; or to foods students bring from home. Students' food choices are influenced by the total eating environment created by schools. This includes the types of foods available throughout the school, point-of-choice nutrition information in the cafeteria and around the school, nutrition education provided in the classroom, and nutrition promotions that reach families and affect the choices of foods brought to school.

Improving the quality of students' dietary intake in the school setting is important because, for many children, meals and snacks consumed at school make a major contribution to their total daily consumption of food and nutrients. National food consumption data collected in 1994 and 1995 show that school foods had the highest saturated fat density of all food outlets.[27] School foods also had higher than recommended levels of sodium—as did other away-from-home foods and at-home foods. Nonetheless, these analyses also showed positive aspects of foods obtained from school. School foods had the highest calcium density of all sources and the highest dietary fiber density of all away-from-home sources. The establishment of an environment that supports a good overall diet would enable school nutrition and food services, in conjunction with students, their families, and other school employees, to make an important contribution to short- and long-term disease prevention and health promotion. In addition, such an environment would foster learning readiness (for example, by encouraging students to consume substantial breakfasts).[66, 67, 68]

19-16. Increase the proportion of worksites that offer nutrition or weight management classes or counseling.

Target: 85 percent.

Baseline: 55 percent of worksites with 50 or more employees offered nutrition or weight management classes or counseling at the worksite or through their health plans in 1998–99.

Target setting method: 55 percent improvement.

Data source: National Worksite Health Promotion Survey, Association for Worksite Health Promotion (AWHP).

Worksites, 1998–99	Offer Nutrition or Weight Management Classes or Counseling		
	Worksite or Health Plan	Worksite	Health Plan
Worksite Size	Percent		
Total (50 or more employees)	55	28	39
50 to 99 employees	48	21	39
100 to 249 employees	51	29	37
250 to 749 employees	59	44	42
750 or more employees	83	70	50

Worksite programs can reach large numbers of employees with information, activities, and services that encourage the adoption of healthy dietary and physical activity behaviors.[69] (See Focus Area 7, Educational and Community-Based Programs and Focus Area 22, Physical Activity and Fitness.) Employer-sponsored programs can be offered onsite or in partnership with community organizations. Examples of such programs include weight management classes, physical activity programs, lunchtime seminars, self-help programs, cooking demonstrations and classes, healthy food service and vending machine selections, point-of-purchase nutrition information, and flexible health benefits that include nutrition-related services.

A recent study of worksite health promotion programs found that specific interventions at the worksite resulted in employees choosing to reduce the amount of fat calories they consumed and eating more fruits, vegetables, and dietary fiber.[70] Worksite health promotion programs may reduce health care costs, including employer costs for insurance programs, disability benefits, and medical expenses.[71, 72]

If possible, nutrition education and weight management programs at the worksite should be part of a comprehensive health promotion program. In addition, employers could reimburse health promotion activities and provide company time for employees to participate in the programs.[73]

Worksite programs should be made available to the family members of employees and company retirees as well as current employees. Also, these programs should be offered in a culturally and linguistically competent manner and any educational materials provided should be culturally and linguistically appropriate.

Primary care providers are well positioned in the health care system to provide preventive services, including nutrition screening and assessment, referral, and counseling. For example, they can screen for age-specific and diagnosis-related nutrition risk factors as a part of routine patient contact. The public views physicians—and registered dietitians in particular—as credible sources of nutrition information.[74] Dietary assessment, counseling, and followup by physicians and qualified nutrition professionals are effective in reducing patient dietary fat intake and serum cholesterol.[75, 76, 77, 78] For many physicians, referring patients to qualified nutrition professionals for nutrition assessment, education, counseling on behavioral change, diet modification, and specialized nutrition therapies represents appropriate clinical practice.

Nutrition counseling by registered dietitians and other qualified nutrition professionals has been found to be cost effective for patients with hyperlipidemia[79, 80] and Type 2 diabetes mellitus.[81] Nutrition services also are a critical component of improved health outcomes for many other diseases and conditions, including obesity, gastrointestinal and hepatic disease, renal disease, cancer, HIV/AIDS, pressure ulcers, burns and trauma, eating disorders, and prenatal care. A 1997 study that evaluated the cost of covering medical nutrition therapy under Medicare part B projected savings to the program of $11 million in 2001 and $65 million in 2004.[82, 83] (See Focus Area 3. Cancer, Focus Area 4. Chronic Kidney Disease, Focus Area 13. HIV, and Focus Area 16. Maternal, Infant, and Child Health.)

Food security means that people have access at all times to enough food for an active, healthy life. It implies that people have nutritionally adequate and safe foods and sufficient household resources to ensure their ability to acquire adequate, acceptable foods in socially acceptable ways—that is, through regular marketplace sources and not through severe coping strategies like emergency food sources, scavenging, and stealing. Hunger in this context refers to the uneasy or painful sensation caused by a lack of food.

While the vast majority of persons in the United States are food secure and have not experienced resource-constrained hunger, both food insecurity and hunger have remained a painful fact of life for too many people.[84, 85] The specific concern is with food insecurity and hunger resulting from inadequate household resources. Other sources of food insecurity (such as illness, child abuse and neglect, or loss of function or mobility) are not included in this definition. Food insecurity and hunger may coexist with malnutrition, but they are not the same thing or even necessarily closely associated. Food insecurity and hunger, however, are believed to have harmful health and behavioral impacts in their own right.[86] These are of particular concern for pregnant women, children, elderly persons, and other nutritionally vulnerable groups.[87]

The United States is committed to increasing food security by working with local leaders as outlined in the U.S. Action Plan on Food Security, through USDA's Community Food Security Initiative, and the Maternal and Child Health Bureau's Healthy Start.[88, 89]

19-17. Increase the proportion of physician office visits made by patients with a diagnosis of cardiovascular disease, diabetes, or hyperlipidemia that include counseling or education related to diet and nutrition.

Target: 75 percent.

Baseline: 42 percent of physician office visits made by patients with a diagnosis of cardiovascu-

lar disease, diabetes, or hyperlipidemia included ordering or providing counseling or education on diet and nutrition in 1997 (age adjusted to the year 2000 standard population).

Target setting method: Better than the best.

Data source: National Ambulatory Medical Care Survey (NAMCS), CDC, NCHS.

Persons With Specific Conditions, 1997	Physician Office Visits That Include Ordering or Providing Diet and Nutrition Counseling or Education			
	19-17. Any of the Three Conditions	Hyper lipidemia*	Cardio-vascular Disease*	Diabetes*
	Percent			
TOTAL	42	65	36	48
Race and ethnicity				
American Indian or Alaska Native	DSU	DSU	DSU	DSU
Asian or Pacific Islander	DSU	DSU	DSU	DSU
Asian	DNC	DNC	DNC	DNC
Native Hawaiian and other Pacific Islander	DNC	DNC	DNC	DNC
Black or African American	46	DSU	40	54
White	41	64	35	47
Hispanic or Latino	DSU	DSU	DSU	DSU
Not Hispanic or Latino	DSU	DSU	DSU	DSU
Black or African American	DSU	DSU	DSU	DSU
White	DSU	DSU	DSU	DSU
Gender				
Female	39	55	34	46
Male	44	73	38	49
Age				
20 to 44 years	45	75	37	49
45 to 64 years	41	62	36	47
65 years and older	33	44	32	45
Family income level†				
Lower income (≤130 percent of poverty threshold)	DNC	DNC	DNC	DNC
Higher income (>130 percent of poverty threshold)	DNC	DNC	DNC	DNC
Disability status				
Persons with disabilities	DNC	DNC	DNC	DNC
Persons without disabilities	DNC	DNC	DNC	DNC

DNA = Data have not been analyzed. DNC = Data are not collected. DSU = Data are statistically unreliable.
Note: Age adjusted to the year 2000 standard population.
*Data for separate conditions are displayed to further characterize the issue.
†A household income below 130 percent of poverty threshold is used by the Food Stamp Program.

Food Security

19-18. Increase food security among U.S. households and in so doing reduce hunger.

Target: 94 percent.

Baseline: 88 percent of all U.S. households were food secure in 1995.

Target setting method: 6 percentage point improvement (50 percent decrease in food insecu-rity; consistent with the U.S. pledge to the 1996 World Food Summit).

Data sources: Food Security Supplement to the Current Population Survey, U.S. Department of Commerce, Bureau of the Census; National Food and Nutrition Survey (beginning in 2001), HHS and USDA.

	Food Secure
U.S. Households, 1995	Percent
TOTAL	88
Race and ethnicity	
American Indian or Alaska Native	78
Asian or Pacific Islander	91
Asian	DSU
Native Hawaiian and other Pacific Islander	DSU
Black or African American	76
White	90
Hispanic or Latino	75
Mexican American	
Not Hispanic or Latino	89
Black or African American	76
White	91
Lower income level (≤130 percent of poverty threshold)*	
All	69
With children (under age 18 years)	59
With elderly persons (aged 65 years and over)	85
Higher income level (>130 percent of poverty threshold)*	
All	94
With children (under age 18 years)	91
With elderly persons (aged 65 years and over)	98
Disability status	
Persons with disabilities	DNC
Persons without disabilities	DNC
Select populations	
Household characteristics	
With children	83
With elderly persons	94

DNA = Data have not been analyzed. DNC = Data are not collected. DSU = Data are statistically unreliable.
*A household income below 130 percent poverty threshold is used by the Food Stamp Program.

RELATED OBJECTIVES FROM OTHER FOCUS AREAS

1. **Access to Quality Health Services**

   1-3.   Counseling about health behaviors

2. **Arthritis, Osteoporosis, and Chronic Back Conditions**

   2-9.   Cases of osteoporosis

3. **Cancer**

   3-1.   Overall cancer deaths

   3-3.   Breast cancer deaths

   3-5.   Colorectal cancer deaths

   3-10. Provider counseling about cancer prevention

4. **Chronic Kidney Disease**

   4-3.   Counseling for chronic kidney failure care

5. **Diabetes**

   5-1.   Diabetes education

   5-2.   New cases of diabetes

   5-6.   Diabetes-related deaths

7. **Educational and Community-Based Programs**

   7-2.   School health education

   7-5.   Worksite health promotion programs

   7-6.   Participation in employer-sponsored health promotion activities

   7-10. Community health promotion programs

   7-11. Culturally appropriate and linguistically competent community health promotion programs

10. **Food Safety**

    10-4. Food allergy deaths

    10-5. Consumer food safety practices

11. **Health Communication**

    11-4. Quality of Internet health information sources

12. **Heart Disease and Stroke**

    12-1.   Coronary heart disease (CHD) deaths

    12-7.   Stroke deaths

    12-9.   High blood pressure

    12-11. Action to help control blood pressure

    12-13. Mean total blood cholesterol levels

    12-14. High blood cholesterol levels

16. **Maternal, Infant, and Child Health**

    16-10. Low birth weight and very low birth weight

    16-12. Weight gain during pregnancy

    16-15. Spina bifida and other neural tube defects

    16-16. Optimum folic acid levels

    16-17. Prenatal substance exposure

    16-18. Fetal alcohol syndrome

    16-19. Breastfeeding

18. **Mental Health and Mental Disorders**

    18-5. Eating disorder relapses

22. **Physical Activity and Fitness**

    22-1.   No leisure-time physical activity

    22-2.   Moderate physical activity

    22-3.   Vigorous physical activity

    22-6.   Moderate physical activity in adolescents

    22-7.   Vigorous physical activity in adolescents

    22-9.   Daily physical education in schools

    22-13. Worksite physical activity and fitness

26. **Substance Abuse**

    26-12. Average annual alcohol consumption

TERMINOLOGY

Anemia: A condition in which the hemoglobin in red blood cells falls below normal. Anemia most often results from iron deficiency but also may result from deficiencies of folic acid, vitamin B12, or copper, or from chronic disease, certain conditions, or chronic blood loss.

Body mass index (BMI): Weight (in kilograms) divided by the square of height (in meters), or weight (in pounds) divided by the square of height (in inches) times 704.5. Because it is readily calculated, BMI is the measurement of choice as an indicator of healthy weight, overweight, and obesity.

Calorie: Unit used for measuring the energy produced by food when metabolized in the body.

Cholesterol: A waxy substance that circulates in the bloodstream. When the level of cholesterol in the blood is too high, some of the cholesterol is deposited in the walls of the blood vessels. Over time, these deposits can build up until they narrow the blood vessels, causing atherosclerosis, which reduces the blood flow. The higher the blood cholesterol level, the greater is the risk of getting heart disease. Blood cholesterol levels of less than 200 mg/dL are considered desirable.

Levels of 240 mg/dL or above are considered high and require further testing and possible intervention. Levels of 200-239 mg/dL are considered borderline. Lowering blood cholesterol reduces the risk of heart disease.

HDL (high-density lipoprotein) cholesterol: The so-called good cholesterol. Cholesterol travels in the blood combined with protein in packages called lipoproteins. HDL is thought to carry cholesterol away from other parts of the body back to the liver for removal from the body. A low level of HDL increases the risk for CHD, whereas a high HDL level is protective.

LDL (low-density lipoprotein) cholesterol: The so-called bad cholesterol. LDL contains most of the cholesterol in the blood and carries it to the tissues and organs of the body, including the arteries. Cholesterol from LDL is the main source of damaging buildup and blockage in the arteries. The higher the level of LDL in the blood, the greater is the risk for CHD.

Coronary heart disease (CHD): The type of heart disease due to narrowing of the coronary arteries.

Dietary fiber: Plant food components, including plant cell walls, pectins, gums, and brans that cannot be digested.

Dietary Guidelines for Americans: A report published by the U.S. Department of Agriculture and U.S. Department of Health and Human Services that explains how to eat to maintain health. The guidelines form the basis of national nutrition policy and are revised every 5 years. This chapter refers mostly to the 2000 guidelines.

Fats/fatty acids: Fats and fatty acids are hydrocarbon chains ending in a carboxyl group at one end that bond to glycerol to form fat. Fatty acids are characterized as saturated, monounsaturated or polyunsaturated depending on how many double bonds are between the carbon atoms. Fatty acids supply energy and promote absorption of fat-soluble vitamins. Some fatty acids are "essential," because they cannot be made by the body.

Saturated fatty acids: Fatty acids with no double bonds between carbon atoms. Levels of saturated fatty acids are especially high in meat and dairy products that contain fat. Saturated fatty acids are linked to increased blood cholesterol levels and a greater risk for heart disease.

Trans-**fatty acids:** Alternate forms of naturally occurring unsaturated fatty acids produced in fats as a result of hydrogenation, such as when vegetable oil becomes margarine or shortening. *Trans*-fatty acids also occur in milk fat, beef fat, and lamb fat. These fatty acids have been associated with increased blood cholesterol levels.

Unsaturated fatty acids: Fatty acids with one or more double bonds between carbon atoms. These fatty acids do not raise blood cholesterol levels.

Polyunsaturated: Fatty acids with more than one double bond between carbon atoms.

Monounsaturated: Fatty acids with one double bond between carbon atoms.

Food Guide Pyramid: A graphic depiction of U.S. Department of Agriculture's current food guide that includes five major food groups in its "base" (grains, vegetables, fruits, milk products, and meats, and meat substitutes) and a "tip" depicting the relatively small contribution that discretionary fat and added sugars should make in U.S. diets. The Food Guide Pyramid provides information on the choices within each group and the recommended number of servings.

Food security: Access by all people at all times to enough food for an active, healthy life. It includes at a minimum (1) the ready availability of nutritionally adequate and safe foods, and (2) an assured ability to acquire acceptable foods in socially acceptable ways.

Food insecurity: Limited or uncertain availability of nutritionally adequate and safe foods or limited and uncertain ability to acquire acceptable foods in socially acceptable ways.

HDL-cholesterol: See cholesterol.

Hunger: The uneasy or painful sensation caused by a lack of food.

Hypertension: High blood pressure.

Hypertriglyceridemia: Elevated levels of triglycerides in the blood.

Iron deficiency: Lack of adequate iron in the body to support and maintain functioning. It can lead to iron deficiency anemia, a reduction in the concentration of hemoglobin in the red blood cells due to a lack of iron supply to the bone marrow.

LDL-cholesterol: See cholesterol.

Linear growth: Increase in length or height.

Medical nutrition therapy: Use of specific nutrition counseling and interventions, based on an assessment of nutritional status, to manage a condition or treat an illness or injury.

Metabolism: The sum total of all the chemical reactions that go on in living cells.

Nutrition: The set of processes by which nutrients and other food components are taken in by the body and used.

Obesity: A condition characterized by excessive body fat.

Osteoporosis: A bone disease characterized by a reduction in bone mass and a deterioration of the bone structure leading to bone fragility.

Overweight: Excess body weight.

Physical activity: Bodily movement that substantially increases energy expenditure.

Registered dietitian: A food and nutrition expert who has met the minimum academic and professional requirements to receive the credential "RD." Many States and Commonwealths also have licensing laws for dietitians and nutrition practitioners.

Sedentary behavior: A pattern of behavior that is relatively inactive, such as a lifestyle characterized by a lot of sitting.

Type 2 diabetes: The most common form of diabetes, which results from insulin resistance and abnormal insulin action. Type 2 diabetes was previously referred to as noninsulin-dependent diabetes mellitus (NIDDM) and adult-onset diabetes.

REFERENCES

1. American Academy of Pediatrics, Work Group on Breastfeeding. Breastfeeding and the use of human milk. *Pediatrics* 100(6):1035–1039, 1997.

2. Frazao, E. The high costs of poor eating patterns in the United States. In: Frazao, E., ed. *America's Eating Habits: Changes and Consequences.* Washington, DC: U.S. Department of Agriculture (USDA), Economic Research Service (ERS), AIB-750, 1999.

3. National Center for Health Statistics (NCHS). Report of final mortality statistics, 1995. *Monthly Vital Statistics Report* 45 (11):Suppl. 2, June 12, 1997.

4. Frazao, E. The American diet: A costly problem. *Food Review* 19:2–6, 1996.

5. National Institutes of Health (NIH). *NIH Consensus Statement: Optimal Calcium Intake.* 12(4), 1994.

6. USDA and U.S. Department of Health and Human Services (HHS). *Dietary Guidelines for Americans.* 5th ed. USDA Home and Garden Bulletin No. 232. Washington, DC: USDA, 2000.

7. USDA. *The Food Guide Pyramid.* USDA Home and Garden Bulletin No. 252. Washington, DC: USDA, 1992.

8. Yip, R. The changing characteristics of childhood iron nutritional status in the United States. In: Filer, Jr., L.J., ed. *Dietary Iron: Birth to Two Years.* New York, NY: Raven Press, Ltd., 1989, 37–61.

9. NCHS. *Healthy People 2000 Review, 1998–99.* DHHS Pub. No. (PHS) 99–1256. Hyattsville, MD: Public Health Service (PHS), 1997.

10. HHS. Recommendations for the use of folic acid to reduce the number of cases of spina bifida and other neural tube defects. *Morbidity and Mortality Weekly Report* 41:1–7, 1992.

11. Lewis, C.J.; Crane, N.T.; Wilson, D.B.; et al. Estimated folate intakes: Data updated to reflect food fortification, increased bioavailability, and dietary supplement use. *American Journal of Clinical Nutrition* 70:198–207, 1999.

12. Flegal, K.M.; Carroll, M.D.; Kuczmarski, R.J.; et al. Overweight and obesity in the United States: Prevalence and trends, 1960–1994. *International Journal of Obesity* 22(1):39–47, 1998.

13. Kuczmarski, R.J.; Carroll, M.D.; Flegal, K.M.; et al. Varying body mass index cutoff points to describe overweight prevalence among U.S. adults: NHANES III (1988–1994). *Obesity Research* 5(6):542–548, 1997.

14. World Health Organization (WHO). *Obesity: Preventing and Managing the Global Epidemic. Report of a WHO Consultation on Obesity, Geneva, 3–5 June 1997.* Geneva, Switzerland: WHO, 1998.

15. NIH. Clinical guideline on the identification, evaluation and treatment of overweight and obesity in adults—The evidence report. *Obesity Research* 6(Suppl. 2):51S–209S, 1998.

16. Troiano, R.P., and Flegal, K.M. Overweight children and adolescents: Description, epidemiology, and demographics. *Pediatrics* 101:497–504, 1998.

17. Wolf, A.M., and Colditz, G.A. Current estimates of the economic cost of obesity in the United States. *Obesity Research* 6(2):97–106, 1998.

18. Centers for Disease Control and Prevention (CDC). Guidelines for school health programs to promote lifelong healthy eating. *Morbidity and Mortality Weekly Report* 45(RR-9):1–33, 1996.

19. Kelder, S.H.; Perry, C.L.; Klepp, K.I.; et al. Longitudinal tracking of adolescent smoking, physical activity,

and food choice behaviors. *American Journal of Public Health* 84(7):1121–1126, 1994.

20. Variyam, J.N.; Blaylock, J.; Lin, B.H.; et al. Mother's nutrition knowledge and children's dietary intakes. *American Journal of Agricultural Economics* 81(2), May 1999.

21. Collins, J.L.; Small, M.L.; Kann, L.; et al. School health education. *Journal of School Health* 65(8):302–311, 1995.

22. Contento, I.; Balch, G.I.; Bronner, Y.L.; et al. Nutrition education for school-aged children. *Journal of Nutrition Education* 27(6):298–311, 1995.

23. Lytle, L., and Achterberg, C. Changing the diet of America's children: What works and why? *Journal of Nutrition Education* 27(5):250-260, 1995.

24. USDA, Food and Nutrition Service (FNS). *Team Nutrition Strategic Plan.* Washington, DC: FNS, 1998.

25. NIH Technology Assessment Conference Panel. Methods for voluntary weight loss and control. Consensus development conference, March 30 to April 1, 1992. *Annals of Internal Medicine* 119(7.2):764–770, 1993.

26. Wilkening, V.L. FDA's regulations to implement the NLEA. *Nutrition Today* 13–20, 1993.

27. Lin, B.H.; Guthrie, J.; and Frazao, E. Nutrient contribution of food away from home. In: Frazao, E., ed. *America's Eating Habits: Changes and Consequences.* Washington, DC: USDA, ERS, AIB-750, 1999.

28. Crane, N.T., Hubbard, V.S.; and Lewis, C.J. National nutrition objectives and the Dietary Guidelines for Americans. *Nutrition Today* 33:49–58, 1998.

29. WHO Expert Committee. *Physical Status: The Use and Interpretation of Anthropometry. Report of a WHO Expert Committee.* WHO Technical Report Series: 854. Geneva, Switzerland: WHO, 1995.

30. Gallagher, D.; Visser, M.; Sepulveda, D.; et al. How useful is body mass index for comparison of body fatness across age, sex, and ethnic groups? *American Journal of Epidemiology* 143(3):228–239, 1996.

31. CDC. *Pediatric Nutrition Surveillance, 1997.* Full report. Atlanta, GA: HHS, CDC, 1998.

32. PHS. *The Surgeon General's Report on Nutrition and Health.* DHHS Pub. No. (PHS) 88050210. Washington, DC: HHS, 1988.

33. National Research Council. *Diet and Health: Implications for Reducing Chronic Disease Risk.* Washington, DC: National Academy Press, 1989.

34. HHS, Food and Drug Administration (FDA). Notice of final rule: Food labeling; health claims and label statements; dietary fiber and cardiovascular disease. *Federal Register* 2552-2605, January 5, 1993.

35. HHS, FDA. Notice of final rule: Food labeling; health claims and label statements; dietary fiber and cancer. *Federal Register* 2537–2552, January 5, 1993.

36. Chief Medical Officer's Committee on Medical Aspects of Food. *Nutritional Aspects of the Development of Cancer.* London, England: Stationery Office, 1998.

37. World Cancer Research Fund, in association with American Institute for Cancer Research. *Food, Nutrition and the Prevention of Cancer: A Global Perspective.* Washington, DC: the Fund, 1997.

38. USDA, Agricultural Research Service (ARS). Unpublished data from the 1994–96 Continuing Survey of Food Intakes by Individuals, February 1998.

39. Morton, J.F., and Guthrie, J.F. Changes in children's total fat intakes and their food sources of fat, 1989–91 versus 1994–95: Implications for diet quality. *Family Economics and Nutrition Review* 11(3):44–57, 1998.

40. Guthrie, J.F., and Morton, J.F. Food sources of added sweeteners in the diets of Americans. *Journal of the American Dietetic Association* 100(1):43–48, 51, 2000.

41. National Heart, Lung, and Blood Institute (NHLBI). *The Report of the Expert Panel on Population Strategies for Blood Cholesterol Reduction. National Cholesterol Education Program of the National Heart, Lung, and Blood Institute.* Washington, DC: HHS, 1990.

42. Lichtenstein, A.H.; Ausman, L.M.; Jalbert, S.M.; et al. Effects of different forms of dietary hydrogenated fats on serum lipoprotein cholesterol levels. *New England Journal of Medicine* 340(25):1933–1940, 1999.

43. Ip, C., and Carroll, K., eds. Proceedings of the workshop on individual fatty acids and cancer. Washington, DC, June 4–5, 1996. *American Journal of Clinical Nutrition* 66(Suppl. 6):1505S-1586S, 1997.

44. Freedman, L.S.; Prentice, R.L.; Clifford, C.; et al. Dietary fat and breast cancer: Where are we? *Journal of the National Cancer Institute* 85(10):764–765, 1993.

45. Allison, D.B.; Egan, S.K.; Barraj, L.M.; et al. Estimated intakes of *trans* fatty and other fatty acids in the U.S. population. *Journal of the American Dietetic Association* 99(2):166–174, 1999.

46. NHLBI. *Sixth Report of the Joint National Committee on Prevention, Detection, Evaluation, and Treatment of High Blood Pressure.* DHHS Pub. No. 98–4080. Washington, DC: HHS, 1997.

47. Elliott, P.; Stamler, J.; Nichols, R.; et al., for the Intersalt Cooperative Research Group. Intersalt revisited: Further analyses of 24 hour sodium excretion and blood pressure within and across populations. *British Medical Journal* 312:1249–1253, 1966.

48. Stamler, J.; Stamler, R.; and Neaton, J.D. Blood pressure, systolic and diastolic, and cardiovascular risks: U.S. population data. *Archives of Internal Medicine* 153(5):598–615, 1993.

49. Kurtz, T.W.; Al-Bander, H.A.; and Morris, R.C. "Salt sensitive" essential hypertension in men: Is the sodium ion alone important? *New England Journal of Medicine* 317 (17):1043–1048, 1987.

50. Mattes, R., and Donnelly, D. Relative contributions of dietary sodium sources. *Journal of the American College of Nutrition* 10(4):383–393, 1991.

51. James, W.P.T.; Ralph, A.; and Sanchez-Castillo, C.P. The dominance of salt in manufactured food in the sodium intake of affluent societies. *Lancet* 1 (8530):426–429, 1987.

52. Institute of Medicine. *Dietary Reference Intakes for Calcium, Phosphorus, Magnesium, Vitamin D, and Fluoride.* Washington, DC: National Academy Press, 1997.

53. Life Sciences Research Office, Federation of American Societies for Experimental Biology. Prepared for the Interagency Board for Nutrition Monitoring and Related Research. *Third Report on Nutrition Monitoring in the United States.* Vol. 1. Washington, DC: U.S. Government Printing Office, 1995, 104–105.

54. Tippett, K., and Cleveland, L. How current diets stack up: Comparison with the dietary guidelines. In: Frazao, E., ed. *America's Eating Patterns: Changes and Consequences.* Washington, DC: USDA, ERS, AIB-750, 1999.

55. Bucher, H.C.; Cook, R.J.; Guyatt, G.; et al. Effects of dietary calcium supplementation on blood pressure. A meta-analysis of randomized controlled trials. *Journal of the American Medical Association* 275:1016–1022, 1996.

56. Allender, P.S.; Cutler, J.A.; Follman, D.; et al. Dietary calcium and blood pressure: A meta-analysis of randomized clinical trials. *Annals of Internal Medicine* 124(9):825–829, 1996.

57. Idjradinata, P., and Pollitt, E. Reversal of developmental delays in iron-deficient anaemic infants treated with iron. *Lancet* 341(8836):1–4, 1993.

58. Lozoff, B.; Jimenez, E.; and Wolf, A.W. Long-term developmental outcome of infants with iron deficiency. *New England Journal of Medicine* 325 (10): 687–694, 1991.

59. Scholl, T.O.; Hediger, M.L.; Fischer, R.L.; et al. Anemia vs iron deficiency: Increased risk of preterm delivery in a prospective study. *American Journal of Clinical Nutrition* 55(5):985–998, 1992.

60. Bruner, A.B.; Joffe, A.; Duggan, A.K.; et al. Randomized study of cognitive effects of iron supplementation in non-anaemic iron-deficient adolescent girls. *Lancet* 348(9033):992–996, 1996.

61. CDC. Recommendations to prevent and control iron deficiency in the United States. *Morbidity and Mortality Weekly Report* 47(RR-3):1–29, 1998.

62. Perry, G.S.; Yip, R.; and Zyrkowski, C. Nutritional risk factors among low-income pregnant U.S. women: The Centers for Disease Control and Prevention (CDC) Pregnancy Nutrition Surveillance System, 1979 through 1993. *Seminars in Perinatology* 19(3): 211–221, 1995.

63. CDC. *Pregnancy Nutrition Surveillance, 1996.* Full report. Atlanta, GA: HHS, CDC, 1998.

64. Looker, A.C.; Dallman, P.R.; Carroll, M.D.; et al. Prevalence of iron deficiency in the United States. *Journal of the American Association* 277:973–976, 1997.

65. USDA, ARS. Data tables: Results from USDA's 1994–96 Continuing Survey of Food Intakes by Individuals and 1994–96 Diet and Health Knowledge Survey. Riverdale, MD: USDA, ARS, Beltsville Human Nutrition Research Center, December 1997. <http://www.barc.usda.gov/bhnrc/foodsurvey/home.htm>January 14, 1998.

66. Devaney, B., and Stewart, E. *Eating Breakfast: Effects of the School Breakfast Program.* Washington, DC: USDA, FNS, 1998.

67. Murphy, J.M.; Pagano, M.E.; Nachmani, J.; et al. The relationship of school breakfast to psychosocial and academic functioning: Cross-sectional and longitudinal observations in an inner-city school sample. *Archives of Pediatric and Adolescent Medicine* 152(9): 899–907, 1998.

68. Pollitt, E. Does breakfast make a difference at school? *Journal of the American Dietetic Association* 95(10): 1134–1139, 1995.

69. PHS. *Worksite Nutrition: A Guide to Planning, Implementation, and Evaluation.* 2nd ed. Washington, DC: American Dietetic Association (ADA) and Office of Disease Prevention and Health Promotion, PHS, HHS, 1993.

70. Sorensen, G.; Stoddard, A.; Hunt, M.K.; et al. The effects of a health promotion-health protection intervention on behavior change: The WellWorks Study. *American Journal of Public Health* 88(11):1685–1690, 1998.

71. Goetzel, R.Z.; Jacobson, B.H.; Aldana, S.G.; et al. Health care costs of worksite health promotion participants and non-participants. *Journal of Occupational and Environmental Medicine* 40(4):341–346, 1998.

72. Shephard, R.J. Employee health and fitness—State of the art. *Preventive Medicine* 12(5):644–653, 1983.

73. Felix, M.R.; Stunkard, A.J.; Cohen, R.Y.; et al. Health promotion at the worksite. I. A process for establishing programs. *Preventive Medicine* 14(1):99–108, 1985.

74. ADA. *The American Dietetic Association 1997 Nutrition Trends Survey.* Chicago, IL: ADA, 1997.

75. Caggiula, A.W.; Christakis, G.; Farrand, M.; et al. The Multiple Risk Factor Intervention Trial (MRFIT). IV. Intervention on blood lipids. *Preventive Medicine* 10(4):443–475, 1987.

76. Geil, P.B.; Anderson, J.W.; and Gustafson, N.J. Women and men with hypercholesterolemia respond similarly to an American Heart Association step 1 diet. *Journal of the American Dietetic Association* 95(4):436–441, 1995.

77. Gambera, P.J.; Schneeman, B.O.; and Davis, P.A. Use of the Food Guide Pyramid and U.S. Dietary Guidelines to improve dietary intake and reduce cardiovascular risk in active-duty Air Force members. *Journal of the American Dietetic Association* 95(11):1268–1273, 1995.

78. Hebert, J.R.; Ebbeling, C.B.; Ockene, I.S. et al. A dietitian-delivered group nutrition program leads to reductions in dietary fat, serum cholesterol, and body weight: The Worcester Area Trial for Counseling in Hyperlipidemia (WATCH). *Journal of the American Dietetic Association* 99(5):544–552, 1999.

79. McGehee, M.M.; Johnson, E.Q.; Rasmussen, H.M.; et al. Benefits and costs of medical nutrition therapy by registered dietitians for patients with hypercholesterolemia. *Journal of the American Dietetic Association* 95:1041–1043, 1995.

80. Sikand, G. Medical nutrition therapy lowers serum cholesterol and saves medication costs in men with hypercholesterolemia. *Journal of the American Dietetic Association* 98:889–894, 1998.

81. Franz, M.J., Splett, P.L.; Monk, A.; et al. Cost-effectiveness of medical nutrition therapy provided by dietitians for persons with non-insulin dependent diabetes mellitus. *Journal of the American Dietetic Association* 95(9):1018–1024, 1995.

82. Sheils, J.F.; Rubin, R.; and Stapleton, D.C. The estimated costs and savings of medical nutrition therapy: The Medicare population. *Journal of the American Dietetic Association* 99(4):428–435, 1999.

83. Johnson, R.K. The Lewin Group Study—What does it tell us and why does it matter? *Journal of the American Dietetic Association* 99(4):426–427, 1999.

84. Bickel, G.; Andrews, M.; and Carlson, S. The magnitude of hunger: In a new national measure of food security. *Topics in Clinical Nutrition* 13(4):15–30, 1998.

85. Food Research and Action Center. *Community Childhood Hunger Identification Project: A Survey of Childhood Hunger in the United States.* Vol. 1. Washington, DC: the Center, 1995.

86. Kendall, A.; Olson, C.M.; and Frongillo, Jr., E.A. Validation of the Radimer/Cornell measures of hunger and food insecurity. *Journal of Nutrition* 125(11): 2793–2801, 1995.

87. Foreign Agricultural Service (FAS), USDA. *U.S. Action Plan on Food Security: Solutions to Hunger.* Washington, DC: USDA, FAS, 1999.

88. USDA. *USDA's Community Food Security Initiative Action Plan.* USDA Community Food Security Initiative, August 1999.

89. Health Resources and Services Administration (HRSA), Maternal and Child Health Bureau. *Community Outreach, The Healthy Start Initiative: A Community-Driven Approach to Infant Mortality Reduction.* Vol. IV. Washington, DC: HRSA, 1996.

GLOSSARY

abortifacient A substance that induces abortion or miscarriage—the premature expulsion of a fetus from the womb.

acrid A sharp, bitter or unpleasantly pungent taste or smell.

adjuvant A substance (usually an herb) added to boost the effect of another substance.

alterative A substance that promotes a gradual change in nutrition or in the body without creating a particular effect of its own.

analgesic A painkiller.

anaphrodisiac A substance that reduces sexual desire and/or potency.

anesthetic A substance used to obliterate sensation, especially of pain.

anodyne A painkiller.

antacid A substance that neutralizes excess acid in the stomach and relieves discomfort and flatulence.

anthelmintic A substance used to kill or expel worms from the intestines.

antiabortive A substance that inhibits a potential abortion or miscarriage.

antiasthmatic A substance that relieves asthma symptoms.

antibiotic A substance that inhibits or destroys bacteria, viruses, amoebas and other microorganisms.

anticatarrhal A substance that thwarts or eliminates the formation of mucus.

anticoagulant A substance that prevents blood clotting.

antiemetic A substance that prevents or alleviates nausea and vomiting.

antihydrotic A substance used to inhibit perspiration.

anti-inflammatory A substance that reduces or fights an area of redness, heat, swelling or pain in the body that characterizes a non-specific immune response to injury or infection.

antilithic A substance that dissolves or diminishes stones or gravel in the urinary tract.

antimicrobial A substance that rids the body of microorganisms that have caused an undesirable effect in the body or on the skin.

antineoplastic A substance that specifically inhibits or fights tumor development.

antiperiodic A substance that counteracts intermittent diseases such as malaria.

antiphilogistic An anti-inflammatory.

antipyretic A substance that reduces fever.

antirheumatic A substance that prevents or relieves rheumatic symptoms.

antiscorbutic A substance containing vitamin C that prevents and cures scurvy.

antiscrofulous A substance that counteracts scrofula, a tuberculous adenitis or swelling of the lymph nodes in the neck.

antiseptic A substance that prevents or counteracts the growth of harmful microorganisms.

antispasmodic A substance that relaxes nervous tension related to digestive or muscular spasms.

antitussive A substance that relieves coughing.

aperient A mild bowel stimulant.

aphrodisiac A substance that stimulates or increases sexual desire and/or potency.

appetizer A substance that stimulates the desire to eat.

aromatic A substance whose fragrance or agreeable odor acts as a relaxant or stimulant.

astringent A substance that reduces secretion or discharges from bodily tissues; a drying agent.

Ayurveda The 6,000 year-old holistic medical science of India, named from two Sanskrit words meaning "life" and "knowledge."

balsam A resinous substance from trees that has soothing and healing action.

bitter One of the characteristic taste sensations (along with salt, sour and sweet) that may be acrid, astringent or disagreeable; a substance that increases appetite and promotes digestion.

botany The study, or science, of plant life.

calmative A substance used as a tranquilizer or sedative.

cardiac A substance that has an effect on the heart.

carminative A substance that relieves griping (severe bowel pains) and intestinal gas.

cathartic A laxative.

caustic A substance capable of corroding or burning bodily tissue.

chologogue A substance that increases the flow of bile into the intestinal tract.

coagulant A substance that promotes the formation of clots, such as blood clots.

counterirritant A substance that irritates one part of the body to counteract irritation in another part.

decongestant A substance that relieves mucus build-up in the respiratory tract.

demulcent A substance that soothes irritated membranes and other tissues.

deodorant A substance that masks or destroys undesirable odors.

depressant A substance that reduces nervous stimulation.

depurative A purifying, cleansing substance, especially for the bloodstream.

detergent A substance that cleanses wounds and removes diseased or necrotic material.

diaphoretic A substance that promotes perspiration.

digestive A substance that promotes the digestion of foods throughout the alimentary tract.

disinfectant An antiseptic.

diuretic A substance that promotes urination.

dysmenorrhea Menstrual pain or disorder.

emetic A substance that induces vomiting.

emmenagogue A substance that encourages menstrual flow.

emollient A softening, soothing agent used externally.

errhine A substance that induces sneezing and nasal discharge.

euphoriant, euphorigen A substance that induces an extraordinary or abnormal sense of happiness, "floating," etc.

expectorant A substance that promotes the expulsion of mucus from the lungs and other respiratory structures.

family The biological reference to a group of related plants or animals; a family is a category above a genus and below an order (e.g., Brassica, the crucifer family).

febrifuge An antipyretic, or fever reducer.

galactagogue A substance that promotes and increases the secretion of mother's milk.

genus A biological classification, in Latin, between family and species.

hallucinogen A substance that induces bizarre visions, apparitions, sounds or other visual or auditory hallucinations.

hemostatic A substance that arrests bleeding.

herb An annual, biennial or perennial plant used for its aromatic, flavoring or medicinal properties.

hepatic A substance that affects the liver.

hydragogue A laxative that promotes copious watery discharge.

hypnotic A sleep-producing agent.

irritant A substance that produces adverse reaction.

laxative A substance that promotes the evacuation of fecal material from the intestines.

lithotriptic A substance that dissolves or eliminates urinary, kidney or biliary gravel and stones.

mucilaginous Gummy or having the consistency of gelatin.

narcotic Therapeutically, a substance that kills pain and induces sleep.

nauseant A substance that creates the desire to vomit.

nephritic A substance that affects the kidneys.

nervine A tranquilizer or sedative.

oxytocic A substance that promotes uterine contraction to aid in childbirth.

parasiticide A substance that kills parasites that have invaded the digestive tract or the skin.

pectoral A remedial substance for chest and lung diseases.

poison A substance that can harm or destroy living tissue.

purgative A substance that promotes a dramatic expulsion of waste materials from the intestines; a strong laxative.

refrigerant A cooling agent; a substance capable of lowering body heat.

restorative A substance capable of reviving consciousness or normal bodily functions.

rubefacient A mild irritant that creates redness of the skin.

sedative A substance that reduces nervous tension.

sialagogue A substance that promotes salivation.

species A biological classification, in Latin, of related organisms under the category of genus.

specific A substance used to affect a particular disease or problem.

stimulant A substance that excites or activates a bodily (including physical and mental) process.

stomachic A substance that fortifies the stomach or promotes healthy stomach activity.

styptic An astringent or hemostatic; a substance that arrests bleeding.

sudorific A diaphoretic, or substance that promotes perspiration.

taeniacide A vermifuge, or agent that destroys tapeworms.

tonic A strengthening agent.

vasoconstrictor A substance that causes blood vessels to narrow and increases blood pressure.

vasodilator A substance that causes blood vessels to expand and lowers blood pressure.

vermicide An anthelmintic; a substance that kills worms in the intestines.

vermifuge A substance that induces the expulsion of intestinal worms.

vesicant A substance that causes blisters.

vulnerary A substance that promotes cell growth and repair in the case of wounds.

BIBLIOGRAPHY

"Active H, Patrick Flanagan's Silica Hydride Supplement from Generations of Health," Synergy. Available on-line URL: http://www.crystalenergy.co.uk/active-h.html. Downloaded April 6, 2003.

Allaby, Michael, ed. *The Concise Oxford Dictionary of Botany.* New York: Oxford University Press, 1992.

American Dietetic Association. "Caffeine: How Much Is Too Much?" Special advertising section, *Time*, November 21, 1994.

———. "Positions of the American Dietetic Association: Enrichment and Fortification of Foods and Dietary Supplements." *Journal of the American Dietetic Association* 94(1994): 661–663.

———. "Position of the American Dietetic Association: Food and Nutrition Misinformation." *Journal of the American Dietetic Association* 102(2002): 260–266.

———. "Position of the American Dietetic Association and Dietitians of Canada: Vegetarian Diets." *Journal of the American Dietetic Association* 103(2003): 748–765.

American Journal of Dentistry 5(1992): 269.

American Medical Association. *AMA Drug Evaluations Subscription.* Chicago, 1992.

American Medical Association. "Caffeine Use Can Lead to Dependence." News release, Department of Science News, Chicago, October 4, 1994.

American Medical Association. "Consumption of Dark Green, Leafy Vegetables Could Lower Risk of Vision Disorder." News release. Department of Science News, Chicago, November 8, 1994.

American Medical Association. "Some Herbal Medications May Cause Liver Injury." News release. Department of Science News, Chicago: February 7, 1995.

Appel, L. J., E. R. Miller 3d, A. J. Seidler, and P. K. Whelton. "Does Supplementation of Diet with 'Fish Oil' Reduce Blood Pressure? A Meta-Analysis of Controlled Clinical Trials." *Archives of Internal Medicine* 153(1993): 1429–1438.

"Appendix A: Resources and Guidelines on Buying and Using Nutraceuticals." Available on-line. URL: http://www.americanutra.com/appendix.html.

Balluz, Lina S., et al. "Vitamin and Mineral Supplement Use in the United States, Results from the Third National Health and Nutrition Examination Survey," *Archives of Family Medicine* 9 (March 2000): 258–262.

Barnett, Robert A. "Can Vitamins Save Your Life?" *Family Circle*, February 1, 1995: 24.

Bartlow, Stephanie. "Drink up! Water Is a Necessity." *The Ocean County Medical News Update*, vol. 1, no. 9, June 1994: 8.

Bellisfield, Dale. "Food as Medicine: An Enlightened Approach to Eating." Siegler Center for Integrative Medicine, Saint Barnabas Ambulatory Care Center, Livingston, N.J., June 2003. Unpublished handout.

Berkow, R., M. B. Fletcher, et al. *The Merck Manual of Diagnosis and Therapy.* 15th ed. Rahway, N.J.: 1987.

Bielory, L., and R. Gandhi. "Asthma and Vitamin C." *Annuals of Allergy* 73(1994): 89–96.

Bittman, Mark. "Eating Well: A Little Cooking Goes a Long Way for Vegetable Nutrients." *New York Times*, August 31, 1994: C4.

Blumenthal, M., ed. *The Complete German Commission E Monographs: Therapeutic Guide to Herbal Medicines.* British Herbal Medicine Association Integrative Medicine Communications, Boston: 1998.

Bourre, Jean-Marie, M. D. *Brainfood: A Provocative Exploration of the Connection Between What You Eat and How You Think.* Boston: Little, Brown and Company, 1990.

Bradley, P., ed. *British Herbal Compendium.* Vol. I. Dorset, Great Britain: British Herbal Medicine Association, 1992.

Braunwald, E., K. J. Isselbacher, R. G. Petersdorf, et al., eds. *Harrison's Principles of Internal Medicine.* New York: McGraw-Hill, 1987.

Brody, Jane E. "Illness Raises Concern on Herbal Preparations." *New York Times*, February 8, 1995.

Brown, H., B. R. Cassileth, J. P. Lewis, and J. H. Renner. "Alternative Medicine—or Quackery?" *Patient Care*, June 15, 1994: 91.

Burg, Dale. "Eat Your Spinach." *New Woman*, February 1994: 144.

Burtis, W. J., L. Gay, K. L. Insogna, et al. "Dietary Hypercalcemia in Patients with Calcium Oxalate Kidney Stones." *American Journal of Clinical Nutrition* 60 (1994): 424–429.

Butler, J. C., et al. "Measles Severity and Serum Retinol (Vitamin A) Concentration Among Children in the United States." *Pediatrics* 91(1993): 1176–1181.

"Buying Vitamins: What's Worth the Price?" *Consumer Reports*, September, 1994.

Canadian Pediatric Society—Société Canadienne de Pédiatrie. "Megavitamin and megamineral therapy in childhood." *Canadian Medical Association Journal* 143 (1990): 1009–1013.

Carroll, L. "Iodine Supplements in Pregnancy May Prevent Cretinism." *Medical Tribune,* February 2, 1995.

Cataldo, Corinne, Linda DeBruyne, and Eleanor Whitney. *Nutrition and Diet Therapy.* 3rd ed. St. Paul: West Publishing Co., 1992.

Chopra, Deepak, M.D. *Perfect Health: The Complete Mind/Body Guide.* New York: Harmony Books, 1991.

Christoffel, K. "A Pediatric Perspective on Vegetarian Nutrition." *Clinical Pediatrics* 20(1981): 632–643.

"Chronic Fatigue Diets Rebuked." *Medical Tribune,* March 1993.

Couturier, Lisa. "Protecting Our Fellow Creatures." *New Woman,* February 1994: 96.

"Cure It with Herbs." *First,* February 27, 1995: 43–47.

Dalsky, G. P. "Exercise: Its Effect on Bone Mineral Content." *Clinical Obstetrics and Gynecology* 30(1987): 820–32.

Davis, Adelle. *Let's Eat Right to Keep Fit.* New York: New American Library, Harcourt Brace Jovanovich, Inc., 1970.

Dickinson, A. *Benefits of Nutritional Supplements.* Washington, D.C.: Council for Responsible Nutrition, 1987.

"Dietary Guidelines for Healthy American Adults," American Heart Association, http://www.americanheart.org/presenter.jhtml?identifier=4561, January 22, 2003.

"Don't Eliminate All Fat from Diet." Your Body: An Owner's Manual column. *Asbury Park Press,* May 10, 1994.

Dorland's Illustrated Medical Dictionary. 28th ed. Philadelphia: W. B. Saunders, 1994.

Drug Information for the Health Care Professional. 14th ed. Taunton, Massachusetts: Rand McNally, 1994.

Eastman, Peggy. "Getting a Better Fix on Supplements," *AARP Bulletin* (May 2003): 16–18.

Elmer-Dewitt, Philip. "Fat Times: What Health Craze? Thanks to Too Much Food and Too Little Sweat, Americans Are Heavier Than Ever." *Time,* January 16, 1995: 58.

Findlay, S. "Nutritional Bodyguards." *Fitness,* March–April 1993: 4–6.

"Fish Oil Reported to Offer No Benefit Against Restenosis." *Cardiology World News,* September 15, 1994: 7.

Forman, A. "Mining for minerals—Zinc Is Worth Its Weight in Gold." *Environmental Nutrition* 17 (1994): 1–6.

Fried, J. *Vitamin Politics.* Buffalo, N.Y.: Prometheus Books, 1984.

Friedman, Max. "Whatever Happened to Hemp?" *Vegetarian Times,* August 1994: 71.

Friend, T. "Zinc Levels May Offer New Theory on Alzheimer's." *USA Today,* September 2, 1994.

"Fruits, Vegetables Provide Folic Acid." Nutrition column. *Asbury Park Press,* February 8, 1994.

Fulder, Stephen. *The Tao of Medicine: Ginseng, Oriental Remedies, and the Pharmacology of Harmony.* New York: Destiny Books, 1980.

Futoryan, T. and B. A. Gilchrest. "Retinoids and the Skin." *Nutrition Reviews* 52(1994): 299–306.

Gamboa, P. M., et al. "Allergic Contact Urticaria from Poppy Flowers (*Papaver rhoeas*)." *Contact Dermatitis* 37, no. 3 (September 1997): 140–141.

Gapinski, J. P., J. V. Van Ruiswyk, G. R. Heudebert, and G. S. Schectman. "Preventing Restenosis with Fish Oils Following Coronary Angioplasty. A Meta-analysis." *Arch Internal Medicine* 153 (1993): 1595–1601.

Garrison, R. H., and E. Somer. *The Nutrition Desk Reference.* 2nd ed. New Canaan, Conn.: Keats Publishing, 1990.

Gilman, A. G., T. W. Rall, A. S. Nies, and P. Taylor, eds. *Goodman and Gilman's The Pharmacological Basis of Therapeutics.* 8th ed. New York: McGraw-Hill, 1990.

Golden, W. E. "Folic Acid for the Prevention of Neural Tube Defects." *Patient Outcomes* July–August 1994: 23–25.

Goldfarb, S. "Diet and Nephrolithiasis." *Annual Review of Medicine* 45(1994): 235–243.

Greenberg, E. R., Baren, J. A., Tosteson, T. D., et al. "A Clinical Trial of Antioxident Vitamins to Prevent Colorectal Adenoma." *New England Journal of Medicine* 331(1994): 141–147.

Gruenwald, J., T. Brendler, and J. Christof. *PDR for Herbal Medicines.* Montvale, N.J.: Medical Economics Company, 1998.

Gutfeld, G. and T. Hanlon. "Choosing Your Best Prostate Prescription." *Prevention,* June 1994: 80, 90–91.

Harrington, Geri. *Real Food, Fake Food and Everything in Between.* New York: Macmillan Publishing Company, Inc., 1987.

Harris, R. "Vitamins and Neural Tube Defects." Editorial. *British Medical Journal* 296(1988): 80–81.

Heinonen, O. P., and D. Albanes. "The Effect of Vitamin E and Beta Carotene on the Incidence of Lung Cancer and Other Cancers in Male Smokers." *New England Journal of Medicine* 330(1994): 1029–1035.

Hendler, S. S. *The Doctor's Vitamin and Mineral Encyclopedia.* New York: Simon and Schuster, 1990.

Herbert, V., and M. S. Subak-Sharpe, eds. *The Mt. Sinai School of Medicine Complete Book of Nutrition.* New York: St. Martin's Press, 1990.

Hertog, M. G. L., et al. "Dietary Antioxidant Flavonoids and Risk of Coronary Heart Disease: The Zutphen Elderly Study." *Lancet* 342 (1993): 1007–1011.

Hoffman, F. A. "Micronutrient Requirements of Cancer Patients." *Cancer* 55(1 Suppl)(1985): 295–300.

Hogan, Mary Ann. "Nutritional Aids: Helping Patients Choose the Right Liquid Dietary Supplement." *Advance for Nurses,* Greater New York/New Jersey (June 9, 2003).

Hrabak, D. "A Fish Oil Story: Omega-3's Return to Fight Heart Disease, Cancer." *Environmental Nutrition* 17(1994): 1–3.

Hu, Frank, B. "The Mediterranean Diet and Mortality—Olive Oil and Beyond," *New England Journal of Medicine* (June 26, 2003): 2595–2596.

Hunter, D. J., et al. "Prospective Study of the Intake of Vitamins C, E, A and the Risk of Breast Cancer." *New England Journal of Medicine* 329(1993): 234.

Hutchens, Alma R. *Indian Herbology of North America.* Boston: Shambhala, 1991.

Jancin, B. "Calcium for Osteoporosis: Little Help, Little Harm." *Family Practice News,* February 15, 1994.

Joslin Diabetes Center. "New Research Suggests Vitamin E May Prevent Vascular Complications." Press release. October 25, 1994.

Kail, K. "Multivitamin-Mineral Complexes: Your Nutritional Insurance Policy." *Health Foods Business,* April 1992: 87–89.

Kanter, M. M., L. A. Nolte, and J. O. Holloszy. "Effects of an Antioxident Vitamin Mixture on Lipid Peroxidation at Rest and Post-exercise." *Journal of Applied Physiology* 74 (1993): 965–969.

Katzman, Shoshanna, and Wendy Shankin-Cohen. *Feeling Light: The Holistic Solution to Permanent Weight Loss and Wellness.* New York: Avon Books, 1997.

Koop, C. Everett, M. D., *The Surgeon General's Report on Nutrition and Health.* Rocklin, Calif.: Prima Publishing and Communications, 1988.

Krause, Marie V., and Kathleen L. Mahan. *Food, Nutrition and Diet Therapy.* 6th ed. Philadelphia: W. B. Saunders Co., 1979.

Kritz, Fran. "Government Taking a Closer Look at Medicinal Plants." *Medical Tribune,* January 19, 1995.

Lad, Vasant. *Ayurveda: The Science of Self-Healing.* Wilmot, Wis.: Lotus Press, 1985.

Lefferts, L. Y. "Run, Radicals, Run." *Nutrition Action Health Letter* 20(1993): 4.

Lieberman, S., and N. Bruning. *The Real Vitamin & Mineral Book.* Garden City Park, N.Y.: Avery Publishing Group, 1990.

Liebman, B. "The Ultra Mega Vita Guide." *Nutrition Action Health Letter.* 20(1993): 7–8.

Lipkowitz, M. A., and T. Navarra. *Allergies A to Z.* New York: Facts On File, 1994.

"Lorenzo's Oil and Lymphocytopenia." *New England Journal of Medicine* 330(1993), no. 8: 577.

Lust, John. *The Herb Book.* New York: Bantam Books, 1974.

Lyons, A. S., and R. J. Petrucelli. *Medicine, An Illustrated History.* New York: Abradale Press, 1987.

Marcuard, S. P., L. Albernaz, and P. G. Khazanie. "Omeprazole Therapy Causes Malabsorption of Cyanocobalamin (Vitamin B_{12}). *Annals of Internal Medicine* 120(1994): 211.

Margen, S., and D. A. Ogar. "Low Calorie Carrot Jewel of a Vegetable." *Asbury Park Press,* September 6, 1994.

Matthews, Karen. "Fungal Tea Mushrooming as Health Fad." *Asbury Park Press,* February 7, 1995: B1.

McAdam, P. "Vitamin D Drug Enhances Psoriasis Therapy." *Medical Tribune,* April 7, 1994.

McAllister-Smart, Joanne. "Antioxidants for the Uninitiated." *Vegetarian Times,* April 1994: 26.

McCann, J. "Antioxidants Show Promise in Cancer Therapy." *Medical Tribune,* April 7, 1994.

McIntyre, Anne. *The Complete Women's Herbal: A Manual of Healing, Herbs and Nutrition for Personal Well-Being and Family Care.* New York: Henry Holt Co., 1994.

McKenna, Dennis J., Kenneth Jones, and Kerry Hughes. *Botanical Medicines: The Desk Reference for Major Herbal Supplements.* 2nd ed. New York: The Haworth Herbal Press, 2002.

Medicine the Year in Review 1992. New York; Medical Tribune, 1993.

Messina, Virginia, Vesanto Melina, and Ann Reed Mangels. "A New Food Guide for North American Vegetarians." *Journal of The American Dietetic Association* 103 (2003): 771–775.

MidLife Women's Network. "Food, Fats & You." *Midlife Woman* 2 (1992): 1–9.

Miller, L. "Twice-a-Day Dose of Vitamin C May Be Key." *USA Today,* October 18, 1994.

Mindell, E. *Vitamin Bible.* New York: Warner Books, 1991.

Morris, M. C., F. Sacks, and B. Rosner. "Does Fish Oil Lower Blood Pressure? A Meta-analysis of Controlled Trials." *Circulation* 88 (1993): 522–533.

"Most Everyone Can Use a Modest Increase in Calcium, Says NIH." *Modern Medicine,* 16 (1995): 11.

National Center for Complementary and Alternative Medicine. "NCCAM Consumer Advisory on Ephedra," NCCAM, National Institutes of Health. Available on-line. URL: http://nccam.nih.gov/health/alerts/ephedra/consumeradvisory.htm. Downloaded October 10, 2003.

"National Institute of Health (NIH)." *World Book Encyclopedia.* Chicago: World Book-Childcraft International 14(1979): 40.

New Jersey Naturally. Resource Directory for Natural Living, Winter/Spring 1995. New York: City Spirit Publications.

"Nutrition." *The New Encyclopedia Britannica, Macropedia.* vol. 13. Chicago: Encyclopedia Britannica, Inc., 1974.

"Nutritional Supplements Shown to Provide Valuable Health Benefits," American Medical Association Science News Media Briefings. Available on-line. URL: http://www.ama-assn.org/ama/pub/print/article/4197-6758.html. Downloaded

"Nutrition Checklist." Washington, D.C.: The Nutrition Screening Initiative, 1992.

Nutrition column. *Asbury Park Press.* February 28, 1994.

"Nutritional Analysis of Kamut Brand Grain," Kamut Association of North America. Available on-line. URL: http://www.kamut.com./index2.html. Downloaded April 6, 2003.

Office of Public Affairs, Department of Health and Human Services, "HHS Acts to Reduce Potential Risks of Dietary Supplements Containing Ephedra," FDA News. Available on-line. URL: http://www.fda.gov/bbs/topics/news/2003/new00875.html. Downloaded October 10, 2003.

Olin, B. R., and S. K. Hebel, et al., eds. *Facts and Comparisons.* St. Louis: J. B. Lippencott Co., 1994.

Pauling, L., and C. Moertel. "A Proposition: Megadoses of Vitamin C Are Valuable in the Treatment of Cancer." *Nutrition Review* 44(1986): 28–32.

Pfeifer, S. "On the Occurrence of Glaudine in Opium and Papaver rhoeas L." *Pharmazie* 20, no. 4 (April 1965): 240.

———, and V. Hanus. "On the Alkaloids from Papaver rhoeas L." *Pharmazie* 20, no. 6 (June 1965): 394.

Physician's Desk Reference. Montvale, N.J.: Medical Economics, 1994.

Pizzorno, Joseph E., Jr., and Michael T. Murray. *Textbook of Natural Medicine.* 2nd ed. Edinburgh, U.K.: Churchill Livingstone, 1999.

"Powerful Ephedrine Eyed for Side Effects, Toxicity." *The Ocean County Medical News Update,* vol. 1, no. 9, June 1994: 16.

Pratt, Steven. "MSG—Is It Harmless or an 'Excitotoxin'?" *Asbury Park Press,* August 3, 1994: B1.

"Problems with Dietary Supplements," *Medical Letter On Drugs and Therapeutics* 44, no. 1140 (September 30, 2002): 84–86.

Prochaska, Hans, Annette Santamaria, and Paul Talalay. "The Rapid Detection of Inducers of Enzymes That Protect Against Carcinogens." The Proceedings of the National Academy of Science, USA, vol. 89, March 1992: 2394–2398.

Quinn, E. Q. and J. R. Meese. "Pseudotumor Cerebri, a Review." *The Female Patient* 19(1994): 16–24.

Recker, R. R. "Common Misconceptions about Calcium Absorption." Lecture. *Gastroenterology Observer,* July–August, 1994.

Rector-Page, Linda G. *Healthy Healing: An Alternative Reference.* Sonora: Calif., Healthy Healing Publications, 1994.

Reid, Ian, M. D., Ruth Ames, N.Z.C.S., Margaret Evans, B.Sc., et al. "The Effect of Calcium Supplementation on Bone Loss in Post-Menopausal Women." *The New England Journal of Medicine,* 328(1993): 460–464.

"Report 8 of the Council on Scientific Affairs (A-99): Review of AMA Recommendations on Folic Acid Supplementation," American Medical Association. Available on-line. URL: http://www.ama-assn.org/ama/pub/print/article/2036-2337.html. Downloaded January 22, 2003.

Retsinas, Greg. "Couple Guilty of Assault in Vegan Case," *New York Times,* 5 April 2003.

Richer, S. P. "Is There a Prevention and Treatment Strategy for Macular Degeneration?" *Journal of the American Optometric Association* 64 (1993): 838–850.

Rivlin, R. S. "Nutrition and Aging." Lecture, University of Medicine and Dentistry of New Jersey, Robert Wood Johnson Medical School. April 27, 1990.

Roberts, H. J.: "Vitamin E and Gynecomastia." Letter. *Hospital Practice* 29 (1994): 12.

Roche Biomedical Laboratories. *Directory of Services.* Stowe, Ohio: Lexi-Comp, 1991.

Rosenbaum, Michael E., M. D., and Dominick Bosco. *Super Fitness Beyond Vitamins: The Bible of Super Supplements.* New York: New American Library Books, 1987.

Rubenstein, E., and D. D. Ferdermann, eds. *Scientific American Medicine.* New York: Scientific American, 1987.

"Salmonella Arizona Infections Associated with Ingestion of Rattlesnake Capsules." Archives of Internal Medicine, 149(1989): 701, 705.

Sambrook, P., et al. "Prevention of Corticosteroid Osteoporosis; a Comparison of Calcium, Calcitriol and Calcitonin." *New England Journal of Medicine* 328(1993): 1747–1752.

Schart, D. "Vitamins 101, How to Buy Them." *Nutrition Action Health Letter.* January/February 1993: 5–6.

Schulz, V., R. Hansel, and V. Tyler. *Rational Phytotherapy: A Physician's Guide to Herbal Medicine.* 3rd ed. Berlin, Germany: Springer, 1998.

Seddon, J. M., and C. H. Hennekens. "Vitamins, Minerals and Macular degeneration. Promising but Unproven Hypothesis." Editorial: comments. *Archives of Ophthalmology* 112 (1994): 176–179.

Severo, Richard. "Linus C. Pauling Dies at 93; Chemist and Voice for Peace." *New York Times,* August 21, 1994: 1.

Shils, M. E., J. A. Olson, and M. Shike, eds. *Modern Nutrition in Health and Disease.* 8th ed. Philadelphia: Lea & Febiger, 1994.

Simpson, Glenn. "A Raid on Your Medicine Chest." *US Weekend,* February 18–20, 1994.

Somer, E. *The Essential Guide to Vitamins and Minerals.* New York: HarperPerennial, 1992.

Soulimani, R., et al. "Behavioral and Pharmaco-toxicological Study of Papaver rhoeas L. in Mice." *J Ethnopharmacol* 74, no. 3 (March 3, 2001): 265–274.

Southgate, D. A., "Minerals, Trace Elements, and Potential Hazards." *American Journal of Clinical Nutrition* 45 (supplement)(1987): 1256–1266.

Spiro, H. M. *Clinical Gastroenterology.* 2nd ed. New York: Macmillan, 1977.

Stähelin, H. B. "Vitamins and Cancer." *Recent Results in Cancer Research* 108(1988): 227–234.

Tadesco, L. Conversations between Myron Lipkowitz with a registered nutritionist. August 1994 to February 1995.

"Taking vitamins—Can They Prevent Disease?" *Consumer Reports,* September 1994; 561–564.

Thomas, Clayton L., ed. *Taber's Cyclopedic Medical Dictionary.* 17th ed. Philadelphia: F. A. Davis Company, 1993.

Thomson, W. A. *Medicines from the Earth: A Guide to Healing Plants.* New York: McGraw-Hill, 1978.

Tierra, Michael. *The Way of Herbs.* New York: Pocket Books, 1990.

Toufexis, A. "The New Scoop on Vitamins." *Time.* April 6, 1992: 54–59.

Tyler, V. *The Honest Herbal: A Sensible Guide to the Use of Herbs and Related Remedies.* 3rd ed. New York: Pharmaceutical Products Press, 1993.

U.S. Code Congressional and Administrative News, 103rd Congress, no. 9, December 1994. St. Paul: West Publishing Co., 108-Stat. 4329.

U.S. Code Service, Food and Drugs, Sections 1–600. Rochester, N.Y.: The Lawyers Co-Operative Publishing Co., 1994, pp. 288–290.

U.S. Department of Health and Human Services/Public Health Service. "Lead Poisoning Associated with Use of Traditional Ethnic Remedies—California, 1991–1992." *Morbidity and Mortality Weekly Report,* vol. 42, no. 27, July 16, 1993.

U.S. Food & Drug Administration. "Folic acid-fortified food." *FDA Medical Bulletin* 24(1994): 9.

———. "The new food label." *FDA Medical Bulletin* 24(1994): 2–3.

———. National Institutes of Health. "Chapter 19: Nutrition and Overweight," Healthy People 2010. Available on-line. URL: http://www.healthypeople.gov/document/html/volume2/19nutrition.htm. Downloaded October 10, 2003.

Ulene, A. *Count Out Cholesterol.* New York: Alfred A. Knopf, 1989.

Ulene, A., and V. Ulene. *The Vitamin Strategy.* Berkeley, Calif.: Ulysses Press, 1994.

United States Pharmacopia. 22nd rev. ed. The United States Pharmacopeial Convention, Inc. Easton, Pa.: Mack Printing Co., 1990.

"Vitamin and Mineral Supplements," American Heart Association. Available on-line. URL: http://www.americanheart.org/presenter.jhtml?identifier=4788. Downloaded January 1, 2003.

"Vitamin E and C Supplements Lower Risk of Coronary Death Among the Elderly." *Modern Medicine* 63(1995): 15.

"Vitamins and Minerals from A to Z Quiz." McMahon Co., 1993.

"Vitamins for Vision." *Nutrition Action Health Letter,* January/February 1994. Original source: *Archives of Ophthalmology* 111(1993): 1246.

"Vitamins linked to immune system." *Asbury Park Press,* September 13, 1994: B3.

Wade, Nicholas. "Method and Madness: Believing in Vitamins." *New York Times Magazine,* May 22, 1994: 20.

Ward, Bernard. *Healing Foods from the Bible.* Boca Raton, Fla.: Globe Communications Corp., 1994.

Ward, John T. "Vitamin Craze." *Asbury Park Press,* April 3, 1994: B1.

Weiss, Gaea, and Shandoe Weiss. *Growing and Using the Healing Herbs.* Emmaus, Pa.: Rodale Press, 1985.

"What Are Dietary Supplements?" National Institutes of Health Office of Dietary Supplements. Available online. URL: http://www.ods.od.nih.gov/whatare/whatare.html. Downloaded January 23, 2003.

Whitehead R. G. "Vitamins, Minerals, Schoolchildren and IQ." Editorial. *British Medical Journal* 302(1991): 548.

Wichtl, M., and Bisset, N. G. (eds)., "Poppy Flowers." In *Herbal Drugs and Phyto-pharmaceuticals.* Stuttgart, Germany: CRC Press, 1994.

York, E. "Diet, Exercise and Bone Mineral Content." Letter. *Annals of Internal Medicine* 102(1985): 418.

ADDITIONAL INTERNET SOURCES

American Dietetic Association, "Your Link to Nutrition and Health!" Available on-line. URL: http://www.eatright.org/. Downloaded January 29, 2003.

Arbor Nutrition guide. Available on-line. URL: http://www.arborcom.com/frame/welcome.htm. Downloaded January 29, 2003.

Center for Food Safety & Applied Nutrition, U.S. Food and Drug Administration. Available on-line. URL: http://vm.cfsan.fda.gov/. Downloaded

Center for Science in the Public Interest. Available on-line. URL: http://www.cspinet.org/. Downloaded January 29, 2003.

Cyberdiet. Available on-line. URL: http://www.cyberdiet.com/reg/index.html. Downloaded January 29, 2003.

Food and Nutrition Information Center. Available on-line. URL: http://www.nalusda.gov/fnic/. Downloaded January 29, 2003.

Holistic Animal Therapy Association. Available on-line. URL: http://www.hataa.asn.av. Downloaded October 28, 2003.

MayoClinic Food & Nutrition Center. Available on-line. URL: http://www.mayoclinic.com/findinformation/conditioncenters/centers.cfm?obje ctid=00085. Downloaded January 29, 2003.

Moberly, Heather K., and Amy L. Paster. "Nutrition and Vegetarianism," Association of College & Research Libraries. Available on-line. URL: http://www.ala.org/acrl/resapr98.html. Downloaded January 29, 2003.

National Institute of Diabetes & Digestive & Kidney Diseases. Available on-line. URL: http://www.niddk.nih.gov/health/nutrit/nutrit.htm. Downloaded January 29, 2003.

NutriBase. Available on-line. URL: http://www.nutribase.com/homepage.shtml. Downloaded January 29, 2003.

Nutrition Navigator, Tufts University. Available on-line. URL: http://navigator.tufts.edu/. Downloaded January 29, 2003.

U.S. Food and Drug Administration. Available on-line. URL: http://www.fda.gov. Downloaded October 28, 2003.

INDEX